Psychodynamic Treatment Approaches to Psychopathology, Vol 2

Editors

RACHEL Z. RITVO
SCHUYLER W. HENDERSON

CHILD AND ADOLESCENT PSYCHIATRIC CLINICS OF NORTH AMERICA

www.childpsych.theclinics.com

Consulting Editor
HARSH K. TRIVEDI

April 2013 • Volume 22 • Number 2

ELSEVIER

1600 John F. Kennedy Boulevard • Suite 1800 • Philadelphia, Pennsylvania, 19103-2899

http://www.theclinics.com

CHILD AND ADOLESCENT PSYCHIATRIC CLINICS OF NORTH AMERICA Volume 22, Number 2
April 2013 ISSN 1056–4993, ISBN-13: 978-1-4557-7072-4

Editor: Joanne Husovski
Developmental Editor: Donald Mumford

Child and Adolescent Psychiatric Clinics of North America (ISSN 1056-4993) is published quarterly by Elsevier Inc., 360 Park Avenue South, New York, NY 10010-1710. Months of issue are January, April, July, and October. Business and Editorial Offices: 1600 John F. Kennedy Boulevard, Suite 1800, Philadelphia, PA 19103-2899. Periodicals postage paid at New York, NY and additional mailing offices. Subscription prices are $297.00 per year (US individuals), $471.00 per year (US institutions), $149.00 per year (US students), $343.00 per year (Canadian individuals), $567.00 per year (Canadian institutions), $189.00 per year (Canadian students), $408.00 per year (international individuals), $567.00 per year (international institutions), and $189.00 per year (international students). International air speed delivery is included in all *Clinics* subscription prices. All prices are subject to change without notice. **POSTMASTER:** Send address changes to *Child and Adolescent Psychiatric Clinics of North America*, Elsevier Health Sciences Division, Subscription Customer Service, 3251 Riverport Lane, Maryland Heights, MO 63043. **Customer Service: 1-800-654-2452 (U.S. and Canada); 314-447-8871 (outside U.S. and Canada). Fax: 314-447-8029. E-mail: JournalsCustomer Service-usa@elsevier.com (for print support) or journalsonlinesupport-usa@elsevier.com (for online support).**

Reprints. For copies of 100 or more of articles in this publication, please contact the Commercial Reprints Department, Elsevier Inc., 360 Park Avenue South, New York, New York 10010-1710 Tel.: (212) 633-3812; Fax: (212) 462-1935, e-mail: reprints@elsevier.com.

Child and Adolescent Psychiatric Clinics of North America is covered in *MEDLINE/PubMed (Index Medicus), ISI, SSCI, Research Alert, Social Search, Current Contents,* and *EMBASE/Excerpta Medica.*

Printed and bound by CPI Group (UK) Ltd, Croydon, CR0 4YY

Transferred to digital print 2013

Contributors

CONSULTING EDITOR

HARSH K. TRIVEDI, MD
Associate Professor of Psychiatry, Vanderbilt University School of Medicine; Executive Medical Director, and Chief of Staff, Vanderbilt Psychiatric Hospital, Nashville, Tennessee

CONSULTING EDITOR EMERITUS

ANDRÉS MARTIN, MD, MPH

FOUNDING CONSULTING EDITOR

MELVIN LEWIS, MBBS, FRCPSYCH, DCH

EDITORS

RACHEL Z. RITVO, MD
Assistant Clinical Professor of Psychiatry and Behavioral Sciences, George Washington University School of Medicine and Health Sciences, Washington, DC

SCHUYLER W. HENDERSON, MD, MPH
Assistant Clinical Professor of Psychiatry, Department of Child and Adolescent Psychiatry, New York University, New York, New York

AUTHORS

JILL BELLINSON, PhD
Private Practice Psychologist and Psychoanalyst; Faculty, William Alanson White Institute, Adelphi University, Institute for Psychoanalytic Training and Research, Metropolitan Institute for Training in Psychoanalytic Psychotherapy, New York, New York; New York Institute for Training in Psychotherapy, Brooklyn, New York; Supervises, Clinical Psychology Doctoral Program, City University of New York, Teachers' College, Columbia University, New York, New York; Associate Editor, Journal of Infant, Child, and Adolescent Psychotherapy

EFRAIN BLEIBERG, MD
Director, Child and Adolescence Psychiatry, Professor and Vice Chair, Menninger Department of Psychiatry and Behavioral Sciences, Baylor College of Medicine; Service Chief, Psychiatry, Texas Childrens Hospital, Houston, Texas

PETER CHUBINSKY, MD
Clinical Instructor, Department of Psychiatry, Harvard Medical School, Boston, Massachusetts; Faculty, Division of Child and Adolescent Psychiatry, Cambridge Health

Alliance, Cambridge, Massachusetts; Faculty, Boston Psychoanalytic Society and Institute, Newton Centre, Massachusetts

PETER FONAGY, PhD, FBA
Research Department of Clinical Educational and Health Psychology, University College London, London, United Kingdom

HORACIO HOJMAN, MD
Clinical Assistant Professor, Department of Psychiatry and Human Behavior, Brown Alpert Medical School, Providence, Rhode Island

ALLAN M. JOSEPHSON, MD
Professor and Chief, Division of Child and Adolescent Psychiatry, CEO, Bingham Clinic, School of Medicine, University of Louisville, Louisville, Kentucky

LEONARDO NIRO NASCIMENTO, MSc, MA
Research Department of Clinical Educational and Health Psychology, University College London, London, United Kingdom

JACK NOVICK, PhD
Training and Supervising Analyst, International Psychoanalytic Association; Former Associate Professor, Department of Psychiatry, University of Michigan Medical School, Michigan

KERRY KELLY NOVICK
Training and Supervising Analyst, International Psychoanalytic Association

ROSE PALMER, BA, PGDip
Research Department of Clinical Educational and Health Psychology, University College London, London, United Kingdom

ERICA WILLHEIM, PhD
Clinical Director, Family PEACE Program, Ambulatory Care Network, New York Presbyterian Hospital, Columbia University Medical Center; Assistant Professional Psychologist, Department of Psychiatry, Columbia University College of Physicians and Surgeons; Parent-Infant Psychotherapy Training Program, Columbia University Center for Psychoanalytic Training and Research, New York, New York

JUDITH A. YANOF, MD
Training and Supervising Analyst in Child, Adolescent, and Adult Psychoanalysis, Boston Psychoanalytic Society and Institute; Instructor, Psychiatry, Harvard Medical School, Boston, Massachusetts

Contents

Preface   ix

Rachel Z. Ritvo and Schuyler W. Henderson

The State of the Evidence Base for Psychodynamic Psychotherapy for Children and Adolescents   149

Rose Palmer, Leonardo Niro Nascimento, and Peter Fonagy

> This article reviews outcomes of psychodynamic psychotherapy (PP) for children and adolescents reported in articles identified by a comprehensive review of the literature on treatment evaluations of psychological and medical interventions for mental disorders in pediatric populations. The review identified 48 reports based on 33 studies. While there is evidence of substantial clinical gains associated with PP, in almost all the studies, when contrasted with family-based interventions, PP fares no better and appears to produce outcomes with some delay relative to family-based therapies. Further rigorous evaluations are needed, but evidence to date suggests that the context in which PP is delivered should be extended from the traditional context of individual therapy and parents should be included in the treatment of children.

Dyadic Psychotherapy with Infants and Young Children: Child-Parent Psychotherapy   215

Erica Willheim

> This article briefly reviews the historical and empiric foundations of dyadic psychotherapy, highlighting the evolution of the central tenet that very young children exist in a relational context. The target of therapeutic intervention must therefore be the caregiver-child relationship. General features of dyadic psychotherapy are discussed, as well as aspects that are unique to the treatment of very young children. An overview of the goals and intervention modalities of Child-Parent Psychotherapy is provided as an example of an evidence-based dyadic intervention that incorporates theoretical principles and techniques of psychodynamic psychotherapy.

Family Intervention as a Developmental Psychodynamic Therapy   241

Allan M. Josephson

> Families are the context for development. One key way families influence developing children is through family experience, which becomes part of the child's inner world. It is through this cognitive template that the child interprets the world and negotiates developmental challenges. This article reviews a continuum of family interventions targeting interactions that shape the child's mind, and offers guidance to the clinician about when to use individual and family approaches.

Play Technique in Psychodynamic Psychotherapy   261

Judith A. Yanof

Imaginary play is often a child's best way of communicating affects, fantasies, and internal states. In play children are freer to express their forbidden and conflicted thoughts. Consequently, one of the best ways for the therapist to enter the child's world is to do so from within the displacement of the play process. For children who cannot play, the therapist's goal is to teach the child to use play as a means of communication and to create meaning. This article present clinical examples to illustrate how the author uses play in the clinical situation.

Games Children Play: Board Games in Psychodynamic Psychotherapy   283

Jill Bellinson

Children of latency age have typically outgrown dramatic play but have not yet developed the ability to talk about their thoughts and feelings in therapy; at this stage they often play structured board games, during their own playtime and during therapy sessions. This article discusses ways to use board-game play therapeutically, by watching the way children stretch and bend the rules to display their psychological self-states, and by interpreting their experiences within the play.

Mentalizing-Based Treatment with Adolescents and Families   295

Efrain Bleiberg

In this article, the process of mentalizing, its components, and role in self-regulation and attachment are reviewed. An examination is presented of the neurodevelopmental changes affecting the adolescent's capacity to mentalize and the role of such compromised mentalizing in the adolescent's vulnerability to adaptive breakdown and psychopathology, in general, and to emerging personality disorders, in particular. The principles, objectives, and core features of mentalizing-based treatment and its application to adolescents and families are discussed.

A New Model of Techniques for Concurrent Psychodynamic Work with Parents of Child and Adolescent Psychotherapy Patients   331

Kerry Kelly Novick and Jack Novick

To address the neglect of the importance of parent work in the psychodynamic psychotherapy of children and adolescents, the authors present a model of concurrent dynamic parent work that has demonstrated success with patients of all ages. The model includes dual goals for all therapies, addresses the challenge of confidentiality by differentiating privacy and secrecy, and emphasizes the importance of parent work throughout treatment.

Psychodynamic Perspectives on Psychotropic Medications for Children and Adolescents   351

Peter Chubinsky and Horacio Hojman

Recent trends in pediatric psychopharmacology have resulted in advances in treatment but also an overly optimistic and, at times, simplistic extension of pediatric psychopharmacology practice. Concerns about these changes in the field are discussed. The authors outline how understanding the meaning of medications to all those involved in the prescribing process can help integrate our thinking about this complex interaction with patients and their families.

Index   **367**

CHILD AND ADOLESCENT PSYCHIATRIC CLINICS

FORTHCOMING ISSUES

Complementary and Integrative Therapies
Deborah Simkin, MD, and
Charles Popper, MD,
Editors

Psychosis
Jean Frazier, MD, and
Yael Dvir, MD, *Editors*

Acute Management of Autism Spectrum Disorders
Matthew Siegel, MD, and Bryan King, MD, *Editors*

RECENT ISSUES

January 2013
Psychodynamic Approaches to Psychopathology, Vol 1
Rachel Z. Ritvo, MD, and
Schuyler W. Henderson, MD, *Editors*

October 2012
Psychopharmacology
Harsh K. Trivedi, MD, and
Kiki D. Chang, MD, *Editors*

July 2012
Anxiety Disorders
Moira Rynn, MD, Hilary Vidair, PhD, and
Jennifer Urbano Blackford, PhD,
Editors

April 2012
Child and Adolescent Depression
Stuart J. Goldman, MD, and
Frances Wren, MD, *Editors*

Preface

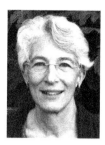

Rachel Z. Ritvo, MD *and* Schuyler W. Henderson, MD, MPH
Editors

This issue of *Child and Adolescent Psychiatric Clinics of North America* is the second in a pair of volumes devoted to providing a view of psychodynamic psychotherapy as it is currently practiced. A century has passed since psychodynamic psychotherapy with children made its debut in the case of "Little Hans," in which the horse phobia of a 5-year-old boy was treated by Freud through consultations and subsequent recommendations to the boy's father.[1] During the following century, child and adolescent psychodynamic psychotherapy flourished when child and adolescent psychiatry focused on fostering development and a healthy adaptation to life circumstances. With the publication of the DSM III, the field shifted toward a focus on diagnosis, with descriptive psychopathology as an organizing rubric. In keeping with this shift, volume 1, "Psychodynamic Approaches to Psychopathology in Children and Adolescents," began with a bow to neuroscience and developmental science and then proceeded to focus on psychodynamic approaches to specific psychopathologies in children and adolescents: anxiety, depression, and eating disorders, and conditions related to trauma and severe medical illness.

In this second volume, we turn our attention to "Psychodynamic Treatment Modalities for Children and Adolescents," as they are currently used. First, in "The State of the Evidence Base for Psychodynamic Psychotherapy," Palmer, Nascimento, and Fonagy present a comprehensive look at the expanding evidence base for psychodynamic psychotherapy for children and adolescents. Although their overview shows that it can be an effective treatment, they also demonstrate that this seminal treatment approach is "clearly understudied," evidence of neglect or a lag in the field of research development. Traditionally, psychodynamic psychotherapy has been identified as an individual therapy mimicking the iconic individual therapy, psychoanalysis. The review of the evidence base presented here suggests that psychodynamic treatment principles might be most efficaciously delivered in nontraditional contexts such as dyadic therapy, where the parent-child dyad is the focus of treatment or family therapy.

Multiple, complementary lines of psychodynamic theoretical inquiry have, over the course of 75 years, contributed to the development of dyadic therapy, reviewed by Willheim in "Dyadic Psychotherapy with Infants and Young Children: Child-Parent Psychotherapy (CPP)." Observational research with infants and caregivers and

Child Adolesc Psychiatric Clin N Am 22 (2013) ix–xi
http://dx.doi.org/10.1016/j.chc.2013.01.002
1056-4993/13/$ – see front matter © 2013 Published by Elsevier Inc.

research on attachment that led to operationalization of attachment status and of reflective function as a measure of mentalization (the ability to hold mental states of self and other in mind) melded with clinical insights of psychodynamic infant psychiatry to produce dyadic therapy. Willheim provides the reader with an introduction to the general and the unique features of dyadic therapy with examples from Child-Parent Psychotherapy, a manualized treatment for dyads who have experienced trauma that has an increasingly robust evidence base.

Next, moving from the dyad to the family, Josephson describes interventions with youths and their families in "Family Intervention as a Developmental Psychodynamic Therapy." A child or adolescent's mental processes, his or her internal working models, are forged in family interactions. Formulating a youthful patient's difficulties requires formulating the influences in the family matrix; subsequent interventions, for child and family, are guided by these formulations.

Individual play therapy remains the core modality of psychodynamic psychotherapy and the skills learned by psychodynamic play therapists are frequently deployed in other therapy settings. Yanof's "Play Technique in Psychodynamic Psychotherapy" brings together classical theory and clinical findings with the latest advances in play technique as it has moved away from an overreliance on interpretation and has added developmental assistance to its repertoire. With ample examples and a minimum of psychoanalytic jargon, Yanof's article is a rich resource for all, from beginners to the most experienced clinicians. This work via play is elaborated on by Bellinson in her contribution, "Games Children Play: Board Games in Psychodynamic Psychotherapy." Bellinson explores the use of board games, which appear to be highly structured, in unstructured dynamic therapy.

A psychodynamic intervention that can be applied in both individual and family settings is mentalizing-based treatment. Bleiberg reviews the components and the process of mentalizing and its role in self-regulation and attachment. Neurodevelopmental changes impact adolescents' capacity to mentalize, making adolescents vulnerable to adaptive breakdown and psychopathology. He presents the principles, objectives, and core features of mentalizing-based treatment and its application to both adolescents and families.

"A New Model of Techniques for Concurrent Psychodynamic Work with Parents of Child and Adolescent Psychotherapy Patients" by the Novicks provides a practical guide to working with parents when providing individual psychodynamic psychotherapy to their offspring. Addressing a frequently neglected topic in child and adolescent psychiatry training programs, this article makes accessible a model of parent work that emphasizes building a therapeutic alliance, maintaining a developmental perspective, assisting parents in mastering the parenting role, and maintaining confidentiality.

Our volume closes with a timely look at "Psychodynamic Perspectives on Psychotropic Medications for Children and Adolescents." Chubinsky and Hojman explore the multifaceted meanings of medication for all those involved in the complex process that results in a prescription. In this era of skyrocketing prescribing and polypharmacy, the authors' hope that integrating psychodynamic thinking (such as an awareness of countertransference, an attuned understanding of a patient's fantasies regarding the medication, and consideration of parents' fears of damaging their child) will lead to more judicious and effective use of psychotropic agents to treat our vulnerable youth.

On a final note, we should add that we are grateful to Dr Trivedi and to the editorial team behind *Child and Adolescent Psychiatry Clinics of North America*; in particular, this was intended as a single volume and the publisher graciously facilitated a second volume when the critical mass of authorial interest, enthusiasm, and quality prose burst the confines of one edition. It is encouraging and inspiring to know that this area of child and adolescent psychiatry is so energetically supported by publishers, authors, budding and established researchers, editors, and readers. It is not uncommon to hear about the fading relevance of psychodynamic psychotherapy, but not only are eulogies premature, these volumes hint that this is one of the few treatment perspectives that is actually standing the test of time.

Rachel Z. Ritvo, MD
George Washington University School
of Medicine and Health Sciences
Washington, DC, USA

Schuyler W. Henderson, MD, MPH
Department of Child and Adolescent Psychiatry
New York University
New York, NY, USA

E-mail addresses:
rzritvomd@gmail.com (R.Z. Ritvo)
schuylermd@yahoo.com (S.W. Henderson)

REFERENCE

1. Freud S. Analysis of a phobia in a five-year-old boy (1909). In: Strachey JE, editor. The standard edition of the complete psychological works of Sigmund Freud, vol. X. London: Hogarth Press; 1955. p. 3–149.

The State of the Evidence Base for Psychodynamic Psychotherapy for Children and Adolescents

Rose Palmer, BA, PGDip, Leonardo Niro Nascimento, MSc, MA,
Peter Fonagy, PhD, FBA*

KEYWORDS

- Psychodynamic • Psychotherapy • Children • Adolescents • Mental health
- Depression • Anxiety

KEY POINTS

- The body of rigorous research supporting psychodynamic therapies for adults for most disorders remains limited.
- There is some evidence to support the use of psychodynamic psychotherapy for children whose problems are either internalizing or externalizing with internalizing symptoms. There is also evidence that the support and inclusion of parents is an important aspect of this treatment.
- There is evidence that effects tend to increase following the end of treatment.
- There is evidence that behavioral problems are more resistant at least to a classical, insight-oriented psychodynamic approach.
- In light of the limitations of CBT in severe disorders in comparison with medication, it behooves us to investigate the effectiveness of alternative treatment approaches.

INTRODUCTION

The requirement for rigorous professional standards and clear accountability for clinical decisions is widely recognized in all branches of health care, and increasingly in mental health.[1] To be guided by empirically substantiated intuition enhances professional accountability as well as the transparency of clinical judgment.[2] It has been robustly argued that evidence-based psychotherapies (EBPs) must replace

Research Department of Clinical Educational and Health Psychology, University College London, London, UK
* Corresponding author. Psychoanalysis Unit, Research Department of Clinical, Educational and Health Psychology, University College London, 1-19 Torrington Place, London WC1E 7HB, UK.
E-mail address: p.fonagy@ucl.ac.uk

Child Adolesc Psychiatric Clin N Am 22 (2013) 149–214
http://dx.doi.org/10.1016/j.chc.2012.12.001
1056-4993/13/$ – see front matter © 2013 Elsevier Inc. All rights reserved.

Abbreviations: Evidence-base for Psychotherapy for Children and Adolescents

Measures		Therapy	
AFI	Adult Functioning Index	ABFT	Attachment-Based Family Therapy
BDI	Beck Depression Inventory	AFT	Adolescent-Focused Individual Therapy
BDI-II	Beck Depression Inventory Revised	BFST	Behavioral Family Systems Therapy
BMI	Body Mass Index	BPP	Brief Psychodynamic Psychotherapy
BSAG	Bristol Social Adjustment Scale	CAT	Cognitive Analytic Therapy
CAPS	Clinician-Administered PTSD Scale	CPP	Child-Parent Psychotherapy
CBCL	Child Behavior Check List	CS	Community Standard Intervention
		EBP	Evidence-Based Psychotherapy
CDI	Child Depression Inventory	EOIT	Ego-Oriented Individual Therapy
CGAS	Children's Goal Assessment Scale	EUC	Enhanced Usual Care
CPSS	Child PTSD Symptom Scale	FBT	Family-Based Treatment
DC: 0-3	Semistructured Interview for Diagnostic Classification 0 to 3	FIPP	Focused Individual Psychodynamic Psychotherapy
EAT	Eating Attitudes Test	GP	Group Psychotherapy
FAD	Family Assessment Device	GCC	Good Clinical Care
GAF	Global Assessment of Functioning	IP	Individual Psychotherapy
GARF	Global Assessment of Relational Functioning	IPCT	Individual Psychodynamic Child Therapy
GAS	Goal Attainment Scales	LTPP	Long-Term Psychoanalytic Psychotherapy
GHQ	General Health Questionnaire		
IBW	Ideal Body Weight	PE-A	Prolonged Exposure Therapy
K-GAS	Kiddie Global Assessment Scale	PHV	Psychoeducational Home Visits
K-SADS	Kiddie Schedule for Affective Disorders	POST	Psychodynamic-Orientated Supportive Therapy
K-SADS-PL	Kiddie Schedule for Affective Disorders Present and Lifetime	PP	Psychodynamic Psychotherapy
MFQ	Moods and Feelings Questionnaire	PPP	Preschooler-Parent Psychotherapy
PARQ	Parent Adolescent Relationship Questionnaire	RPT	Reciprocal Play Therapy
PSCR	Psychic and Social Communicative Findings Report	SEPP	Supportive Expressive Play Psychotherapy
RCBC	Revised Child Behavior Checklist	SFT	Structural Family Therapy
SCID-II	Structured Clinical Interview for DSM-IV Axis II Disorders	SIFT	Systems Integrative Family Therapy
SCL- 90-R	Symptoms Checklist-90 Revised	STPP	Short-Term Psychoanalytic Psychotherapy
SFSR	Structural Family Systems Ratings	TAU	Treatment as Usual
SIQ-JR	Suicide Ideation Questionnaire – Junior	TLDP	Time-Limited Dynamic Therapy
SOFAS	Social and Occupational Functioning Assessment Scale		
TAT	Thematic Apperception Test	**Others**	
TCS	Target Complaint Scales	AN	Anorexia Nervosa
TRF	Teacher Report Form	ASD	Autistic Spectrum Disorder
WISC	Wechsler Intelligence Scale for Children	BPD	Borderline Personality Disorder
WISC-III	Wechsler Intelligence Scale for Children 3rd Edition	CAMHS	Child and Adolescent Mental Health Service
Y-OQ-SR	Youth Outcome Questionnaire Self-Report	DBD	Disruptive Behavior Disorders
YSR	Youth Self-report Form	f	Female
		m	Male
		NC	Nonmaltreated Comparison
		OCD	Obsessive Compulsive Disorder
		ODD	Oppositional Defiant Disorder
		PTSD	Posttraumatic Stress Disorder

treatment as usual (TAU) in everyday clinical care (eg, see Clark[3]). Many, particularly those from a psychodynamic or systemic orientation, have raised significant objections to this.[4,5] Much of the debate focuses on the external validity of findings from randomized controlled trials (RCTs) because (1) the demographic and clinical characteristics of the patients included in trials differ in terms of severity and comorbidity; (2) the timing of dosage and concomitant treatments in trials correspond poorly to the treatment regimens normally available, even in relation to normal clinical application of EBPs; (3) the settings in which EBPs are administered in empirical studies tend to be more highly specialized and incorporate a superior level of care; and (4) the outcomes normally used are argued to be of limited relevance to ordinary clinical practice.

At the heart of these questions on external validity is the issue recently raised eloquently by Cartwright and Munro.[6] These investigators point to the increasing reliance in health care policy on RCTs. The basic logic of RCTs is that of John Stuart Mill's "method of difference,"[7] which attempts to locate differences in the probability of a particular outcome with or without the treatment intervention in two groups with identical characteristics in relation to factors associated with the likelihood of change. RCTs are placed at the top of the hierarchy from the point of view of the clarity of causal association between intervention and change.[8] Cartwright and Munro[6] question this assumption in relation to supporting policy decision making. They formulate their doubt about RCTs in relation to "stable capacities" (p. 262). This concept is introduced in place of the notion of external validity. External validity may indeed be too narrow to bear the burden of meaning in relation to the question decision makers are faced with. A successful RCT demonstrates that the intervention works somewhere, but "will it work for us?" (p. 265). This question points to the need for further research in relation to those treatments that appear to be effective in some contexts but not in others. Multisystemic Therapy, for example, can boast of successful trials in the United States and Norway, but failed replication in Sweden and Canada.[9–21]

To extract ourselves from this quandary, further evidence is required in relation to understanding how a treatment achieves the desired outcome, and what conditions are necessary for these outcomes to be realistic. Evidence concerning moderating factors, as well as the impact of concurrent processes, for example, medication, must be available to judge the applicability of an RCT to a particular setting. Alan Kazdin, in his exploration of the gap in research concerning disease and therapeutic mechanisms, came to a similar conclusion.[22] For a treatment to be considered evidence-based, more than RCTs are required.

This argument, however, has often been taken to imply that RCTs can be replaced by methods that do not comply with Mill's "method of difference."[7] In particular, often those favoring a psychoanalytic model use arguments concerning the limitations of RCTs to argue for "practice-based evidence," the replacement of causal arguments with a correlational, observational approach. We accept that evidence from RCTs is not necessarily the only base for determining what constitutes EBP. The American Psychological Association's Presidential Task Force on evidence-based practice (2006) explicitly proposed requiring evidence from clients' values and preferences, and clinicians' real-world observations, in addition to research evidence, as a basis for establishing EBP. So, some argue that not only are RCTs for psychotherapy flawed (see previously) but also that there are alternative ways of establishing psychotherapy as "evidence-based." However, the denial of RCTs as a key part of establishing the validity of a therapeutic modality is misguided. The history of medicine is littered with interventions that did remarkable duty as therapies and yet when subjected to RCT methodology were shown to have no benefit over alternative treatments or, in fact, to prevent the patient from benefiting from a superior intervention, in terms of either effect size (ES) or speed. Perhaps the most dramatic example is the RCT that ended 100 years of radical mastectomies for breast carcinoma only 30 years ago. The study showed that half a million women, who had been subjected to disabling, horrendously mutilating operations performed with the best of intentions, on the basis of a fallacious theory about the way in which carcinoma spread, could have had equally good outcomes with lumpectomies.[23]

RCTs are necessary but not sufficient. This is a problem because RCTs consume money, time, and energy. Rawlins[24] reminds us that of 153 pharmaceutical RCTs performed between 2005 and 2006, the median cost was more than £5 million, with the interquartile range stretching to £10.5 million. As we have pointed out before, RCTs are an imperfect tool; almost certainly their results are best seen as one part of a research cycle.[25]

Empirical knowledge is multifaceted and complex, and in line with this, the practice of EBP requires sophistication in relation to the scrutiny of empiric data. Uncontrolled trials, such as single case studies, open trials, or time-series studies have a contribution to make to the knowledge base, particularly in relation to telling us about the feasibility of an intervention, its likely acceptance by a patient, and its potential for effectiveness. RCTs are the "gold standard," but there are a number of issues to consider in evaluating RCT investigations, including the design, the size, the characteristics of the sample, the outcome measures used, the clinicians implementing the psychotherapy, data analyses, and qualitative assessment of unintended consequences, both positive and negative. For example, factors such as the quality of randomization, are known to reflect outcome, but clinicians are generally not well situated to make judgments concerning technical details, such as the exact timing of randomization. This is why critical reviews that summarize and synthesize a body of research are of great value. Sadly, for the field of psychotherapy research, the number of reviews in a range of areas exceeds the number of original studies, probably because of the expense of RCTs and the relatively low cost of reviewers' time.[26]

Further, narrative reviews have major limitations. They rely on the statistical significance of a study to determine the efficacy of an intervention, but statistical significance is determined in large part by sample size. Meta-analyses pool results from multiple studies and thus bypass the low statistical power that handicaps psychotherapy research. Because of the relationship between statistical significance and sample size, studies need to be evaluated in terms of observed effect sizes to determine whether they are likely to be of clinical significance. Effect sizes tend to be grouped, with those below an r of 0.15 (or d of 0.3) being considered small and those above an r of 0.35 (or d of 0.75) considered large.[27] Meta-analyses aggregate effect sizes arithmetically, giving an indication of the size of the effect that one might expect if the RCTs on which the analysis is based are representative. Such aggregation is possible if RCTs are sufficiently homogeneous in terms of the target population and the treatment method and outcome measures. Sadly, the literature on psychodynamic interventions for children does not include a sufficient number of studies evaluating the same treatment with the same or similar set of measures to permit valid and meaningful aggregation. In this review, therefore, we will compromise between providing a simple narrative review of findings and providing a systematic assessment of study quality and effect sizes on primary outcome measures.

AIMS OF THIS REVIEW

This review aimed to identify, describe, and review studies evaluating the efficacy and/ or effectiveness of psychodynamic treatment for children and adolescents with mental health problems. We also aimed to evaluate the quality of the studies identified by performing a qualitative review, and using the Randomized Controlled Trial Psychodynamic Quality Rating Scale (RCT-PQRS)[28] for RCTs and quasi-randomized studies.

METHOD OF THIS REVIEW

We have attempted to ensure a systematic process by searching the literature on children and adolescents with most mental disorders, using an exhaustive algorithm to identify treatment trials. This was part of our comprehensive review of pediatric mental health outcome literature,[29] for which we have reviewed more than 15,000 references. In our computer search of all major databases (PubMed, PsychInfo, Cochrane, Medline, and Embase), we used 100 terms referring to different aspects of child and adolescent mental health and combined these with 11 terms describing psychotherapy (the search algorithms are available on request from the authors).

The computer search identified 1212 abstracts, which were reviewed. A hand search of bibliographies, key journals, and publicly available reports also identified 51 abstracts. All 1263 references were screened, and from this a corpus of 48 articles reporting on 33 primary studies was identified. The search covered the period up to May 2012 (**Fig. 1**).

To be included in the review, articles had to meet the criteria of relevance, outcome, and design.

Relevance: Studies that reported evaluations of psychodynamic interventions with children and/or adolescents (aged 0–18) with mental health problems

Outcome: Studies were selected only if they reported outcomes that were either directly related to a disorder (eg, symptom reduction) or to intermediary variables. In the latter case, the reviewers had independent evidence of an impact on mental health associated with the outcome or an impact on mental health was plausible.

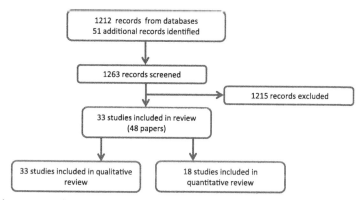

Fig. 1. Literature review.

Design: The review focused on studies with an experimental or quasi-experimental design. Observational studies, such as cohort or case studies, were also considered, but possible effects of bias are indicated throughout the article. This was a necessary relaxation of exclusion criteria because a preliminary exploration of evidence suggested that excluding poorly controlled studies would severely limit the available evidence. We have reviewed all available evidence, highlighting in the review the methodological shortcomings and cautioning readers to interpret the results with appropriate care.

Inclusion criteria were:

1. A clear description was provided of the patient population in the study, in terms of either diagnosis or specific problems addressed in the treatment.
2. Psychodynamic psychotherapy (PP) or a therapy sharing a substantial number of features with the psychodynamic approach was used as a treatment (see later in this article for an elaboration of this point).
3. Participants were children and adolescents.
4. The study was reported in the English language.
5. There was a systematic effort to measure the outcome, using a standardized measure, at least at pre- and post-test.

Although the review that this subsample draws from considered all mental health interventions for children and adolescents, here we were interested only in studies that included a therapy with a substantial psychodynamic component. We define "psychodynamic," following Fonagy and Target,[30] as a stance taken to human subjectivity that is comprehensive, and aimed at a comprehensive understanding of the interplay between aspects of the individual's relationship with her or his environment, external and internal. Freud's great discovery "where id was, there ego shall be,"[31(p80)] often misinterpreted, points to the power of the conscious mind to radically alter its position with respect to aspects of its own functions, including the capacity to end its own existence through killing the body. Psychodynamic, as elaborated by Fonagy and Target,[30] refers to this extraordinary potential for dynamic self-alteration and self-correction, seemingly totally outside the reach of nonhuman species. We therefore define the "psychodynamic approach" in terms of 8 basic postulates that encapsulate this self-correcting process[30]:

1. The notion of psychological causation (mental disorder can be conveniently thought about as "caused" by the mental activity [eg, thoughts, feelings, wishes])
2. That there are limitations on consciousness, and nonconscious mental states have influence
3. The assumption of the internal representations of interpersonal relationships
4. The ubiquity of psychological conflict as one of the drivers of psychopathology
5. The assumption of psychic defenses to moderate experiences of distress
6. The assumption of complex (multiple) psychological meanings of experience
7. An emphasis on the therapeutic relationship in models of change
8. That a developmental perspective on both pathology and treatment is vital

Unlike many previous reviews, in this summary of the literature, we consider as psychodynamic treatments studies exploring the effectiveness of therapies that integrate significant psychodynamic components into a multimodal package. We feel justified in doing this because the boundary between what is and is not within a particular modality has been growing increasingly fuzzy over recent years. Thirty-five years ago, psychoanalysis could be readily distinguished from behavior therapy in terms of its model of the mind, its theory of change, and its clinical methods.[32] In the twenty-first century, changes in both cognitive behavioral approaches and psychodynamic theory and technique have led to an increasing convergence of both understanding and clinical method. The work of McCullough,[33] Ryle and Kerr,[34] Weissman and colleagues,[35] Young,[36] Safran,[37] and others has occupied a conceptual space in between psychodynamic and non-psychodynamic domains. It is justifiable to review some of the findings from this boundary domain, as it bears on the validity of the psychodynamic approach. Throughout the review we consider traditional psychodynamic alongside integrative dynamic approaches.

Quality Rating

While all persons may be created equal, the studies of psychotherapy they in turn create are certainly not. Similarly, standards for reviewing these studies are often not as transparent as they could be, giving rise to further heterogeneity. To meet this challenge, in this review the quality of the studies was judged using the RCT-PQRS.[28] This scale, which was created by the *Ad Hoc Subcommittee for Evaluation of the Evidence Base for PP of the APA Committee on Research on Psychiatric Treatments* to evaluate the quality of RCTs, consists of 24 items relating to study design, reporting, and execution. The items cover the domains of description of subjects, definition and delivery of treatment, outcome measures, data analysis, treatment assignment, and overall quality of the study. Each item is rated on a scale from 0 to 2, with 0 being a poor description, execution or justification, 1 being a brief description or either a good description or an appropriate criteria but not both, and 2 being a well-described, executed and, where necessary, justified design element. A 25th item is an omnibus rating on a scale ranging from 1 (exceptionally poor study) to 7 (exceptionally good study). Two raters independently scored each article and achieved high interrater reliability on the total scores across 13 studies ($r = 0.97$). Where there was disagreement between the 2 raters, we aggregated the scores. We include the total RCT-PQRS rating with each RCT (please see **Table 1**) and draw attention to particular problems in relation to each study.

Data Extraction

For all RCTs and quasi-randomized controlled trials, a quantitative analysis was performed. Using data provided in the articles, between-group and pre-post effect sizes (r) on primary outcome measures were calculated.

REVIEW

The best and most comprehensive review of outcome studies of psychodynamic approaches to child and adolescent mental health problems is the recent excellent article by Midgley and Kennedy,[38] which covers very similar ground to the current review, although perhaps arrives at slightly different conclusions. Other reviews in books and chapters by our group[29,30] provide less systematic but helpful summaries. Overall, the literature is sparse. In comparison with other modalities, PP has been poorly served by empiric investigations. Scholarly and clinical reviews of psychosocial treatments reflect the cumulative impact of repeated statements of the mantra that "the absence of evidence does not indicate evidence for the absence of effectiveness." Sadly, whereas 10 to 15 years ago, reviews of evidence-based psychosocial treatments would have included psychodynamic treatments to ensure comprehensive coverage (eg, Hibbs[39] and Weiscz[40]), more recent compilations (eg, Weiscz and Kazdin,[41] Kazdin,[42] and Kazak and

Table 1
RCT-PQRS ratings of the quality of studies

Article	Randomized Controlled Trial Psychodynamic Quality Rating Scale Item																									Total
	1	2	3	4	5	6	7	8	9	10	11	12	13	14	15	16	17	18	19	20	21	22	23	24	25	
Chanen et al,[80] 2008	2	1	0	2	2	2	2	2	0	2	2	2	1	2	2	2	2	1	2	2	2	2	2	2	6	41
Diamond and colleagues,[70] 2010	2	1	2	2	2	2	1	2	1	2	2	0	2	1	2	2	2	1	2	2	2	2	2	2	6	41
Gilboa-Schechtman et al,[57] 2010	2	1	2	2	2	2	1	2	2	2	2	2	2	2	1	2	1	2	2	2	2	2	1	2	7	41
Kronmuller et al,[50] 2010	2	1	0	0	1	2	2	0	0	1	2	0	0	2	0	2	1	1	0	1	2	1	2	1	3	24
Lieberman et al,[75] 2005	2	1	1	0	1	1	1	2	0	2	2	2	2	2	2	2	1	0	0	2	2	2	1	2	4	32
Lock et al,[67] 2010	2	1	2	2	2	1	1	1	2	2	2	2	2	2	2	2	1	2	2	2	2	2	2	2	6	41
Moran et al,[87] 1991	2	2	0	0	2	1	2	2	1	2	2	2	1	2	0	2	1	0	0	1	1	0	2	2	3	30
Muratori et al,[46] 2002	2	2	2	2	2	2	2	2	0	2	2	2	2	2	0	0	0	1	1	2	2	1	0	1	4	33
Robin et al,[59] 1999	2	2	2	2	2	2	2	0	2	2	2	0	2	2	1	2	1	1	0	2	2	2	2	2	5	39
Smyrnios and Kirby,[44] 1993	1	1	0	1	2	0	2	0	0	1	2	2	0	2	1	2	0	0	1	0	2	2	2	2	3	26
Szapocznik et al,[54] 1989	2	0	0	2	2	2	2	1	2	2	1	1	1	2	0	2	0	2	2	1	2	2	2	2	5	34
Trowell et al,[48] 2002	2	1	0	2	2	1	0	1	2	2	2	0	0	2	2	2	2	1	0	1	2	2	1	2	4	32
Trowell et al,[55] 2007	2	2	1	2	2	0	1	0	2	2	1	0	0	2	2	1	1	1	2	2	2	2	2	2	5	35

Items 1–24 are rated 0 (poor description, execution, or justification of a design element), 1 (brief description or either a good description or an appropriate method/criteria but not both), or 2 (well-described, executed, and, where necessary, justified design element). Item 25 is rated from 1 (exceptionally poor study) to 7 (exceptionally good study).

Description of subjects
1. Diagnostic method and criteria for inclusion and exclusion
2. Documentation or demonstration of reliability of diagnostic methodology
3. Description of relevant comorbidities
4. Description of numbers of subjects screened, included, and excluded

Definition and delivery of treatment
5. Treatment(s) (including control/comparison groups) are sufficiently described or referenced to allow for replication
6. Method to demonstrate that treatment being studied is treatment being delivered (only satisfied by supervision if transcripts or tapes are explicitly reviewed)
7. Therapist training and level of experience in the treatment(s) under investigation
8. Therapist supervision while treatment is being provided
9. Description of concurrent treatments (eg, medication) allowed and administered during course of study (if patients on medication are included, a rating of 2 requires full reporting of what medications were used; if patients on medications are excluded, this alone is sufficient for a rating of 2)

Outcome measures

10. Validated outcome measure(s) (either established or newly standardized)

11. Primary outcome measure(s) specified in advance (though does not need to be stated explicitly for a rating of 2)

12. Outcome assessment by raters blinded to treatment group and with established reliability

13. Discussion of safety and adverse events during study treatment(s)

14. Assessment of long-term post-termination outcome (should not be penalized for failure to follow comparison group if this is a wait-list or nontreatment group that is subsequently referred for or active treatment)

Data Analysis

15. Intent-to-treat method for data analysis involving primary outcome measure

16. Description of dropouts and withdrawals

17. Appropriate statistical tests (eg, use of Bonferroni correction, longitudinal data analysis, adjustment only for a priori identified confounders)

18. Adequate sample size

19. Appropriate consideration of therapist and site effects

Treatment Assignment

20. A priori relevant hypotheses that justify comparison group(s)

21. Comparison group(s) from same population and time frame as experimental group

22. Randomized assignment to treatment groups

Overall quality of the study

23. Balance of allegiance to types of treatment by practitioners

24. Conclusions of study justified by sample, measures, and data analysis, as presented (note: useful to look at conclusions as stated in study abstract)

Total

25. Overall Score

colleagues[43]) do not have any coverage of PP. Time may be running out for dynamic psychotherapy for children.

There are relatively few randomized trials of PP, and most of those that are available have, as we discuss in this article, contrasted PP with another evidence-based treatment rather than providing comparison with a genuine control condition. In this article, we consider quasi-randomized methods separately, as well as studies using matched cases, non-matched control groups, and open trials. Notwithstanding the shortcomings of RCTs, we give most space in this review to studies in which patients were randomized at baseline and fidelity to treatment protocol could be examined in relation to an explicitly detailed manual. **Table 2** summarizes each study and is found at the end of this article.

RCTs

Comparison with TAU

Smyrnios and Kirkby[44] performed one of the first RCTs of PP (n = 30) comparing time-limited psychotherapy, time-unlimited psychotherapy, and a minimal contact group in Australia. Children were randomly divided into 3 groups of 10: 1 group received "time-unlimited" psychoanalytic therapy using a Kleinian model (on average 28 sessions, with a range from 3 to 62 sessions); 1 group received short-term therapy (on average 10.5 sessions, with a range from 5 to 12 sessions); and 1 group was offered a 3-session consultation. Participants were 5-year-old to 9-year-old children with a diagnosis of emotional disturbance specific to childhood. Assessment took place at baseline, at end of treatment and at 4-year follow-up. Measures included the Goal Attainment Scales, Target Complaint Scales, Van der Veen Family Concept Inventory and Bristol Social Adjustment Scale. All 3 groups showed significant improvements from pretest to posttest on a number of individual and family ratings, but the effect size was greatest for the time-unlimited treatment. At 4-year follow-up, the effect sizes for target complaints were no longer significantly different from the control group, who were likely to have had other treatments. In line with this, the consultation group caught up with the treated groups and reported significant improvement relative to posttreatment on follow-up, severity of target problems, and measures of family functioning. All groups improved significantly on therapist measures of goal attainment from pretest to 4-year follow-up, but only the minimal contact group reported significant improvements on severity of target problems and measures of family functioning. This study, admittedly with a very small sample size, but with random allocation to the minimal contact, time-limited, and time-unlimited groups, appears to show a reverse dose-response effect, with those in treatment for longest and most intensively showing relatively less gain. There was substantial attrition from the trial and the last observed value carried forward analysis used is a poor technique for dealing with missing data points in an RCT. With almost half of the participants missing for follow-up, the study was dramatically underpowered and there were no significant interaction effects between group and time-only differences between the patterns of significant differences across groups. The severity of presentations was mild, and in other studies the benefit of long-term intensive intervention was observed only for children with relatively severe emotional problems (multiple diagnoses with low level of functioning).[45] In brief, the study holds no implications for the "stable capacity" of PP.

Muratori and colleagues[46] performed a small random-allocation study (n = 30) of children (aged 6–11) with "severe emotional disorders" (pure emotional disorders [International Classification of Diseases, Tenth Revision (ICD-10)] n = 17, mixed emotional disorders [ICD-10] n = 13). Although the study used an inadequate method of treatment allocation, based on treatment vacancies, there is no reason to assume that the allocation was not at least quasi-random. Fifteen children who underwent Brief Dynamic Psychotherapy (BDP) (11 sessions, child-only and parent–child sessions) were compared with matched controls (n = 15) who received other types of treatment in community services. Both groups were evaluated at baseline, 6 months, and 18 months using the Children's Global Assessment Scale (CGAS) and Child Behavior Checklist (CBCL). There was a positive change in the experimental group (total problems). Both groups improved on the CGAS scale, but the BDP group did better at both 6- and 18-month follow-up. The investigators also report better outcomes for children younger than 9 and for those with a diagnosis of "pure emotional disorder." The conclusions we can draw from this study are limited by its small sample size, lack of random assignment, and because children in the control group did not receive homogeneous treatment.

Adding to the participants so that the study was adequately powered, the investigators reported on a follow-up with a larger sample size.[47] In both reports, at end of treatment, the between-group effect sizes were small. Unusually for trials of psychotherapy, treatment effects increased during the 2-year follow-up period (the so-called "sleeper effect"), including a move into the nonclinical range for the average child with internalizing problems (in the psychodynamically treated group only).[47] There were no significant differences between treatments on the CBCL at end of treatment. The experimental group showed greater improvement in the CGAS at end of treatment as well as at follow-up, with a medium between-group effect size reported at 6 and 12 months. Although the comparison group also showed improvement, at follow-up, only the BDP group's mean moved to the functional range. Between baseline and follow-up only, the treatment group improved significantly on all 3 scales of the CBCL, but improvement was more marked on the emotional than the externalizing subscale. Pre-post effect sizes for the PP were generally large for the symptom scores but small for changes in social competence. At 2-year follow-up, 34% of the PDP-treated group were in the clinical range on symptomatic measures, compared with 65% of the TAU controls. The conclusions from this trial are limited because of the small sample size and the lack of random allocation; however, it is encouraging that patients receiving PP sought mental health services at a significantly lower rate than those in the TAU comparison condition over the 2-year follow-up period and the study weakly confirms the stable capacity of PP.

Trowell and colleagues[48] compared an individual and a psychoeducational group psychotherapy in terms of the outcomes for traumatized, sexually abused girls (aged 6–14). The girls were randomly assigned to 30 sessions of individual psychotherapy (n – 35) or up to 18 sessions of group psychotherapy (n – 30). Both treatments were manualized and both included parent work. Assessment took place before therapy and 1 year and 2 years after. The measures used included the Orvaschel posttraumatic stress disorder (PTSD) scale, the Kiddie Schedule for Affective Disorders and the Kiddie Global Assessment Scale (K-GAS). These young people presented with a range of psychiatric problems, most commonly PTSD and depression. At baseline, the main Diagnostic and Statistical Manual Mental Disorders, Fourth Revision (DSM-IV) diagnoses were mixed: PTSD (73%), major depressive disorder (MDD) (57%), general anxiety disorder (GAD) (37%), and separation anxiety disorder (58%). Both treatment groups showed a substantial reduction in psychopathology, and there were no differences between the 2 treatments on the K-GAS. Pre-post K-GAS effect sizes were very large ($r > 0.70$) at all time points. Psychodynamic treatment was somewhat superior to psychoeducation, but the difference was not as marked as might be expected. Superiority was particularly evident in relation to

PTSD and GAD. Depression, however, was relatively less likely to improve, as was separation anxiety. Individual therapy led to a greater improvement on measures of the manifestations of PTSD, particularly on the reexperience of the traumatic event and persistent avoidance of stimuli dimensions of the PTSD scale. GAD was the most likely to remit; of the 26 participants who had this disorder at baseline, 81% no longer had it at 1-year follow-up; 69% of those with MDD and 50% of those with separation anxiety disorder no longer had these disorders at 1-year follow-up. A subsequent report underscored the importance of the mother's support for the therapy as a predictor of improvement in the children and the benefit that the mothers gained in terms of their own mental health from the child's treatment.[49] Thus, although there were some indications of the superiority of individual treatment, the differences appear to be relatively small. Little support can be harnessed from this study for the psychodynamic approach in general, despite the very impressive effect size, because the psychoeducational group comparison probably had few features of the psychodynamic arm and was crucially lacking the individual interpretative therapeutic interventions.

Kronmuller and colleagues[50] performed a prospective study in 2 stages: the first was an RCT examining the efficacy of short-term PP compared with a wait-list control, and the second was a naturalistic study to assess the effectiveness of long-term psychoanalysis with no control group. Seventy-one patients (aged 6–18 years) with externalizing and internalizing problems received an average of 82 therapy sessions. The therapies were performed using a manual. In the context of this study, instruments were developed or translated and psychometrically evaluated. Compared with the wait-list control, patients receiving short-term psychotherapy showed a significantly greater reduction in the Psychic and Social Communicative Findings Report (PSCR) total score. For longer-term treatment, there were significant improvements on all of the PSCR subscales. Long-term treatment effect sizes were higher than for short-term treatment. The study had a relatively small sample, which was heterogeneous, and the long-term treatment was performed without a control. Nevertheless, the short-term treatment results indicate the benefits of psychodynamics for a mixed neurotic condition.

A very small RCT (n = 30) of adolescents showed a surprisingly strong statistically significant benefit from 10 sessions of PP in a school setting in India. The vast majority of young people improved in PP (more than 90%, reported effect size 1.8).[51] Notably, young people with externalizing problems were specifically excluded from this sample. Therapy outcome was independently, but not blindly, assessed by teachers. No implications can be drawn from this report for PP.

Active treatment comparisons

In its traditional formulations, a great deal of significance has been attached to the 1:1 relationship between therapist and patient in the mechanisms of change in psychodynamic child therapy.[52,53] A number of studies have been performed to test the validity of this assumption by contrasting individual dynamic therapy with other models to a lesser or greater extent informed by psychoanalytic ideas.

Individual psychodynamic child therapy, structural family therapy, recreational control group Szapocznik and colleagues[54] performed an RCT (n = 69) comparing Individual Psychodynamic Child Therapy (IPCT; n = 26), Structural Family Therapy (SFT; n = 26), and a Recreational control group (n = 11) in a sample of Hispanic boys (aged 6 through 12) with behavioral and emotional problems (32% oppositional defiant disorder [ODD], 30% anxiety disorder, 16% conduct disorder [CD]). All subjects received weekly sessions of 50 to 90 minutes. Five types of measure were used:

1. Revised Child Behavior Checklist (RCBC)
2. Revised Behavior Problem Checklist (BPC-R)
3. Child Depression Inventory (CDI)
4. Children's Manifest Anxiety Scale
5. Psychodynamic Child Rating Scale (PCRS)

Structural family systems ratings Assessment took place at baseline, end of treatment, and 1-year follow-up. Both treatments were found to be effective in reducing both behavioral and emotional problems relative to a no-treatment control group. The improvements were maintained at 1-year follow-up. There was significantly greater attrition in the control group (43%) than in the SFT (16%) and the IPCT conditions (4%). Final data analyses were performed only on subjects who had completed treatment. Four times as many families were lost from family therapy than individual therapy, but family functioning improved following family therapy and deteriorated following individual PP. It is not clear whether the uneven attrition might have contributed to the apparently greater deterioration of family functioning in the individual psychotherapy group.[54] This strongly supports the acceptability of PP but is equivocal in relation to its effectiveness.

Individual psychodynamic psychotherapy, systemic family therapy Trowell and colleagues[55] performed a multicenter experimental study to assess the effectiveness of focused individual PP (FIPP) and systems integrative family therapy (SIFT) in a sample of children and young adolescents aged between 9 and 15 years (mean 12 years) with moderate and severe depression. Participants were randomized to 1 of 2 active treatments, based on caseness (FIPP, n = 35; SIFT, n = 37). Treatment was performed over 9 months and participants received a mean of eleven 90-minute sessions of family therapy or a mean of twenty-five 50-minute sessions of individual therapy plus parallel sessions of therapy for parents. Assessment took place at baseline, end of therapy, and at 6-month follow-up. At the end of treatment, 74.3% of the FIPP group and 75.7% of the SIFT group were no longer clinically depressed. At 6-month follow-up, the rates of depression had decreased further; 100% of cases in the SIFT group and 81% of cases in the FIPP group were no longer clinically depressed, suggesting a "sleeper effect" for family therapy as well as individual dynamic therapy. The FIPP was effective for MDD, dysthymia, and double depression, and there were no relapses in the follow-up period. There was also a reduction in comorbid conditions across the study.[56] The results are consistent with the suggestion that SIFT may achieve its results more quickly than FIPP, but by 6 months posttreatment there were no substantial differences between the groups. Methodologically, this is a relatively well-designed study, but is limited by the attrition at follow-up and particularly by the lack of a TAU or waiting-list comparison group. It suggests that PP may be an effective intervention for depression but unlikely to be more effective than systemic family therapy.

Prolonged exposure therapy for adolescents, active controlled time-limited dynamic therapy In a pilot RCT, Gilboa-Schechtman and colleagues[57] examined the efficacy and maintenance of developmentally adapted prolonged exposure therapy for adolescents (PE-A) compared with active controlled time-limited dynamic therapy (TLDP-A). Thirty-eight 12-year-olds to 18-year-olds with PTSD related to a single traumatic event were randomly assigned to 1 of 2 treatment arms. Both groups reported decreases in PTSD symptoms and improvements in general functioning; however, the changes were greater for adolescents in the prolonged exposure therapy group. Participants in this arm reported larger mean decreases in posttraumatic symptom scores and depression scores, and greater increases in adaptation. At the end of treatment, 68.4% of the adolescents in the PE-A group and 36.8% of those in the TDLP-A group no longer met diagnostic criteria for PTSD. At 6-month and 17-month follow-up, treatment gains and group differences were maintained. In summary, exposure treatment was more effective than individual psychotherapy. However, the pre-post effect size in the TDLP-A group was substantial, although in the absence of a no-treatment control condition, it is hard to assess whether this is attributable to a spontaneous process of recovery. Methodologically, the study is clearly of high quality, but limitations of sample size (only 19 per arm) of this pilot investigation preclude definitive conclusions in relation to PP. Further, there is considerable heterogeneity even in this small sample, notwithstanding the primary diagnosis of PTSD as an inclusion criterion. However, there is no support from this study to suggest that PP should be used in preference to exposure-based therapies in the treatment of PTSD.

Behavioral family systems therapy, ego-oriented individual therapy An RCT of behavioral family systems therapy (BFST) aimed to contrast BFST with an "inert" treatment, ego-oriented individual therapy (EOIT), a specially designed treatment with a clear psychodynamic basis.[58,59] In this small RCT, 37 adolescent female patients (aged 12–19) with anorexia (DSM-III) who received either BFST or ego-oriented individual therapy (EOIT) were compared. Both groups received treatment for 12 to 18 months. BFST patients received weekly 72-minute therapy sessions, whereas EOIT patients met weekly for 45 minutes and bimonthly with parents for 54 minutes. Subjects were assessed on a variety of physical and psychological measures at baseline, posttreatment, and 1-year follow-up. Each patient received 10 to 16 months of therapy and was assessed post therapy and followed up at 1.0, 2.5, and 4.0 years. Both treatments were effective; two-thirds of the girls reached their target weights by the end of treatment, and at 1-year follow-up, 80% of those receiving family therapy and 69% of those treated individually had reached their target weights (a difference that was not statistically significant). On body mass index (BMI), both the BFST and EOIT groups improved, but the BFST group improved more (mean change = 4.7) than the EOIT group (mean change = 2.3). As is often found, the nonpsychodynamic approach produced changes faster, but in this instance carried the cost of a somewhat higher rate of hospitalization. Both therapies produced equally large improvements in attitudes to eating and depressed affect and family functioning.[58] Robin and colleagues[58] concluded that parental involvement was essential to the success of their interventions for younger adolescents with anorexia nervosa, but that family dynamics could still be influenced without requiring the adolescent and her parents to be in the room together for all therapy sessions. In other reports, the difference between therapies (group vs individual and family) were small, but therapy of whatever kind is clearly better than no treatment.[60] These studies support the use of PP in the treatment of anorexia, albeit not in preference to family-based interventions, but perhaps to be offered to patients as alternative approaches as part of showing respect for treatment preference.

Family therapy, individual therapy in anorexia and eating disorders The comparability of the effectiveness of family and individual approaches in the aforementioned studies contrasts with findings showing the long-term superiority of family therapy for a younger age group of patients with anorexia when family therapy was compared with a psychodynamic approach.[61–65] In these studies at the Maudsley hospital, individuals who were relatively older appeared to benefit more from individual treatment, whereas younger individuals benefited more from family-based approaches. A follow-up of individuals treated with individual PP also showed the effectiveness of the psychodynamic approach with eating-disordered patients.[66]

In an attempt to resolve these conflicting observations, Lock and colleagues[67] contrasted individual therapy and family-based treatment (FBT) for individuals meeting criteria for anorexia nervosa. Adolescent-focused therapy (AFT) assumes that adolescents confuse self-control with meeting biologic needs. The treatment encourages separation-individuation and the enhancement of tolerance of negative affect. At the end of treatment, 23% of the AFT group and 42% of the FBT group had achieved full remission but the difference between the 2 groups was not significant; however, the difference was maintained and even increased in terms of the percentage of those who met criteria for full remission, showing FBT to be superior to AFT. Treatment effects were greater for the FBT group on a number of measures but the difference between the groups disappeared on the self-report measure of eating attitudes. This is a very good-quality study, perhaps the best in this body of RCTs. It suggests that family therapy may be the treatment of choice for anorexia when compared with PP but that PP achieves good results with these patients; however, the absence of a TAU control group does not allow us to conclude that individual dynamic therapy is an effective treatment. It should be recognized that, given the nature of the disorder and the current state of knowledge, anything other than an effective therapy comparison would be unethical for this diagnostic group.

Integrative (nontraditional) applications of the psychodynamic model of therapy

Suicidal behavior in adolescents Although not strictly speaking individual PP, the approach proposed by Diamond and Josephson[68] to address suicidal behavior in adolescents is relatively close to PP in implementation. Attachment based family therapy (ABFT) focuses on strengthening the attachment bonds between the adolescent and parent to produce a protective and secure base from which the adolescent can develop. It is based on attachment theory, which is a psychoanalytic model in its origin and, in the view of many, in its current applications.[69] An RCT in the United States compared this attachment-based family therapy (n = 35) with enhanced usual care (EUC; n = 31) for suicidal adolescents aged 12 to 17 years.[70] Outcome measures were the suicidal ideation questionnaire (SIQ-JR),[71] the Scale for Suicidal Ideation (SSI),[72] and the Beck Depression Inventory Revised.[73] The adolescents were assessed at baseline, 6 weeks, 12 weeks, and 24 weeks. Compared with EUC, the ABFT group showed a significantly greater rate of improvement on the SIQ-JR, SSI, and Beck Depression Inventory during the treatment period. On the SIQ-JR at 6, 12, and 24 weeks, 69.7%, 87.1%, and 70% of the ABFT group and 40.7%, 51.7%, and 34.6% of the EUC group, respectively, no longer reported suicidal ideation at the clinical level. The SSI demonstrated similar responses. In addition, 58.1% of the ABFT group and 38.5% of the EUC group showed clinically meaningful change in depression scores. Dropout was notably lower in the ABFT group. This is an important study because suicidal ideation is a powerful predictor of suicide attempts and a reduction in suicidal ideation may be a key outcome.[74] Although we note that there was consistency across self-report, clinician ratings, and depression diagnosis, there was no objective assessment of outcome by blinded assessors. Effects could be observed at 24 weeks, but there is no evidence that these outcomes were maintained in the long term. Nevertheless, the study constitutes preliminary evidence for the value of PP implemented as a family intervention for this group of severely impaired young people.

Children exposed to marital violence Another family intervention with children with emotional disorders was reported by Lieberman and colleagues.[75] Again, this was a treatment that is undoubtedly psychodynamic in its conception, but nontraditional in its implementation. In a hallmark RCT of dyadic therapy, Lieberman and colleagues[75] studied 75 dyads of mothers and preschool-aged children (39 girls and 36 boys; age mean = 4.06, SD = 0.82). The selection criteria included high-risk status, embodied in exposure to marital violence but where the perpetrator was no longer in the home. They were randomized to either child–parent psychotherapy (CPP) or monthly case management plus referral to community services (which could include individual therapy). The therapy was relatively long term, with fifty 1-hour sessions that focused on the mother's own history and the way this interacted with her perception of her child. Assessments were performed at intake, post therapy, and 6-month follow-up. The primary outcome was the CBCL and a structured interview covering emotional and behavioral problems and PTSD symptoms (Semi-structured Interview for Diagnostic Classification 0 to 3 [DC: 0–3]). Children in the group assigned to CPP improved significantly more than those assigned to TAU; at the end of treatment, they showed decreased behavioral problems and PTSD symptoms. The CPP children were also less likely to be diagnosed with PTSD after treatment. Mothers in the CPP group showed significantly less PTSD avoidance symptoms than those in the control group. On the whole, pre-post differences were significant for the child psychotherapy group, but not for the TAU condition. From point of view of the quality of the report, the study was rated moderate-good. The limitations included a relatively small sample size, which was selected on a risk-experience rather than a presenting symptom or disorder, and the treatment fidelity not being comprehensively reported. Further, the TAU condition is poorly described. Nevertheless, it joins a group of therapies in which PP is effectively implemented in the family context.

Children exposed to traumatic and stressful life events Ghosh-Ippen and colleagues[76] grouped the sample from the Lieberman and colleagues'[75] study according to the quantity of traumatic and stressful life events (TSEs) they had experienced (low risk <4 vs high risk 4+). Among high-risk children, those in the CPP group showed significantly more improvement than children in the comparison group. High-risk CPP children also showed greater reductions in PTSD (5% vs 53%) and depression, number of co-occurring diagnoses, and behavioral problems. Among the low-risk children, the CPP group showed significant improvement in PTSD symptoms, whereas the comparison group did not. The investigators also report that CPP may be especially efficacious for mothers of high-risk children; CPP mothers showed significant reductions in PTSD and depression, whereas comparison mothers did not show the same improvements. At follow-up, the high-risk group showed significant improvements in the children's behavior and reductions in maternal depression, whereas the comparison group did not. This study needs replication but points in the direction of important potential moderators for dyadic implementation of PP for families that experience trauma.

Maltreated children The model of dyadic intervention with young children turns out to be a powerful application of the psychodynamic model for early intervention. In a unique trial of PP designed to compare the efficacy of preventive dyadic interventions for maltreated children, Toth and colleagues[77] randomized 87 mothers and their preschoolers into 3 groups. Participants received preschooler–parent psychotherapy

(PPP; n = 23), psychoeducational home visitation, which was a didactic model of intervention directed at parenting skills (PHV; n = 34), or community standard intervention (CS; n = 30). A further group (NC; n = 35) with no history of maltreatment was used as comparison. The PPP model consisted of 60 minutes a week of dyadic interventions with a clinical psychologist, and was designed to provide the mother with "corrective emotional experience" in relation to her own experiences of deprivation and maltreatment. This toddler–parent psychotherapy has as its focus assisting the mother to change her behavior in relation to the child and modify the child's expectations of the mothers' behavior. A narrative story-stem task was used to measure the effect of maltreatment in the internal representations. In the task, the chosen narratives depicted moral dilemmas or conflicts and emotionally charged events in the context of parent–child and family relationships. Assessment was made at baseline and 1 year after recruitment. PPP had a better pre-post effect size in each of the 4 items assessed (maladaptive maternal representations, negative self-representations, positive self-representations, and mother–child relationship expectations). There was no significant difference among the 3 other groups (PHV, CS, and NC) in terms of change scores. There was a significant change in mother–child relationship expectations of PPP children. Children became more positive over the course of the intervention in comparison with NC and PHV children. This attachment-theory–informed PP intervention appeared as more effective at improving representations of self and of caregivers than an intervention based on parenting skills, which is often the recommended therapy for this age group. The study is of good methodological quality and provides evidence for recommending dyadic PP for children with maltreatment histories.

Attachment in children of mothers with MDD A similar study was designed to prevent the risk of insecure attachment in children of mothers with severe affective disorder. The development of insecure attachment relationships in the offspring of mothers with MDD may initiate a negative trajectory loading to future psychopathology.[78] Toth and colleagues[79] designed an attachment-theory–guided intervention to promote secure attachment in children of mothers who had experienced MDD since their child's birth. A total of 130 mothers were recruited and randomly assigned to toddler–parent psychotherapy (DI, n = 66) or to a control group (DC, n = 64). There was a further comparison group of nondepressed mothers with no current or history of major mental disorder. Children from that group were also recruited to serve as a nondepressed comparison group (NC; n = 68). The mean age of the children was 20.34 months at the initial assessment. Insecure attachment was significantly higher in both clinical groups (DI and DC) at baseline compared with the group of children without maternal psychopathology. Postintervention assessment was at 3 years (36 months). Insecure attachment remained high in the DC group but the rate of secure attachment had increased substantially in the DI group and was significantly higher than that for the DC group. It was also higher than for the NC group, in which there was little maternal psychopathology, although the group was demographically comparable to both the clinical groups. These results offer strong evidence to support the efficacy of toddler–parent psychotherapy in fostering secure attachment relationships in young children of depressed mothers. This is one of the best-controlled studies of integrative dynamic therapy, but, along with the study of maltreatment, it addresses an at-risk rather than a diagnosed population and therefore may not be included in many reviews in which the presence of a clinical diagnosis represents an entry criterion for the review.

Children with borderline personality disorder Cognitive analytic therapy (CAT) is another nontraditional implementation of psychodynamic ideas integrated with cognitive therapy. In an RCT, Chanen and colleagues[80] compared the effectiveness of up to 24 sessions of CAT and manualized good clinical care (GCC) for outpatients who fulfilled between 2 and 9 DSM-IV criteria for BPD, including self-harm. Eighty-six participants were randomized, and follow-up data were gathered for 41 participants in the CAT group and 37 in the GCC group. Primary outcomes were reduction in psychopathology (Structured Clinical Interview for DSM-IV Axis II Disorders, Youth Self Report [YSR]), parasuicidal behavior (semistructured interview), and improvement in global functioning (Social and Occupational Functioning Assessment Scale). The median number of therapy sessions received was 13 for the CAT group and 11 for the GCC group. Both treatment groups demonstrated improvements over the 2-year period from baseline to final follow-up. There were no significant differences between the 2 conditions at posttreatment; both conditions showed substantial improvement. This study is important because self-harm, when accompanied by depression, is an important predictor of suicidal behavior in adolescence. A strong point of the study is that treatments were delivered as intended to be delivered in real-world services and there was a rigorous control condition. To control for therapist effects, the same therapists were used for both interventions; this could have caused a "leakage" effect (being trained in one orientation impacts on the manner in which the other intervention is delivered), but adherence to the models was rated as excellent. The sample size was small to show a difference between 2 active treatments. Part of the reason why there may have been no difference observed is because the control condition was "rigorously implemented" in a well-structured design with many of the "nonspecific" features of the experimental treatment. Nevertheless, no support for the use of PP in treatment of self-harm can be gained from the study.

Summary

This review of RCTs has provided stronger support for the use of PP as implemented in a family context rather than as classically envisioned as an individual therapy. In comparison with other individual therapies, there is little evidence to recommend PP perhaps with the exception of emotional disorders in younger children. Beyond this, older adolescents with anorexia have been shown to benefit. In other contexts, family interventions appear quicker and as or more effective. However, there is an accumulating body of evidence that a dyadic, parent-child implementation of PP may be quite efficacious in a range of contexts, particularly those involving maltreatment or family trauma. It should be noted also that in some studies, retaining families in treatment and research appeared to be more difficult than in individual therapy. This was not the case for studies in which family based-dyadic treatment was offered to mothers and younger children.

Quasi-experimental and Comparison Group Studies

Although opportunities abound, few studies have appeared in the literature to show the effects of PP compared with an appropriate comparison population. The yield of such studies is primarily in providing practice-based evidence (to answer the "Will it work for me?" question after an RCT has demonstrated treatment effects because of the intervention).

Comparison with TAU

A naturalistic longitudinal study[81] examined the effectiveness of individual psychotherapy for adolescents (aged 12–18) with a range of severe mental illnesses diagnosed according to DSM-IV criteria. Forty participants were offered psychoanalytic psychotherapy once or twice weekly for 4 to 12 months; 40 other participants were offered TAU. A variety of outcome measures were used: CBCL, YSR, Family Assessment Device (FAD), Global Assessment of Functioning (GAF), and the Global Assessment of Relational Functioning (GARF). Assessment took place at baseline and 12 months. At 12 months, psychotherapy was associated with a greater reduction in depressive, social, and attentional problems compared with TAU. Psychotherapy was associated with increases on the GAF and FAD; however, the greater effectiveness of the treatment depended on the level of psychopathology at baseline. Almost half the participants offered PP did not engage (17 of 20) and there was a high rate of attrition in the TAU group at 1-year follow-up (24 of 40 were not followed up). Taking these considerations together, there is little in this study to support PP as an intervention for adolescents with severe mental disorder.

A series of reports of the Tavistock study of children in the care system[82–85] provided a systematic investigation of PP for children in care. The study aimed to assess whether these severely deprived children could benefit from psychotherapy. The research had a secondary aim to devise a methodology suitable for evaluating PP. In all, 38 children received PP (7 drop-outs). The comparison group consisted of 13 cases in which therapy was recommended but refused. Although the refusal was not necessarily based on the child but on circumstances beyond the child, nevertheless, comparability between the groups would be hard to assume. At baseline, there were few differences between the 2 groups. At 2-year follow-up, most showed improvement in their relationships with adults and with friends, changes in inner representations, and improvements in learning and thinking processes. Although improved self-image was seen, the change came slowly and not as easily as in other domains.[82–85] The study also produced interesting qualitative data on the therapists' thoughts about therapy and its outcomes. The study did not use established outcome measures, making it hard to interpret the effect size of change; however, the individual psychotherapy offered to these children was found to improve the objective indicators of the quality-of-life circumstances in which these children lived, namely, more permanent placements and less disruption of care. The findings were supported by a further study with a single case experimental design.[82] In addition, the results mainly depended on the therapists' assessments and could therefore be seen as low in objectivity; however, some of the ratings were done by blinded external raters. On the whole, there is indication here, that were RCTs available on the PP treatment of children in care, the likelihood is that the effects might generalize to ordinary clinical contexts (show stable capacity).

There is a tradition of psychodynamic work with individuals with chronic physical conditions, such as asthma and diabetes.[86] Trial data are hard to come by, however. The work of George Moran and colleagues[87] with diabetic children is one of the only counterexamples. One small trial demonstrated psychoanalytic psychotherapy to be effective in reducing glycosylated hemoglobin levels relative to a comparison group. The study compared the effects of psychoanalytic treatment plus routine care and routine care in 22 (aged 6–18) diabetic children and adolescents with grossly abnormal blood glucose profiles requiring repeated hospital admissions. Participants in the treatment group were offered psychoanalytic psychotherapy 3 to 4 times a week on the hospital ward; those in the control group received routine medical care and minimal psychological intervention. Assessment was conducted at baseline, 3 months, and 1 year. The treatment was highly effective in improving the diabetic control of children (measured by glycosylated hemoglobin concentration [Hb1Ac]) and this was maintained at 1-year follow-up. Hb1Ac concentration fell to a clinically acceptable range for diabetes in 6 of the treated subjects. None of the untreated group showed such an improvement (P<.025). At follow-up, 9 of the patients in the experimental group remained below their preadmission average HbA1c levels, whereas only 3 of those in the comparison group did so. In a series of experimental single case studies, individual PP was found to improve several growth parameters probably associated with improvement of diabetic control.[88] An earlier study of day-to-day variations of diabetic control of a young girl in child analysis showed an association between the discussion of material in the analytic session and subsequent improvements in diabetic control.[89] These studies deserve consideration because outcomes were measured not by psychological assessment, but by standard measures for diabetes control (M-value and HbA1c). Yet, as pointed out by the investigators themselves, the small group size limits the conclusions that could be drawn. Although this appeared to be a promising approach, particularly given the robust nonreactive measure of treatment outcome, it has sadly not been followed up by subsequent investigations of somatic problems and therefore it is not possible to recommend PP for somatic disorders on the basis of one poorly controlled study (however innovative).

In a further small-scale study, Apter and colleagues[90] reported on 8 adolescents with obsessive-compulsive disorder (OCD) who were inpatients in a psychiatric hospital in Israel. Four cases were allocated to intensive psychodynamically oriented psychotherapy and 4 to supportive educational therapy. Response to nonspecific psychotherapy and milieu therapy was surprisingly good; 7 of the 8 patients were much improved within 3 to 4 months (in terms of checking, cleaning, ruminations, slowness symptoms) and 4 of 8 were completely symptom free. The study suggests that observational data of improvement alone may exaggerate the apparent impact of PP for OCD. The conclusions of this study are limited by its small sample size and lack of randomization.

Comparison with convenience sample
Slonim and collegues[91] reported a study of a group of adolescents (n = 30, aged 15–18) with mixed diagnoses in outpatient clinics in Jerusalem, who were treated with psychoanalytic psychotherapy. The control group consisted of 42 participants with similar ages and demographic backgrounds, studying in the same school as the treated patients. Assessment occurred at the beginning of treatment or school year, and after 12 months. Outcome was measured by the Youth Outcome Questionnaire Self-Report (Y-OQ-SR) and Target Complaint Scales (TCS). The main goal of the study was to correlate rigidity (assessed with the Core Conflictual Relationship Theme method) with treatment outcome. The treatment group showed significant changes in rigidity over the course of a year of psychotherapy, whereas no such changes were detected in the community group. The results of the outcome measures indicate that the treatment group improved significantly more than the community group between baseline and end of treatment (ES = 0.27 for Y-OQ and 0.78 for TCS), and that this improvement was significantly correlated with a decrease in symptoms within the treatment group. However, the comparison group does not protect from the bias of regression to the mean as the 2 groups differed substantially at baseline and greater changes would be expected from the group with higher initial mean scores. The evidence from this study cannot therefore be interpreted as supporting PP in the context of community mental health care.

Deakin and Nunes[92] examined the effectiveness of child psychoanalytic psychotherapy in a clinical outpatient sample of 55 children in Brazil aged 6 to 11 years with mixed diagnoses. The Rorschach, Bender, and Wechsler Intelligence Scale for Children, Third Edition (WISC III) were administered to 23 children aged 6 to 11 years, and the CBCL was completed by the parents at baseline and after 12 months of intervention. The control group was a heterogeneous group of 22 matched children from a local school who did not receive any intervention. In the intervention group, the children showed significant reductions in behavioral and emotional problems. CBCL effect sizes between groups at 12 months were small on the internalizing scale, negligible on the externalizing scale, and insignificant overall. This was a controlled observational study, performed at a clinic with no research culture. There was a high dropout rate (54%) and no manual was used for individual child psychoanalytic psychotherapy (ICPP), so it was not possible to ensure that the therapy was performed as intended. Although offering little solid basis for recommending PP, the greater impact on internalizing than externalizing problems of PP reflects other findings from correlational designs.

Active treatment comparisons
Scholte and van der Ploeg[93] performed a quasi-experimental study (n = 105) with adolescents (mean age 14.9 years) admitted to 4 different residential programs in the Netherlands aiming to treat severe behavioral and emotional difficulties. The following treatment methods were used: behavioral modification, psychodynamic treatment, structured community living, and adventurous learning. The treated children were also compared with a dropout control group (n = 22). Outcome measurement (with CBCL) and assessment took place 1 month into the treatment and at the end of treatment. All programs produced positive outcomes on all 3 domains of the CBCL (internalizing, externalizing, and total problems). The psychodynamically treated group's pre-post effect size was large. This group showed greater improvement than the behavioral modification group, but not quite as large as the structured community living and adventurous learning groups; however, only a small portion of patients moved to a nonclinical condition after 1 year, and thus treatment often had to be extended. The use of dropouts as a control condition and the lack of randomization introduce a bias that has probably increased the apparent effect sizes of the treated groups precluding valid conclusions in relation to PP. Outcomes based entirely on CBCL scores may create concerns about the reactive nature of the assessment approach, as the context of the therapy (individual vs community) may have moderated the way youths and/or informants completed the measures.

A classic study, for many years one of the only studies that considered the issue of intensity of psychological therapy, focused on specific learning difficulties as a target of therapy.[94,95] In the first study, 8 boys received psychoanalytic treatment; 4 received therapy once a week, and the others received therapy 4 times a week. At the end of treatment, the children seen 4 times a week showed greater improvement in adaptation compared with those receiving treatment once a week. This study had a small sample and used unvalidated measures. In the second study, 12 boys (mean age 9 years) presenting with attention-deficit/hyperactivity disorder (ADHD) were split into 3 groups that received different intensities of psychoanalytic psychotherapy. The treatments given to the groups were once weekly psychoanalytic psychotherapy for the first year and then 4 times a week for the rest of the therapy (total duration 36 months); once a week throughout the whole therapy (27 months); and 4 times a week throughout the whole therapy (28 months). All boys made improvements, but those seen more frequently (4 times a week for 1 or 2 years) showed greater improvements in self-esteem, capacity for relationships, frustration tolerance, and flexible adaptation. The study is limited by its small sample size, but suggests that more frequent sessions trigger qualitative process variables, and that quantitative measurement is not always enough to understand improvements after psychotherapy. Without an untreated control group, it is not possible to say whether the improvement would not have occurred spontaneously, except that there was a dose-response relationship that became apparent over the 2 years after treatment. The 8 children who had received more intensive help (more sessions per week) showed increasing benefits in terms of self-esteem, the capacity to form relationships, and the capacity to work, including frustration tolerance.

Summary

Surprisingly, quasi-experimental studies have not been as productive in the field of PP testing as in the case of other psychotherapy investigations. Notwithstanding the problems of interpretation that can bedevil these studies, they potentially provide evidence in relation to the replicability of size of effects observed in RCTs. The studies reviewed in this section have not provided conclusive data in relation to the value of PP for outpatient or institutional treatment contexts.

Observational Studies

Controlled trials teach us a great deal about a therapy, but we can learn much from follow-along or observational studies too. The learning in these instances is less from the size of the improvement of the group overall, but rather from comparisons within the sample potentially identifying the subgroups that benefit most from a treatment.

Clinic-based studies

Community-based psychoanalytic psychotherapy service for young people In a series of articles, Baruch and colleagues[96–98] report the evaluation of a community-based psychoanalytic psychotherapy service for young people between 12 and 25 years old. In the initial report,[99] 106 participants with multiple difficulties are described. They were assessed at intake, at 3 months, 6 months, 1 year, and annually thereafter. The median number of weeks in treatment was 17. The adolescents and young adults in the sample had a median number of 3 diagnoses and 4 significant psychosocial stressors. After 3 months, there was significant improvement ($P<.01$) in Internalizing Problem scores and Total Problem scores on the YSR. The investigators report that externalizing problems appeared more difficult to treat with PP. Twice as many participants improved if they had internalizing disorders, which was a statistically significant difference. Comorbidity with emotional problems increased the likelihood of externalizing problems responding to psychodynamic treatment, as did more frequent treatment. Detailed analysis revealed that participants who improved for externalizing problems also improved for internalizing problems. Most subjects who reported deterioration for externalizing problems did not deteriorate for internalizing problems. Similar conclusions emerged from a report of follow-up of 61 participants from the same study.[97]

Baruch and Fearon[99] reported a 1-year follow-up of 151 participants from the same service. According to self-report data, participants showed an improvement in mean scores on the YSR, fewer participants were in the clinical range, and the participants demonstrated significant reliable change in level of adaptation. Rate of improvement did, however, drop significantly over time. The sample of young people who were reached on follow-up, however, appeared to be unrepresentative of the overall population who received therapy from the service. In a further study,[98] the focus was on the difficulty in collection of observational data, with levels of attrition at 12-month follow-up for self, significant other, and therapist reports being 19.4%, 10.3%, and 16.0%, respectively.

Psychodynamic treatments for varying diagnostic groups The Anna Freud centre (AFC) retrospective study provided information concerning the relative benefits obtained from psychodynamic treatments of varying intensity for a number of diagnostic groups.

Emotional disorders Using data from this study, Target and Fonagy[45] examined the efficacy of psychoanalysis for children with emotional disorders. They compared 254 children and adolescents who underwent full psychoanalysis (4–5 times a week) with 98 children and adolescents treated with psychoanalytic psychotherapy (1–3 times a week) for an average of 2 years. Treatment outcome was assessed with CGAS at referral and termination. There was only very preliminary evidence that PP may be effective in the treatment of anxiety disorders.[45] In this chart review study, children with anxiety disorders (with or without comorbidity) showed greater improvements than those with other conditions, and greater improvements than would have been expected on the basis of studies of untreated outcome. More than 85% of 299 children with anxiety and depressive disorders no longer suffered any diagnosable emotional disorder after an average of 2 years of treatment. Looking in more detail at specific diagnostic groups, it was found that phobias (n = 48), separation anxiety disorders (n = 58), and overanxious disorder (n = 145) were resolved in approximately 86% of cases. OCD was more resistant, ceasing to meet diagnostic criteria in only 70% of cases. There are serious limitations to a retrospective study, and there was no control group or follow-up; however, these rates of improvement appear to be above the level expected from longitudinal studies. For emotional disorder diagnoses, less severe principal diagnosis, better initial adaptation, and younger age were significant predictors of good outcome. A further finding was that children with severe or pervasive symptomatology, such as Generalised Anxiety Disorder (GAD), or multiple comorbid disorders, required more frequent therapy sessions, whereas more circumscribed symptoms, such as phobias, even if quite severe, improved comparably with once-weekly sessions.

Dysthymia and/or major depression The AFC chart review study[100] included 65 children and adolescents with dysthymia and/or major depression, who had been treated for an average of 2 years. By the end of therapy, more than 75% showed reliable improvement in functioning and no depressive symptoms; however, the episodic course of depression means that these pre-post findings with no control group or follow-up cannot be taken as evidence of efficacy. A clearer finding was that children and adolescents with depressive disorders appeared to benefit more from intensive (4–5 sessions per week) than from nonintensive (1–2 sessions per week) therapy, after controlling for length of treatment and level of impairment at referral. This is of some interest, given that the depressed cases were mostly adolescents who generally did not gain additional benefit from frequent sessions.

In the AFC retrospective study,[101] although children and young people treated for major depression were likely to improve even if they remained in the dysfunctional range after treatment, diagnoses related to conduct problems (CD and ODD) appeared particularly resistant to PP. Children with ODD benefited more than those with CD. The difference was mostly explained by premature termination of treatment. Children and young people with disruptive disorder who also had an anxiety disorder diagnosis were more likely to benefit.[101] As noted previously, individual child psychotherapy is now rarely performed in practice without family work. In the AFC retrospective study, concurrent work with parents was a predictor of good outcome.[45]

Outcomes of child psychotherapy in adulthood In a smaller sample from the AFC long-term follow-up, Schachter and Target[102] examined the outcomes of child psychotherapy in adulthood. Thirty-four former child patients treated at the AFC between 1952 and 1991 participated. The subjects took part in a comprehensive interview process comprising 3 or 4 sessions, each lasting between 2.0 and 2.5 hours. The results of 5 different measures were synthesized into a single index, the Adult Functioning Index (AFI). Overall, participants treated as children were not characterized by severe impairment or poor functioning in adulthood. Most reported that they had at least one significant support figure, had experienced relatively low levels of adversity during their adult lives, had few severe life events in recent years, had good health, and had made minimal use of medical services. There was a strong association between positive adult outcome and secure attachment status. Correlation and regression analyses between assessment (pretreatment), termination (conclusion of treatment), and adult outcome showed that the best predictor of adult outcome was the child's overall level of functioning, assessed on the Hampstead Child Adaptation Measure (HCAM) score (Schneider T. Measuring adaptation in middle childhood: the development of the Hampstead Child Adaptation Measure. University College London: Unpublished dissertation, 2000) before receiving treatment. Although this is a unique study, there is little expectation on the part of the investigators of representativeness. Clearly, in the case of long-term follow-up, those with the least difficulty in their current lives may indeed be those who are most readily reached.

Midgley and Target[103,104] looked at the outcome of child psychoanalysis from the perspective of the patient. This study was also part of the AFC long-term follow-up study. The investigators examined the memories of adults who received psychoanalysis as children. Two-thirds of those who took part felt that the therapy had been helpful to them at the time, despite difficulty in assessing how their lives might have been different if they had not received it. There was a range of different ways, both positive and negative, in which the participants felt that psychotherapy had affected their lives. In both articles, the investigators report that many participants emphasized the value of being able to talk and be listened to. The investigators report that those who remembered psychoanalysis in a positive way tended to be in treatment as quite young children.[104] About a quarter of patients remembered child therapy predominantly in relation to their lack of engagement with the process. The study's length of follow-up is unique and it produced an interview protocol for the assessment of long follow-ups.

Case series studies
Outpatient therapy for anorexia nervosa Vilsvik and Vaglum[66] performed a small naturalistic study, following the outcome of 17 adolescents (ages 13–17) with anorexia nervosa who participated in an outpatient program of individual psychotherapy for 1 to 9 years (mean 4 years). The average duration of treatment was 11 months, with weekly sessions. Outcome was measured by weight gain, menstrual status, and analysis of case notes. The investigators report that at follow-up, all patients had improved significantly medically and socially; 9 had recovered fully and 6 had minor anorectic symptoms. However, the conclusions are limited by the small sample size, the lack of a control group, and because referring agencies may have selected an unrepresentative sample. The investigators also recognize that the younger age and stable family situation of the subjects may have helped produce the positive outcome.

Autism Nondirective play is often used to promote communication skills in children with autism.[105] Although such interventions have common components, they are not specifically psychodynamic. The Tavistock Clinic has developed a specialized psychodynamic approach to the treatment of individuals with autism.[106] The approach has some similarities with the intensive emotional support–oriented approach taken by Wieder and Greenspan[107] in the United States, and the Mifne method in Israel.[108] These approaches aim to strengthen nonautistic aspects of the child's functioning, working in a family context as much as possible. Vorgraft and colleagues[109] demonstrated significant improvement in 23 children carefully diagnosed as suffering from autistic disorder and treated at the Mifne Institute. They found a modest but statistically significant change at 6-month follow-up of an intensive 3-week treatment. Despite these findings, outcome data are rather sparse in this area, and the retrospective chart review study at the AFC indicated that psychoanalysis was not helpful with this diagnosis.[110] However, follow-up of these psychoanalytically treated individuals into adulthood identified some individuals with symptoms of pervasive developmental disorder, generally Asperger syndrome, who showed a surprisingly high level of functioning in adulthood.[111]

Violence Pynoos and colleagues[112,113] have developed a program for adolescents who experienced or witnessed violence. The University of California Los Angeles School-Based Trauma/Grief Intervention Program for children and adolescents includes a systematic method for screening students, a manualized 16-week to 20-week group psychotherapy protocol, which addresses current stresses and conflicts not limited to the trauma exposure, and adjunctive individual and family therapy. As a package, the protocol is a skills-based cognitive behavioral therapy (CBT) program and is very far from a prototypical unfocused insight-oriented group psychotherapy, but the attention to developmental considerations and the model of traumatic stress within which the treatment is rooted[113] make the intervention deserving of consideration under a general psychodynamic heading. Two uncontrolled studies of this approach[114,115] found that participation was associated with improvements in trauma-related symptoms and in academic performance. The same group assessed a modification of this protocol for 55 war-traumatized Bosnian adolescents. There was an observed reduction in psychological distress and positive associations between distress reduction and improved psychosocial adaptation.

Severe trauma or deprivation Heede and colleagues'[116] prospective uncontrolled study examined the effect of 3 psychodynamic milieu therapeutic institutions for children aged 6 to 15 years suffering from severe trauma or early deprivation. Over 4 years, 24 Danish-speaking children were included in the research project. Measurement points were baseline and after 2 years of treatment. The study's objective was to give a qualified estimation of whether the child's personality structure had changed during the course of psychodynamic milieu therapy. The investigators reported improvements in the children's cognitive and emotional functioning, self-confidence, and capacities for self-reflection, based on the WISC[117] and psychometric tests (Rorschach ad modum)[118] and Thematic Aperception Test (scored by systems developed by Western[119] and Cramer).[120] The therapy was not as effective in terms of the children's interpersonal relations; however, the lack of a control group limits the conclusions that can be drawn from these results in relation to the potential of PP. Moreover, we do not know whether the measure chosen was sensitive to therapeutic change.

Disruptive behavior disorder Eresund[121] reported on a study performed in Sweden examining a long-term supportive expressive play psychotherapy for children and parents. The participants were 9 boys aged 6 to 10 years with disruptive behavior disorder, and their parents. All the boys had a DSM-IV diagnosis of ODD, and some had comorbid ODD, CD, and DAMP (dysfunction of attention, motor control, and perception). The boys received therapy for their problems twice weekly initially; this was reduced to once a week after 1.5 to 2.0 years. Parents had sessions of their own with the child's therapist every second week (sometimes every week). Treatment lasted between 2 and 5 years, with a median of 2.5 years. At the end of treatment, only one boy still fulfilled DSM-IV ODD criteria. Parents (CBCL) and teachers (TRF) reported better social function after therapy. Improvements were less marked in boys who, in addition to initial diagnoses of ODD or CD, had ADHD. At 1-year follow-up, parent-reported improvements were maintained. This study had a very small sample and no control group; however, this study is important in underscoring the potential of long-term PP in helping children with conduct problems.

Mixed diagnoses Odhammar and colleagues[122] report on an observational study that was part of the Erica Process and Outcome Study (EPOS). The EPOS evaluates goal-formulated, time-limited psychotherapy in conjunction with parallel work with parents. The study aimed to investigate whether children's global functioning improves after PP. Thirty-three children (aged 5–10) with mixed diagnoses (29 children had at least one DSM-IV diagnosis and 15 children had comorbid conditions) underwent PP once or twice a week, with parallel work with parents, for 6 months to 2.5 years. Subjects were assessed with the CGAS and HCAM before and after treatment. A significant difference was found between CGAS before and after treatment ($P<.001$), which had a large effect size. A similar result was found for the HCAM. The 4 subscales of the HCAM that showed the largest changes were general mood, and variability of mood; ability to tolerate frustration and control impulses; development of confidence and self-esteem; and ability to cope with very stressful events. The investigators also undertook qualitative analyses of 2 patients, which highlighted the difficulty of capturing and understanding change processes using quantitative measures. The clear limitation of the study design, which compromises the conclusions that can be made in relation to PP, is that psychotherapists themselves rated the children's global functioning with the CGAS.

Carlberg and colleagues[123] explored children's expectations and experiences of PP in a small subsample of participants from the EPOS study. The participants were children aged between 6 and 10 years who had at least one DSM-IV diagnosis at the start of psychotherapy; the most common was ADHD (n = 6). Seven of the children had more than one diagnosis. The children's attitudes were assessed at the start and end of treatment through semistructured interviews using self-rating instruments, drawing materials, and toys. According to the self-ratings, the children showed a moderate degree of improvement in their problems. The children were able to communicate their expectations and experiences, and most were positive about their expectations and their experiences of therapy after termination.

LIMITATIONS AND SUMMARY

Although we aimed at exhaustive coverage, key contributions may have been missed for a range of administrative and practical reasons. Studies not published in the English language were not accessible to review. Anecdotal case reports, which represent a large proportion of the psychodynamic literature, were not included. We did not aggregate the studies using meta-analytic methods; there are too few studies using genuinely comparable treatment procedures for aggregation to be justified.

The body of rigorous research supporting psychodynamic therapies for adults for most disorders remains limited, particularly relative to research supporting pharmaceutical treatments and even other psychosocial approaches, such as CBT.[124–127] There are both practical and theoretical difficulties in mounting trials of dynamic therapies, which go some way to explaining the lack of evidence (eg, the bias against research by many practitioners of psychodynamic therapies and their epistemological problems with accepting the canons of modern scientific studies, the reluctance of funding bodies to invest in research on clinical problems considered to be "solved" by a combination of drug and cognitive behavioral treatments, the expense of mounting trials sufficiently powered to yield information on what treatments are appropriate for which disorder, or the failure to tightly manualize psychodynamic treatments).

Currently there is some evidence to support the use of PP for children whose problems are either internalizing or mixed but with an element of anxiety and emotional disorder. There is also evidence that the support and inclusion of parents is an important aspect of this treatment. There is some evidence that effects tend to increase following the end of treatment. There is evidence that behavioral problems are more resistant at least to a classical, insight-oriented psychodynamic approach. The distinction between family approaches and individual psychodynamic approaches is narrowing. This is particularly clear in the treatment of young children and adolescents with eating disorders, in which it seems that combinations of these 2 approaches are as effective as any other kind of treatment. In line with the grouping together of family and individual approaches, the evidence is stronger for younger children, where parents are almost always included in treatment, and where a dyadic therapeutic model exploring the dynamics of the parent–child relationship may be especially helpful. In our view, it is probably an error to confound the mode of treatment delivery (individual long-term insight-oriented psychotherapy) with the psychological ideas that underpin formulations of pathology and cure which have their origin in that approach. It is, in our view, more than possible that PP has not yet found the best setting and the most efficacious mode of delivering its therapeutic aims. Much of what we had noted as nontraditional applications of psychoanalytic therapy may actually end up as the most commonly used methods for delivering these therapeutic ideas. And why not?

On a separate note, a group of studies in which nonreactive measures of outcome were used (cognitive ability, physiologic indications of compliance with medical treatment) yielded surprisingly large effect sizes, which suggests that researchers of PP need to be willing to look beyond the field of psychological symptoms for the effects of treatment. Those who argue (correctly in our view) for continued investment in this approach point to the limitations of the evidence base supporting CBT (eg, Weston and colleagues[128]) or pharmacologic approaches (eg, Whittington and colleagues[129]). Notwithstanding the general weakness of the evidence base of mental health treatments for children, this weakness is particularly pronounced for psychodynamic treatments, and the shortage of research studies needs to be addressed urgently. In the light of the limitations of CBT in severe disorders in comparison with medication,[130–132] it behooves us to investigate the effectiveness of alternative treatment approaches. Ultimately, however, such a negative case cannot persuade policy makers and funders, and, without intense research on the effectiveness of the method deeply rooted in and shaped by psychological models of pathology, the long-term survival of this orientation is not assured.[8] This is not to say that the techniques that have evolved as part of this approach will not survive (they are effective, and clinicians, being pragmatic people, will continue to discover and use them), but they will be increasingly absorbed into alternative models, and the unique approach pioneered by Freud and outlined in this issue might then not continue.

Table 2
Summary of psychodynamic psychotherapy studies

Authors	Trial Details	Inclusion Criteria	Exclusion Criteria	Participants	Interventions	Primary Outcome Measures	Effect Sizes	Results
Smyrnios and Kirby,[44] 1993	Year: 1993 Design: RCT Follow-up: 4 y Country: Australia	• Diagnostic of "disturbance of emotions specific to childhood" • Age 5–9 y • Assessed by an independent senior child psychiatry consultant as being in need of treatment	• In psychotherapy in the previous year, diagnosis of childhood psychosis • Mental retardation • Severe learning difficulty	Problem/s: Diagnosis of "Disturbance of emotions specific to childhood" N: 30 Sex: 25m, 5f Age: 5–9	• Time-Limited Psychotherapy • Time-Unlimited Therapy • Minimal Contact Group	• Goal Attainment Scales (GAS) • Target Complaint Scales (TCS) • Van der Veen Family Concept Inventory • Bristol Social Adjustment Scale (BSAG)	Pre-post (Time Unlimited) BSAG: r = 0.05 GAS: r = 0.49 Pre-4 y (Time Unlimited) BSAG: r = 0.3 GAS: r = 0.51 Pre-Post (Time Limited) BSAG: r = 0.2 GAS: r = 0.59 Pre-4 y (Time Limited) BSAG: r = 0.53 GAS: r = 0.66 Pre-Post (Minimal Contact) BSAG: r = 0.05 GAS: r = 0.47 Pre-4 y (Minimal Contact) BSAG: r = 0.11 GAS: r = 0.68	• All groups improved from pretest to post-test • Changes in parental measures of family functioning reported by the minimal contact group were significantly greater than those of the time unlimited group • All groups improved significantly on therapist measures of goal attainment from pretest to 4-year follow-up • Only the minimal contact group reported significant improvements on severity of target problems and measures of family functioning

Muratori et al,[46] 2002	Year: 2002
	Design: quasi-randomized controlled study
	Follow-up: 6 and 18 mo
	Country: Italy
		• Age: 6–11
		• Recently emerged symptoms of "emotional disorders"
		• Limited number of life events
		• IQ above 90
			• Children of adoptive families
			• Divorced parents who were in conflict
			
			Problem/s:
			Emotional Disorders
			N: 30
			Sex: 20m, 10f
			Age: 6.3–10.9
				• Brief psychodynamic psychotherapy (BPP)
				• Community services
				
				• CGAS
				• CBCL
				• Social competence
					Between groups
					CGAS
					Post: r = 0.346
					2 y: r = 0.253
					CBCL Total
					Post: r = −0.079
					2 y: r = 0.277
					Pre-post (BPP)
					CGAS: r = 0.64
					CBCL Total: r = 0.15
					Social Competence:
					  r = 0.08
					Pre-2 y (BPP)
					C-GAS: r = 0.62
					CBCL Total: r = 0.58
					Social Competence:
					  r = 0.06
						• There was a positive change in the experimental group between baseline and 18-mo follow-up for total problems
						• Both groups improved on the CGAS scale, but BPP did better both at 6-mo and at 18-mo follow-up
						• Better outcomes for children younger than 9 and for those with a diagnosis of "pure emotional disorder"

(continued on next page)

Table 2
(continued)

Authors	Trial Details	Inclusion Criteria	Exclusion Criteria	Participants	Interventions	Primary Outcome Measures	Effect Sizes	Results
Muratori et al,[47] 2003	Year: 2003 Design: quasi-randomized controlled study Follow-up: 6 mo, 18 mo Country: Italy	• DSM-IV diagnosis of depressive or anxiety disorder, classified as ID. • Symptoms and difficulties for at least 1 y. • CGAS >70	• IQ below 90 • Adoptive families • Families with active divorce process	Problem/s: Depressive or Anxiety Disorder N: 58 Sex: 36m, 22f Age: 6.3–10.9	• Brief psychodynamic psychotherapy • Community Services	• KSADS • CBCL • C-GAS	Between groups CGAS Post: r = 0.391 2 y: r = 0.34 CBCL Total Post: r = 0.019 2 y: r = 0.29 Pre-post (BPP) CGAS: r = 0.7 CBCL Total: r = 0.12 Pre-18 mo (BPP) CGAS: r = 0.68 CBCL Total: r = 0.45	• The experimental group showed great improvement in the CGAS scale both in short as in long-term. • Medium effect size between groups at 6 mo and at follow-up • At follow-up only the experimental group's mean had moved to the functional range • There were no significant differences between treatments on the CBCL between baseline and end of treatment • Between baseline and follow-up, only the treatment group improved significantly on all 3 scales of the CBCL

Study	Characteristics	Inclusion criteria	Problem/s	Intervention	Measures	Results	
Trowell et al,[48] 2002	Year: 2002 Design: RCT Follow-up: 1 and 2 y Country: UK	• Sexual abuse occurred on the basis of balance of probabilities verified by social services and/or court procedure • Girls aged 6–14 • Consent given by legal guardian • Symptoms of emotional or behavioral disturbance • Abuse disclosed within 2 y before referral	Problem/s: Sexual abuse N: 71 Sex: 71f Age: 6–14 • Severe developmental delay • Psychosis • Lack of reasonable confidence that further abuse would not occur • Necessity for hospitalization at initial evaluation	• Individual psychotherapy (IP) • Group psychotherapy (GP)	• Orvachel PTSD scale • K-SADS • K-GAS	Between Group K-GAS 1-y: r = 0.03 2-y: r = −0.02 Exit: r = −0.01 Reexperience of traumatic event 1-y: r = 0.26 2-y: r = 0.37 Exit: r = 0.28 Persistent avoidance of stimuli 1-y: r = 0.21 2-y: r = −0.14 Exit: r = 0.2 Pre-1 y (IP) K-GAS: r = 0.77 Pre –2 y (IP) K-GAS: r = 0.79 Pre-Exit (IP) K-GAS: r = 0.76	• Both groups showed a substantial reduction in psycho-pathology • No differences between the 2 treatments on the KGAS • Individual therapy led to a greater improvement in manifestations of PTSD • Generalized anxiety disorder was the most likely to remit
Kronmuller et al,[50] 2010	Year: 2010 Design: prospective study Follow-up: no Country: Germany	• Outpatients from the Heidelberg Institute with ICD-10 mental disorders	Problem/s: Externalizing and internalizing N: 71 Sex: 43f, 28m Age: 6–18 • Psychotic disorders • Addiction • Serious suicidal tendencies	• Short-term psychoanalytic psychotherapy (STPP) • Wait-list control • Long-term psychoanalytic psychotherapy (LTPP)	• PSCR • WISC • Rorschach ad modum • TAT	Between-Group PSCR Total Score Post: r = 0.502 Pre-post (STPP) Pre-post (LTPP) PSCR (total): r = 0.24	• Compared with the wait list control, patients receiving short-term psycho-therapy showed a significantly greater reduction in the PSCR total score • For longer-term treatment, there were significant improvements on all of the PSCR subscales. Long-term treatment effect sizes

(continued on next page)

Table 2
(continued)

Authors	Trial Details	Inclusion Criteria	Exclusion Criteria	Participants	Interventions	Primary Outcome Measures	Effect Sizes	Results
Sinha and Kapur,[51] 1999	Year: 1999 Design: RCT Follow-up: 5 wk Country: India	• Emotionally disturbed boys in school based -sample	• Externalizing problems	Problem/s: Emotional disturbance N: 30 Sex: 30m Age: 14–15	• Psychodynamic-Orientated Supportive Therapy (POST) • No treatment control	• GHQ • YSR		• The vast majority of young people improved in psychodynamic psychotherapy
Szapocznik et al,[54] 1989	Year: 1989 Design: RCT Follow-up: 1 y Country: USA	• Had 2-parent families (both parents Hispanic) • Had lived in the United States for 3 or more years	• No history of mental retardation • Organic dysfunction • Mental health care • Psychoactive medication • Suicidal ideation	Problem/s: Mixed N: 69 Sex: M Age: 6–12	• Individual Psychodynamic Child Therapy (IPCT) • Structural Family Therapy (SFT) • Recreational control	• Revised Child Behavior Checklist (RCBC) • PCRS • Structural Family Systems Ratings	Between groups (IPCT and SFT) RCBC POST: r = −0.3 1 y: r = 0.01 PCRS POST: r = −0.07 1 y: r = 0.07 SFSR POST: r = 0.01 Pre-post (IPCT) RCBC: r = 0.2 PCRS: r = 0.56 SFSR: r = 0.04 Pre-follow-up (IPCT) RCBC: r = 0.37 PCRS: r = −0.53 SFSR: r = 0.35	• SFT group had the most improved scores on the RCBC. • SFT group had significantly better outcomes than IPCT (P<.05), but neither was significantly better than the control • SFT and IPCT both also significantly better than the control condition on the PCRS (P<.05) • Individual therapy was found to be worse than FT at supporting family functioning • Improvements were maintained at 1 year follow-up.

Study	Design	Inclusion criteria	Exclusion criteria	Sample	Intervention	Measures	Results	Findings

Trowell et al,[55] 2007	Year: 2007
	Design: RCT
	Follow-up: 6 mo
	Country: UK and Finland
		• Score >13 at CDI in conjunction with criteria for Major Depressive Disorder (MDD) and/or Dysthymia on the Kiddie-SADS
		• Living with at least one biologic parent
		• Any psychotropic medication had to have been stopped at least 4 wk before commencement of therapy
			• Depressive disorders
			• Meriting urgent hospitalization
			• Bipolar and Schizoaffective Disorder
			• Severe conduct disorder
			• Parents with psychotic disorder or severe personality disorder
				Problem/s: PTSD
				N: 72
				Sex: 45m, 27f
				Age: 9–15
					• Focused individual psychodynamic psychotherapy (FIPP)
					• Systems integrative family therapy (SIFT)
						• CDI
						• K-SADS
						• Moods and Feelings Questionnaire (MFQ)
							Between Groups
							CDI
							POST: r = −0.251
							6 mo: r = −0.046
							MFQ
							POST: r = −0.145
							6 mo: r = −0.065
							C-GAS
							POST: r = 0.035
							6 mo: r = 0.149
							Pre-Post
							  (individual)
							CDI: r = 0.4
							MFQ: r = 0.42
							C-GAS: r = 0.62
							Pre-6 mo
							  (individual)
							CDI: r = 0.68
							MFQ: r = 0.59
							C-GAS: r = 0.76
								• At the end of treatment, 74.3% of the FIPP group and 75.7% of the SIFT group were no longer clinically depressed
								• At 6 mo follow-up the rates of depression had decreased further; 100% of cases in the SIFT group and 81% of cases in the FIPP group were no longer clinically depressed
								• The FIPP was effective for major depressive disorder, dysthymia and double depression
								• Reduction in comorbid conditions across the study

(continued on next page)

Table 2
(continued)

Authors	Trial Details	Inclusion Criteria	Exclusion Criteria	Participants	Interventions	Primary Outcome Measures	Effect Sizes	Results
Gilboa-Schechtman et al,[57] 2010	Year: 2010 Design: RCT Follow-up: 6 and 17 mo Country: Israel	• Age 12 to 18 y • A primary diagnosis of PTSD related to a single traumatic event • Fluency in Hebrew.	• Organic brain damage • Mental retardation • An on-going trauma-related threat • Suicidal ideation posing imminent danger • Current substance dependence • Pending legal issues • Initiation of treatment with psychotropic medication within the previous 6 wk • Ongoing psychological treatment	Problem/s: PTSD N: 38 Sex: 24f, 14m Age: 12–18	• Prolonged exposure therapy (PE-A) • Time limited dynamic therapy (TLDP)	• K-SADS-PL • CGAS • CPSS • BDI	Between Group CPSS POST: r = −0.23 6 mo: r = −0.25 17 mo: r = −0.11 CGAS POST: r = 0.31 6 mo: r = 0.3 Pre-post (TDLP) CPSS: r = 0.41 BDI: r = 0.71 CGAS: r = 0.37 Pre–17 mo (TDLP) CPSS: r = 0.42 BDI: r = 0.35	• Both groups reported decreases in PTSD symptoms and improvements in general functioning • Changes were greater for adolescents in the PE-A group. • At 6 mo and 17 mo follow-up treatment gains were maintained.

Robin et al,[59] 1999	Year: 1999 Design: RCT Follow-up: 1 y Country: USA	• DSM-III-R criteria for anorexia nervosa • Residing at home with 1 or both parents	• n/a	Problem/s: Anorexia Nervosa N: 37 Sex: 37f Age: 12–19	• EOIT (Ego-Oriented Individual Therapy) • BFST (Behavioral Family Systems Therapy)	• BMI • Target Weight • Resumption of Menstruation • Psychological • Eating Attitudes Test • Ego Functioning • BDI • YSR • CBCL • PARQ	Between groups BMI Post: r = −0.25 1 y: r = −0.15 Pre-post (EOIT) EAT, Teen: r = 0.4 BDI: r = 0.28 CBCL internalizing, Teen: r = 0.47 Pre–1 y (EOIT) EAT, Teen: r = 0.45 BDI: r = 0.38 CBCL internalizing, Teen: r = 0.43	• On BMI, both groups improved, but the BFST group improved more than the EOIT group • Both groups improved similarly on target weight, eating attitudes, depressive affect measures and family relations • Neither showed significant change in ego functioning. • More hospitalizations in the BFST group

(continued on next page)

Table 2
(continued)

Authors	Trial Details	Inclusion Criteria	Exclusion Criteria	Participants	Interventions	Primary Outcome Measures	Effect Sizes	Results
Lock et al,[67] 2010	Year: 2010 Design: Randomized Clinical Trial Follow-up: 6 and 12 mo Country: USA	• Between ages of 12 and 18 y • Living with their parents or legal Guardian • Met the DSM-IV criteria for anorexia nervosa excluding the amenorrhea criterion.	• Current psychotic disorder • Dependence on drugs or alcohol • Physical condition known to Influence eating or weight (eg, diabetes mellitus, pregnancy) • Previous treatment with FBT or AFT	Problem/s: Anorexia nervosa N: 121 Sex: 121f Age: 12–18	• Adolescent Focused Individual Therapy (AFT) • Family-Based Treatment (FBT)	• Full remission: defined as normal weight (≥95% of expected for age, sex and height), and a global Eating Disorder Examination score within 1 SD of published norms • Expected ideal body weight (IBW) • BMI	NOT AVAILABLE	• The 2 therapies were similarly effective in producing full remission: 23% of the AFT group and 42% of the FBT group. • The difference between the 2 groups was not significant. Treatment effects were maintained at follow-up. However, the levels of full remission were significantly higher for the FBT group than the AFT group • At 6-mo and 12-mo follow-up the full remission rates were 18% and 23% for the AFT group and 40% and 49% for the FBT group.

Diamond and colleagues,[70] 2010				
Year: 2010 Design: RCT Follow-up: 6, 12, 24 wk Country: USA	• Scores above 31 on the Suicidal Ideation Questionnaire (SIQJR) and above 20 (ie, moderate depression) on the Beck Depression Inventory (BDI-II) • (1) Needed psychiatric hospitalization, (2) were recently discharged from a psychiatric hospital, (3) had current psychosis, or (4) had mental retardation or history of • Borderline intellectual functioning	Problem/s: Depression N: 66 Sex: 55f, 11m Age: 12–17	• Intervention: Attachment-Based Family Therapy (ABFT) • Enhanced Usual Care (EUC)	• SIQJR, BDI-II	SIQJ-R (rate of change between groups): End of treatment (12 wk): $r = 0.393$ Follow-up (24 wk): $r = 0.399$ SSI (rate of change between groups): 12 wk: $r = 0.268$ 24 wk: $r = 0.276$ BDI-II (rate of change between groups): 12 wk: $r = 0.164$ 24 wk: $r = 0.098$ • Compared with EUC, the ABFT group showed a significantly greater rate of improvement on the SIQ-JR, SSI and BDI during the treatment period • On the SIQ-JR at 6, 12, and 24 wk, 69.7%, 87.1% and 70.0% of the ABFT group and 40.7%, 51.7% and 34.6% of the EUC group, respectively, no longer reported suicidal ideation at clinical level. • The SSI demonstrated similar responses • 58.1% of the ABFT group and 38.5% of the EUC group showed clinically meaningful change in depression scores • Drop out was notably lower in the ABFT group.

(continued on next page)

Table 2
(continued)

Authors	Trial Details	Inclusion Criteria	Exclusion Criteria	Participants	Interventions	Primary Outcome Measures	Effect Sizes	Results
Lieberman et al,[75] 2005	Year: 2005 Design: RCT Follow-up: no Country: USA	• 3–5 y old • Exposed to marital violence • Father figure perpetrating marital violence no longer resided in the home.	• Documented abuse of the target child • Current substance abuse and homelessness • Mental retardation • Psychosis • Autistic spectrum disorder	Problem/s: PTSD N: 75 Sex: 39f, 36m Age: 3–5	• Child-parent psychotherapy (CPP) • Monthly case managements plus referral to community services (TAU)	• DC: 0-3 for Clinicians • CBCL • SCL-90-R • Life Stressor Checklist-Revised • CAPS	Between Group DC 0-3 TSD POST: r = 0.29 CBCL Total Score POST: r = 0.113 CAPS Total Mothers POST: r = 0.2 Pre-post (CPP) DC 0-3 TSD: r = 0.48 CBCL: r = 0.23	• Children in the group assigned to CPP improved significantly more than those assigned to TAU • They showed decreased behavioral problems and TSD symptoms • The CPP children were also less likely to be diagnosed with PTSD after treatment. • Mothers in the CPP group showed significantly less PTSD avoidance symptoms than those in the control group

| Ghosh-Ippen et al,[76] 2011 | Year: 2011
Design: RCT
Follow-up: 6 mo
Country: USA | • 3–5 y old
• Exposed to marital violence
• Father figure perpetrating marital violence no longer resided in the home. | • Documented abuse of the target child
• Current substance abuse and homelessness
• Mental retardation
• Psychosis
• Autistic spectrum disorder | Diagnosis: PTSD
N: 75
Sex: 39f, 36m
Age: 3–5 | • Child-parent psychotherapy (CPP)
• Monthly case managements plus referral to community services (TAU) | • DC: 0-3 for Clinicians
• CBCL
• SCL-90-R
• CAPS | Pre-post (CPP for high-risk children)
CBCL Total Score: $r = 0.32$
PTSD symptoms: $r = 0.57$
Depression symptoms; $r = 0.36$
Pre-post (CPP for low-risk children)
CBCL Total Score: $r = 0.06$
PTSD symptoms: $r = 0.17$
Depression symptoms; $r = 0.11$ | • Among high-risk children, those in the CPP group showed significantly more improvement than children in the comparison group
• High-risk CPP children also showed greater reductions in PTSD and depression, number of co-occurring diagnoses and behavioral problems.
• Among the low-risk children, the CPP group showed significant improvement in PTSD symptoms, but comparison group did not. |

(continued on next page)

Table 2
(continued)

Authors	Trial Details	Inclusion Criteria	Exclusion Criteria	Participants	Interventions	Primary Outcome Measures	Effect Sizes	Results
Saltzman et al,[114] 2001	Year: 2001 Design: uncontrolled tudy Follow-up: Country: US	• Severe exposure, posttraumatic stress disorder (PTSD) • Functional impairment		Diagnosis: PTSD N: 26	• School-based trauma/grief focused group psychotherapy			• Participation was associated with improvements in trauma-related symptoms and in academic performance
Layne et al,[112,115] 2001	Year: 2001 Design: Country: Bosnia			Problem/s: PTSD N: 55 Sex: 45f, 10m Age: 15–19		• Self-report measures of posttraumatic stress • Depression symptoms • Grief symptoms • Psychosocial adaptation • Group satisfaction		• The investigators reported an observed reduction in psychological distress and positive associations between distress reduction and improved psychosocial adaptation

| Toth et al,[77] 2002 | Year: 2002 Design: Randomized controlled study Follow-up: 1 y, 3 y Country: UK | • Maltreated children • Low income | • Non-maltreating families who were identified as maltreating after baseline evaluation | Problem/s: Maltreatment N: 122 mother-infant dyads Age: 4 y | • Preschooler–parent psychotherapy (PPP) • Psycho-educational home visitation (PHV) • Community standard intervention (CS) • Non-maltreated comparison (NC) | • Story stem narratives | • PPP had a better pre-post effect size in each of the 4 items assessed (Maladaptive maternal representations, Negative and Positive Self-representations, and Mother-child relationship expectations) • There was no significant difference among the 3 other groups (PHV, CS, and NC) in terms of change scores • There was a significant change in mother-child relationship expectations of PPP children—children became more positive over the course of the intervention in comparison with NC and PHV children. |

(continued on next page)

Table 2
(continued)

Authors	Trial Details	Inclusion Criteria	Exclusion Criteria	Participants	Interventions	Primary Outcome Measures	Effect Sizes	Results

Chanen et al,[80] 2008	Year: 2008
	Design: RCT
	Follow-up: 12, 24 mo
	Country: Australia
		• Fluent in English
		• Two to 9 DSM–IV criteria for borderline personality disorder (BPD)
		• One or more of the following in childhood:
		  ○ Any personality disorder symptom
		  ○ Any disruptive behavior disorder symptom
		  ○ Low socio-economic status
		  ○ Depressive symptoms
		  ○ History of abuse or neglect.
			• Learning disability
			• Psychiatric disorder due to a general medical condition
			• Pervasive developmental disorder
			• Severe primary Axis I disorder that should be the principal focus of treatment
			• Receiving more than 9 sessions of specialist mental health treatment in the previous 12 mo
				Problem/s: Emerging BPD
				N: 78
				Sex: 59f, 19m
				Age: 15–18
					• Cognitive analytic therapy (CAT)
					• Good Clinical Care (GCC)
						• SCID-II
						• KSADS-PL
						• YSR
						• SOFAS
							Between-Group
							BPD Total Score
							6 mo: r = −0.1
							1 y: r = −0.05
							2 y: r = 0.03
							SOFAS
							6 mo: r = 0.1
							1 y: r = −0.01
							2 y: r = −0.14
							Pre-6 mo (CAT)
							BPD: r = 0.12
							SOFAS: r = 0.35
							Externalizing:
							  r = 0.25
							Internalizing:
							  r = 0.28
							Pre-1 y (CAT)
							BPD: r = 0.18
							SOFAS: r = 0.31
							Externalizing:
							  r = 0.46
							Internalizing:
							  r = 0.42
							Pre-2 y (CAT)
							BPD: r = 0.25
							SOFAS: r = 0.47
							Internalizing:
							  r = 0.56
							Externalizing:
							  r = 0.55
								• Both groups demonstrated improvements baseline to 2-y follow-up
								• No significant differences between the 2 conditions at posttreatment

Tonge et al,[81] 2009	• Young people with serious mental illness consecutively presenting to the CAMHS inpatient service	Problem/s: Mixed	• IPP + TAU	• YSR	Between-group	• At 12 mo, psychotherapy was associated with a greater reduction in depressive, social and attentional problems compared with TAU only
Year: 2009	• Insufficient English to complete the assessment	N: 80	• TAU	• CBCL	YSR withdrawn depressed	
Design: Naturalistic longitudinal study		Sex: 32f, 48m		• Family Assessment Device (FAD)	Post: r = 0.046	• Psychotherapy was associated with increase on the GAF and FAD
Follow-up: 1 y		Age: 12–18		• GAF	Pre-post (IPP + TAU)	
Country: Australia				• GARF	YSR: r = 0.1	• The greater effectiveness of the treatment depended on the level of psychopathology at baseline
					GAF: r = 0.28	• Almost half the participants offered PP did not engage and there was a high rate of attrition in the TAU-only group at 1-y follow-up

(continued on next page)

Table 2
(continued)

Authors	Trial Details	Inclusion Criteria	Exclusion Criteria	Participants	Interventions	Primary Outcome Measures	Effect Sizes	Results
Lush et al,[83] 1991 Boston and Lush,[84] 1994 Lush et al,[82] 1998 Boston et al,[85] 2009	Tavistock Study of Children in the Care System Design: Controlled Observational Study, single case study Follow-up: 6 mo, 1 y Country: UK	• Severely deprived children in residential or foster care or adopted		Diagnosis: mixed N: 20–51 Age: 2–18	• PP • No treatment control	• Clinician questionnaire • Semistructured questionnaire • Qualitative interviews		• Most Children showed improvements in relationships with adults and peers and in learning and thinking

Moran et al,[87] 1991 Fonagy and Moran,[88] 1990 Moran and Fonagy,[89] 1987	Design: quasi-randomized controlled trial, single case studies Follow-up: 1 y Country: UK	• Age range 6–18 y • IDDM of at least 2 y duration • Diagnosis of brittle diabetes according to specific criteria • The absence of psychotic disorder or severe learning difficulties	• Psychotic disorder • Severe learning difficulties	Diagnosis: dangerously uncontrolled insulin dependent diabetes N: 22 Sex: n/a Age: 6–18	• Psychoanalytic treatment plus TAU • TAU	• M-value and glycosylated hemoglobin (HbA1c) concentration • Insulin	Between group M-Value Post: r = 0.58 Insulin Post: r = 0.39 Pre-post (psychoanalytic group) M-Value: r = 0.65 Insulin: r = 0.09	Moran et al, 1991 • The treatment was highly effective in improving the diabetic control of children and this was maintained at 1-y follow-up. • Hb1Ac concentration fell to a clinically acceptable range for diabetes in 6 of the treated subjects • At follow-up, 9 of the experimental group patients and 3 of comparison group remained below their pre-admission average HbA1c levels Fonagy and Moran, 1990 • In a series of experimental single case studies, individual psychodynamic therapy was found to improve several growth

(continued on next page)

Table 2
(continued)

Authors	Trial Details	Inclusion Criteria	Exclusion Criteria	Participants	Interventions	Primary Outcome Measures	Effect Sizes	Results
								parameters probably associated with improvement of diabetic control Moran and Fonagy, 1990 • There was an association between the discussion of material in the analytic session and subsequent improvements in diabetic control
Apter et al,[90] 1984	Year: 1984 Design: Case Series Follow-up: Different for each patient: from 4 mo to 2.5 y Country: Israel	• Inpatients with OCD on the adolescent unit at the Geha Psychiatric Hospital • Severe symptoms and inability to function irrespective of diagnosis		Problem/s: OCD (DSM-III) N: 8 Sex: 5m, 3f Age: 10–16	• Psycho-dynamically orientated therapy with chlormipramine or phenelzine	• Severity rating for OCD • K-GAS		• Seven of the 8 patients were much improved within 3–4 mo and 4 of 8 were completely symptom free

| Slonim et al,[91] 2011 | Year: 2011
Design: non-randomized, naturalistic controlled study
Follow-up: No
Country: Israel | • Adolescents who required psychotherapy
• Mixed diagnoses | • Adolescents who came in for crisis intervention following severe trauma
• Psychosis
• Drug abuse
Problem/s: mixed diagnoses
N: 72
Sex: 44f, 28m
Age (mean): 15–18 (16.3 SD = 0.91) | • PP
• No treatment group from the same school | • Y-OQ-SR
• Target Complaint Scales (TCS) | Pre-post (PP)
Y-OQ: r = 0.27
TCS: r = 0.75
Pre-post (control)
Y-OQ: r = 0.14
TCS: r = 0.43 | • Groups not comparable as very different at baseline
• The treatment group showed significant changes in rigidity over the course of a year of psychotherapy, whereas no such changes were detected in the community group
• The treatment group improved significantly more than the community group between baseline and end of treatment |

(continued on next page)

Table 2
(continued)

Authors	Trial Details	Inclusion Criteria	Exclusion Criteria	Participants	Interventions	Primary Outcome Measures	Effect Sizes	Results
Deakin and Nunes,[92] 2009	Year: 2009 Design: Controlled Observational Study Follow-up: No Country: Brazil	• Aged 6–11 • Referred for psychological treatment	• Pervasive developmental disorders • IQ <80	Diagnosis: Mixed Diagnoses N: 45 Sex: 27f, 18m Age: 6–11 (mean 8.3)	• Individual psychoanalytic psychotherapy (IPP) • No treatment control	• CBCL • Rorschach (only treatment group) • Bender (only treatment group) • WISC III (only treatment group)	Between groups CBCL 12 mo: r = 0.006 CBCL pre-post (IPP): Treatment r = 0.23	• Symptomatic and behavioral positive changes observed for the treatment group • Decrease in anxiety associated with reduction of school problems. • More effective for females presenting internalizing disorders • Not so for males with externalizing: early drop out.

Scholte and van der Ploeg,[93] 2006	Year: 2006 Design: quasi-experimental study Follow-up: no Country: Netherlands	• Adolescents admitted to 4 different residential programs aiming to treat severe behavioral and emotional difficulties	• n/a	Diagnosis: Mixed N: 105 Sex: 79m, 26f Age: 14.9	• Behavior modification • Psychodynamic treatment • Adventurous learning • Structured community living • No treatment control	• CBCL	Between groups (Comparing group to non-treated)* CBCL Total Problems 1 y* Behavior Modification: ES = 0.49* Psychodynamic treatment: ES = 0.68* Structured Community Living: ES = 0.91* Adventurous living: ES = 0.81*	• All programs produced positive outcomes on all 3 domains of the CBCL • The psychodynamic treated group showed greater improvement than the behavioral modification group, but worse than the structured community living and adventurous learning groups • Only a small portion of patients moved to a nonclinical condition after 1 y, and thus treatment had to be extended.
Heinicke,[94] 1965	Year: 1965 Design: Observational Study Follow-up: 1, 2 y Country: US	• 6–10 y of age • Referred due to learning disability related to psychological disturbance • Suitable for psychoanalytic psychotherapy	• IQ <91 • Early drop outs or nonagreed terminations	Diagnosis: Mixed N: 10 Sex: 10m Age: 6–10	• PP 4 times a week • PP once a week	• Stanford Binet, Form L • The Wide Range Achievement Test • Rorscharch • TAT • Michigan Picture test • Draw a Person test		• At the end of treatment the children seen 4 times a week showed greater improvement in adaptation, reading, and flexibility, compared with those receiving treatment once a week

(continued on next page)

Table 2
(continued)

Authors	Trial Details	Inclusion Criteria	Exclusion Criteria	Participants	Interventions	Primary Outcome Measures	Effect Sizes	Results
Heinicke and Ramsay Klee,[95] 1986	Year: 1986 Design: Comparative study Follow-up: 1 y Country: USA	• Children referred for learning disturbance		Problem/s: Mixed N: 12 Sex: males Age: 7–10	• PP of varying intensities	• IQ • Reading Ability • The Diagnostic Profile		• All boys made improvements • Those seen more frequently (4 times a week for 1 or 2 years) showed greater improvements in self-esteem, capacity for relationships, frustration tolerance, and flexible adaptation

Baruch,[96] 1995 Baruch and Fearon,[97] 1998 Baruch and Fearon,[99] 2002 Baruch and Vrouva,[98] 2010	Design: Open non-controlled trial Follow-up: 1 y Country: UK	• Referrals to the Brandon Center, UK	Problem/s: Mixed N: 61–151 Age: 12–25	• Community-based psychoanalytic psychotherapy	• YSR • GAF	Baruch 1995 • After 3 mo, there was significant improvement (P<.01) in Internalizing Problem scores and Total Problem scores on the YSR • Externalizing problems appeared more difficult to treat Baruch, 1998 • Similar conclusions emerged in the report of a follow-up of 61 participants from the same study Baruch and Fearon, 2002 • In the 2002 article that followed 151 participants, they found an improvement in mean scores on the YSR, fewer participants were in the clinical range, and the participants demonstrated significant

(continued on next page)

Table 2
(continued)

Authors	Trial Details	Inclusion Criteria	Exclusion Criteria	Participants	Interventions	Primary Outcome Measures	Effect Sizes	Results
								reliable change in level of adaptation • Rate of improvement dropped significantly over time Baruch, 2010 • Levels of attrition at 12-mo follow-up for self, significant other, and therapist reports were 19.4%, 10.3%, and 16.0%, respectively

Target and Fonagy,[45] 1994 Target and Fonagy,[100] 1994 Fonagy and Target,[110] 1996	Anna Freud Center Chart Review Study Year: 1994 Design: Retrospective Study Country: UK	• Former child patients with the diagnostic of DBD treated at the Anna Freud Center between 1952 and 1991	• Psychosis • Pervasive developmental disorder	Problem/s: Mixed N: Subgroups selected from 763 treatment files	• Psychoanalysis (4–5 times a wk) • PP (1–3 times a wk)	• Children with anxiety disorders (with or without comorbidity) showed greater improvements than those with other condition • More than 85% of 299 children with anxiety and depressive disorders no longer suffered any diagnosable emotional disorder after an average of 2 y of treatment • Phobias, separation anxiety disorders and overanxious disorder were resolved in approximately 86% of cases. • OCD was more resistant, ceasing to meet diagnostic criteria in only 70% of cases • Of those with dysthymia or MDD, more than 75% showed reliable improvement in functioning and

(continued on next page)

Table 2
(continued)

Authors	Trial Details	Inclusion Criteria	Exclusion Criteria	Participants	Interventions	Primary Outcome Measures	Effect Sizes	Results
								no depressive symptoms • Children and adolescents with depressive disorders appeared to benefit more from intensive (4–5 sessions per week) than from nonintensive (1–2 sessions per week) therapy • Predictors of good and poor outcomes were different for the 3 age groups • Diagnoses related CD and ODD appeared particularly resistant to psychodynamic therapy • Children with ODD benefited more than those with CD

Study	Design	Sample	Comorbidity	Problem/s	Intervention	Measures	Findings
Schachter and Target,[102] 2009	Year: 2009 Design: Non-controlled retrospective study Follow-up: Country: UK	• Former child patients treated at the Anna Freud Center between 1952 and 1991	• Mental retardation • Autism psychotic illnesses	Problem/s: Mixed Diagnoses N: 34 Sex: n/a Age: n/a	• Psychoanalytic Child Psychotherapy	• Adult Functioning Index (AFI) • Adult Attachment Interview	• At follow up participants treated as children were not characterized by severe impairment nor poor functioning in adulthood • There was a strong association between positive adult outcome and secure attachment status • The best predictor of adult outcome was the child's overall level of functioning before receiving treatment
Midgley and Target,[104] 2005 Midgley et al,[103] 2006	Design: Non-controlled retrospective Study Follow-up: 18–42 y Country: UK	• All current adults who were referred as children to intensive analysis to the Anna Freud Center between 1952 and 1980	• n/a	Problem/s: Mixed Diagnoses N: 27 Sex: 11m, 16f Age: 5 y 11 mo—16	• Psychoanalytic Psychotherapy	• Qualitative analysis (Interview)	• In both articles the authors report that many participants emphasized the value of being able to talk and be listened to • Those who remember psychoanalysis in a positive way tended to be in treatment as

(continued on next page)

Table 2
(continued)

Authors	Trial Details	Inclusion Criteria	Exclusion Criteria	Participants	Interventions	Primary Outcome Measures	Effect Sizes	Results
								quite young children • There was an emphasis on being accepted and listened to • About a quarter of patients remember child therapy predominantly in relation to their lack of engagement with the process

Vilsvik and Vaglum,[66] 1990	Year: 1989
	Design: Naturalistic study
	Follow-up: 1–9 y
	Country: Norway
		• Evidence of weight phobia and/or distorted body image
		• Pervasive sense of inadequacy
		• One of the following
		  ○ self-induced starvation
		  ○ Weight below 2.5 percentile
			• n/a	Diagnosis: anorexia nervosa
				N: 17
				Sex: f
				Age: 13–17.5
					• Outpatient individual psychodynamic pychotherapy	• Weight gain
						• Menstrual status
						• Analysis of case notes.
								• At follow-up, all patients had improved significantly medically and socially

Vorgraft et al,[109] 2007	Year: 2007 Design: Retro-spective Evaluation Follow-up: 6 mo Country: Israel	• PDD/ASD • Under 5 y		Diagnosis: PDD N: 23 Sex: 15m, 8f Age: 38–49 mo	• Reciprocal play therapy (RPT)	• Childhood Autism Rating Scale • Social Behavior Rating Scale		• Significant improvement in the participants

Heede et al,[116] 2009	Year: 2009 Design: prospective uncontrolled study Follow-up: no Country: Denmark	• Children in a treatment institution • Severe trauma and early deprivation	Diagnosis: Mixed N: 24 Age: 6–15	• Psychodynamic milieu-therapy for 2 y	• TAT • WISC III • Rorschach	• Improvements in the children's cognitive and emotional functioning, self-confidence, capacities for self-reflection • The therapy was not as effective in terms of the children's interpersonal relations
Eresund,[121] 2007	Year: 2007 Design: Non-controlled observational study Follow-up: Country: Sweden	• Boys • With behavior problems • Meeting criteria for DSM-IV ODD	Problem/s: ODD N: 9 Sex: 9m Age: 6–10	• Psychodynamic Supportive Expressive Play therapy (SEPP)	• WISC III • CBCL • TRF • Draw a man test	• At the end of treatment, only one boy still fulfilled DSM-IV ODD criteria • Parents (CBCL) and teachers (TRF) reported better social function after therapy • Improvements less marked in boys who in addition to initial diagnoses of ODD or CD had attention-deficit/hyperactivity disorder • At 1-y follow-up, parent reported improvements were maintained

(continued on next page)

Table 2
(continued)

Authors	Trial Details	Inclusion Criteria	Exclusion Criteria	Participants	Interventions	Primary Outcome Measures	Effect Sizes	Results
Odhammar et al,[122] 2011	Data from the Erica Process and Outcome Study Year: 2011 Design: Non-controlled observational study Follow-up: No Country: Sweden			Problem/s: Mixed N: 33 Sex: 22m, 11f Age: 5–10	• PP	• CGAS • HCAM		• A significant difference was found between CGAS before and after treatment (P<.001) • The 4 subscales of HCAM that showed the largest changes were in general mood, and variability of mood; ability to tolerate frustration and control impulses; development of confidence and self-esteem; and ability to cope with very stressful events • A qualitative analysis highlighted the difficulty of capturing and understanding change processes using quantitative measures

| Carlberg et al,[123] 2009 | Erica Process and Outcome Study (EPOS)
Year: 2009
Design: Qualitative Study
Follow-up: 2 y
Country: UK | • Data from at least one DSM-IV diagnosis | • n/a | Problem/s: Mixed
N: 10
Age: 6–10 | • PP | • Therapist's description of turn point
• Questionnaire with basic information | • The children were able to communicate their expectations and experiences and most were positive in their expectations and their experiences of therapy after termination
• On self-ratings, the children showed a moderate degree of improvement in their problems |

Abbreviations: See list of abbreviations at the beginning of the article; n/a, not applicable.

* These effect sizes are taken from the paper.

REFERENCES

1. President's New Freedom Commission on Mental Health. Achieving the promise: transforming mental health care in America. Final report. Report No. SMA- 03-3832. Rockville (MD): Department of Health and Human Services; 2003.
2. Weisz JR, Kazdin AE, editors. Evidence based psychotherapies for children and adolescents. 2nd edition. New York: Guilford; 2010.
3. Clark DM. Implementing NICE guidelines for the psychological treatment of depression and anxiety disorders: the IAPT experience. Int Rev Psychiatry 2011;23(4):318–27.
4. Stratton P. Formulating research questions that are relevant to psychotherapy. Mental Health and Learning Disabilities Research and Practice 2007;4(2):83–97.
5. Leichsenring F, Rabung S. The role of efficacy vs effectiveness research in evaluating psychotherapy. Mental Health and Learning Disabilities Research and Practice 2007;4(2):125–44.
6. Cartwright N, Munro E. The limitations of randomized controlled trials in predicting effectiveness. J Eval Clin Pract 2010;16(2):260–6.
7. Mill JS. On the definition of political economy and on the method of philosophical investigation in that science reprinted in collected works of John Stuart Mill, vol. IV. Toronto: University of Toronto Press; 1836 [1967].
8. Gabbard GO, Gunderson JG, Fonagy P. The place of psychoanalytic treatments within psychiatry. Arch Gen Psychiatry 2002;59(6):505–10.
9. Borduin CM, Mann BJ, Cone LT, et al. Multisystemic treatment of serious juvenile offenders: long-term prevention of criminality and violence. J Consult Clin Psychol 1995;63:569–78.
10. Borduin C, Schaeffer C. Multisystemic treatment of juvenile sexual offenders: a progress report. J Psychol Hum Sex 2001;13:25–42.
11. Henggeler SW, Melton GB, Smith LA. Family preservation using multisystemic therapy: an effective alternative to incarcerating serious juvenile offenders. J Consult Clin Psychol 1992;60:953–61.
12. Henggeler SW, Melton GB, Brondino MJ, et al. Multisystemic therapy with violent and chronic juvenile offenders and their families: the role of treatment fidelity in successful dissemination. J Consult Clin Psychol 1997;65:821–33.
13. Henggeler SW, Pickrel SG, Brondino MJ. Multisystemic treatment of substance-abusing and -dependent delinquents: outcomes, treatment fidelity, and transportability. Ment Health Serv Res 1999;1:171–84.
14. Henggeler SW, Halliday-Boykins CA, Cunningham PB. Juvenile drug court: enhancing outcomes by integrating evidence-based treatments. J Consult Clin Psychol 2006;74:42–54.
15. Ogden T, Hagen KA. Multisystemic treatment of serious behaviour problems in youth: sustainability of effectiveness two years after intake. Child Adolesc Ment Health 2006;11:142–9 (follow up paper).
16. Rowland MD, Halliday-Boykins CA, Colleen A, et al. A randomized trial of multisystemic therapy with Hawaii's Felix class youths. J Emot Behav Disord 2005;13:13–23.
17. Timmons-Mitchell J, Bender MB, Kishna MA. An independent effectiveness trial of multisystemic therapy with juvenile justice youth. J Clin Child Adolesc Psychol 2006;35:227–36.
18. Borduin CM, Schaeffer CM, Heiblum N. A randomized clinical trial of multisystemic therapy with juvenile sexual offenders: effects on youth social ecology and criminal activity. J Consult Clin Psychol 2009;77(1):26–37.

19. Schoenwald SK, Chapman JE, Sheidow AJ, et al. Long-term youth criminal outcomes in MST transport: the impact of therapist adherence and organizational climate and structure. J Clin Child Adolesc Psychol 2009;38(1):91–105.

20. Butler S, Baruch G, Hickey N, et al. A randomized controlled trial of multisystemic therapy and a statutory therapeutic intervention for young offenders. J Am Acad Child Adolesc Psychiatry 2011;50(12):1220–1235.e2.

21. National Institute for Health and Clinical Excellence. Antisocial personality disorder: treatment, management and prevention. London: NICE; 2010.

22. Kazdin AE. Understanding how and why psychotherapy leads to change. Psychother Res 2009;19(4–5):418–28.

23. Fisher B, Wolmark N, Redmond C, et al. Findings from NSABP Protocol No. B-04: comparison of radical mastectomy with alternative treatments. II. The clinical and biologic significance of medial-central breast cancers. Cancer 1981; 48(8):1863–72.

24. Rawlins M. De Testimonio: on the evidence for decisions about the use of therapeutic interventions. London: Royal College of Physicians (The Harveian Oration); 2008.

25. Roth A, Fonagy P, Parry G. Psychotherapy research, funding, and evidence-based practice. In: Roth A, Fonagy P, editors. What works for whom? A critical review of psychotherapy research. New York: Guilford Press; 1996. p. 37–56.

26. Fonagy P, Target M, Cottrell D, et al. What works for whom? A critical review of treatments for children and adolescents. New York: Guilford; 2002.

27. Cohen J. Statistical power analysis for the behavioural sciences. 2nd edition. Hillsdale (NJ): Erlbaum; 1988.

28. Gerber AJ, Kocsis JH, Milrod BL, et al. A quality-based review of randomized controlled trials of psychodynamic psychotherapy. Am J Psychiatry 2011; 168(1):19–28.

29. Fonagy P, Cottrell D, Philips J, et al. What works for whom? A critical review of treatments for children and adolescents. 2nd edition. New York: Guilford; in press.

30. Fonagy P, Target M. Psychodynamic treatments. In: Rutter M, Bishop D, Pine D, et al, editors. Rutter's child and adolescent psychiatry. 5th edition. Oxford (United Kingdom): Blackwell; 2008. p. 1079–91.

31. Freud S. New introductory lectures on psychoanalysis. In: Strachey J, editor. The standard edition of the complete psychological works of Sigmund Freud. London: Hogarth Press; 1933. p. 1–182.

32. Wachtel P. Psychoanalysis and behaviour therapy: toward an integration. New York: Basic Books; 1977.

33. McCullough JP Jr. Treatment for chronic depression using cognitive behavioral analysis system of psychotherapy (CBASP). J Clin Psychol 2003;59(8):833–46.

34. Ryle A, Kerr IB. Introducing cognitive analytic therapy: principles and practice. Chichester (United Kingdom): J. Wiley; 2002.

35. Weissman MM, Markowitz JC, Klerman GL. Clinician's quick guide to interpersonal psychotherapy. New York: Oxford University Press; 2007.

36. Young JE, Klosko JS, Weishaar M. Schema Therapy: A Practitioner's Guide. New York: Guilford Publications; 2003.

37. Safran JD. The relational turn, the therapeutic alliance, and psychotherapy research: strange bedfellows or postmodern marriage? Contemp Psychoanal 2003;39:449–75.

38. Midgley N, Kennedy E. Psychodynamic psychotherapy for children and adolescents: a critical review of the evidence base. J Child Psychother 2011;37(3): 232–60.

39. Hibbs ED, Jensen PS, editors. Psychosocial treatments for child and adolescent disorders: empirically based strategies for clinical practice. 2nd edition. Washington, DC: American Psychological Association; 2004.

40. Weisz JR. Psychotherapy for children and adolescents: evidence-based treatments and case examples. Cambridge (United Kingdom): Cambridge University Press; 2004.

41. Weisz JR, Kazdin AE. Evidence-based youth psychotherapies for children and adolescents. 2nd edition. New York: Guilford; 2010.

42. Kazdin AE. Mediators and mechanisms of change in psychotherapy research. Annu Rev Clin Psychol 2007;3:1–27.

43. Kazak AE, Hoagwood K, Weisz JR, et al. A meta-systems approach to evidence-based practice for children and adolescents. Am Psychol 2010; 65(2):85–97.

44. Smyrnios KX, Kirkby RJ. Long-term comparison of brief versus unlimited psychodynamic treatments with children and their parents. J Consult Clin Psychol 1993;61(6):1020–7.

45. Target M, Fonagy P. Efficacy of psychoanalysis for children with emotional disorders. J Am Acad Child Adolesc Psychiatry 1994;33(3):361–71.

46. Muratori F, Picchi L, Casella C, et al. Efficacy of brief dynamic psychotherapy for children with emotional disorders. Psychother Psychosom 2002;71(1):28–38.

47. Muratori F, Picchi L, Bruni G, et al. A two-year follow-up of psychodynamic psychotherapy for internalizing disorders in children. J Am Acad Child Adolesc Psychiatry 2003;42(3):331–9.

48. Trowell J, Kolvin I, Weeramanthri T, et al. Psychotherapy for sexually abused girls: psychopathological outcome findings and patterns of change. Br J Psychiatry 2002;180:234–47.

49. Rushton A, Miles G. A study of a support service for the current carers of sexually abused girls. Clin Child Psychol Psychiatr 2000;5(3):411–26.

50. Kronmuller K, Stefini A, Geiser-Elze A, et al. The Heidelberg study of psychodynamic psychotherapy for children & adolescents. In: Tsiantis J, Trowell J, editors. Assessing change in psychoanalytic psychotherapy of children and adolescents. London: Karnac; 2010. p. 115–38.

51. Sinha UK, Kapur M. Psychotherapy with emotionally disturbed adolescent boys: outcome and process study. NIMHANS Journal 1999;17(2):113–30.

52. Fonagy P, Target M. Mentalization and the changing aims of child psychoanalysis. Psychoanalytic Dialogues 1998;8:87–114.

53. Higgitt A, Fonagy P. The psychotherapeutic treatment of borderline and narcissistic personality disorder. Br J Psychiatry 1992;161:23–43.

54. Szapocznik J, Rio A, Murray E, et al. Structural family versus psychodynamic child therapy for problematic Hispanic boys. J Consult Clin Psychol 1989; 57(5):571–8.

55. Trowell J, Joffe I, Campbell J, et al. Childhood depression: a place for psychotherapy—an outcome study comparing individual psychodynamic psychotherapy and family therapy. Eur Child Adolesc Psychiatry 2007;16(3): 157–67.

56. Garoff FF, Heinonen K, Pesonen AK, et al. Depressed youth: treatment outcome and changes in family functioning in individual and family therapy. J Fam Ther 2012;34(1):4–23.

57. Gilboa-Schechtman E, Foa EB, Shafran N, et al. Prolonged exposure versus dynamic therapy for adolescent PTSD: a pilot randomized controlled trial. J Am Acad Child Adolesc Psychiatry 2010;49(10):1034–42.

58. Robin AL, Siegel PT, Moye A. Family versus individual therapy for anorexia: impact on family conflict. Int J Eat Disord 1995;17:313–22.
59. Robin AL, Siegel PT, Moye AW, et al. A controlled comparison of family versus individual therapy for adolescents with anorexia nervosa. J Am Acad Child Adolesc Psychiatry 1999;38:1482–9.
60. Crisp AH, Norton KR, Gowers SG, et al. A controlled study of the effect of therapies aimed at adolescent and family psychopathology in anorexia nervosa. Br J Psychiatry 1991;159:325–33.
61. Dare C, Eisler I, Russell G, et al. Psychological therapies for adults with anorexia nervosa: randomised controlled trial of out-patient treatments. Br J Psychiatry 2001;178:216–21.
62. leGrange D, Eisler I, Dare C, et al. Evaluation of family treatments in adolescent anorexia nervosa: a pilot study. J Eat Disord 1992;12:347–57.
63. Russell GF, Szmukler G, Dare C, et al. An evaluation of family therapy in anorexia nervosa and bulimia nervosa. Arch Gen Psychiatry 1987;44:1047–56.
64. Eisler I, Dare C, Hodes M, et al. Family therapy for adolescent anorexia nervosa: the results of a controlled comparison of two family interventions. J Child Psychol Psychiatry 2000;41:727–36.
65. Eisler I, Dare C, Russell GF, et al. Family and individual therapy in anorexia nervosa: a 5-year follow-up. Arch Gen Psychiatry 1997;54(11):1025–30.
66. Vilsvik SO, Vaglum P. Teenage anorexia nervosa: a 1–9 year follow up after psychodynamic treatment. Nordic Journal of Psychiatry 1990;44(3):249–55.
67. Lock J, Le Grange D, Agras WS, et al. Randomized clinical trial comparing family-based treatment with adolescent-focused individual therapy for adolescents with anorexia nervosa. Arch Gen Psychiatry 2010;67(10):1025–32.
68. Diamond G, Josephson A. Family-based treatment research: a 10-year update. J Am Acad Child Adolesc Psychiatry 2005;44(9):872–87.
69. Fonagy P. Attachment theory and psychoanalysis. New York: Other Press; 2001.
70. Diamond GS, Wintersteen MB, Brown GK, et al. Attachment based family therapy for adolescents with suicidal ideation: a randomized controlled trial. J Am Acad Child Adolesc Psychiatry 2010;49(2):122–31.
71. Reynolds WM. Professional manual for the suicidal ideation questionnaire. Odessa (FL): Psychological Assessment Resources; 1988.
72. Beck AT, Kovacs M, Weissman A. Assessment of suicidal intention: the Scale for Suicide Ideation. J Consult Clin Psychol 1979;47(2):343–52.
73. Beck A, Steer R, Brown G. The Beck depression inventory—second edition. San Antonio (TX): Psychological Corporation; 1996.
74. Hawton K, James A. Suicide and deliberate self harm in young people. Br Med J 2005;330:891–4.
75. Lieberman AF, Van Horn P, Ippen CG. Toward evidence-based treatment: child-parent psychotherapy with preschoolers exposed to marital violence. J Am Acad Child Adolesc Psychiatry 2005;44(12):1241–8.
76. Ghosh-Ippen C, Harris WW, Van Horn P, et al. Traumatic and stressful events in early childhood: can treatment help those at highest risk? Child Abuse Negl 2011;35(7):504–13.
77. Toth SL, Maughan A, Manly JT, et al. The relative efficacy of two interventions in altering maltreated preschool children's representational models: implications for attachment theory. Dev Psychopathol 2002;14(4):877–908.
78. Murray L, Cooper PJ, Wilson A, et al. Controlled trial of the short- and long-term effect of psychological treatment of post-partum depression: 2. Impact on the mother-child relationship and child outcome. Br J Psychiatry 2003;182:420–7.

79. Toth SL, Rogosch FA, Manly JT, et al. The efficacy of toddler-parent psychotherapy to reorganize attachment in the young offspring of mothers with major depressive disorder: a randomized preventive trial. J Consult Clin Psychol 2006;74(6):1006–16.
80. Chanen AM, Jackson HJ, McCutcheon LK, et al. Early intervention for adolescents with borderline personality disorder using cognitive analytic therapy: randomised controlled trial. Br J Psychiatry 2008;193(6):477–84.
81. Tonge BJ, Pullen JM, Hughes GC, et al. Effectiveness of psychoanalytic psychotherapy for adolescents with serious mental illness: 12 month naturalistic follow-up study. Aust N Z J Psychiatry 2009;43(5):467–75.
82. Lush D, Boston M, Morgan J, et al. Psychoanalytic psychotherapy with disturbed adopted and foster children: a single case follow-up study. Clin Child Psychol Psychiatr 1998;3(1):51–69.
83. Lush D, Boston M, Grainger E. Evaluation of psychoanalytic psychotherapy with children: therapists' assessments and predictions. Psychoanal Psychother 1991;5(3):191–234.
84. Boston M, Lush D. Further considerations of methodology for evaluating psychoanalytic psychotherapy with children: reflections in the light of research experience. J Child Psychother 1994;20(2):205–29.
85. Boston M, Lush D, Grainger E. Evaluation of psychoanalytic psychotherapy with fostered, adopted and 'in care' children. In: Midgely N, Anderson J, Grainger E, et al, editors. Child psychotherapy and research new approaches, emerging findings. London: Routledge; 2009. p. 117–28.
86. Shaw RJ, Palmer L. Consultation in the medical setting: a model to enhance treatment adherence. In: Steiner H, editor. Handbook of mental health interventions in children and adolescents. San Francisco (CA): Jossey-Bass; 2004. p. 917–41.
87. Moran G, Fonagy P, Kurtz A, et al. A controlled study of the psychoanalytic treatment of brittle diabetes. J Am Acad Child Adolesc Psychiatry 1991;30:926–35.
88. Fonagy P, Moran GS. Studies on the efficacy of child psychoanalysis. J Consult Clin Psychol 1990;58:684–95.
89. Moran G, Fonagy P. Psycho-analysis and diabetic control: a single-case study. Br J Med Psychol 1987;60:357–72.
90. Apter A, Bernhout E, Tyano S. Severe obsessive compulsive disorder in adolescence: a report of eight cases. J Adolesc 1984;7(4):349–58.
91. Slonim DA, Shefler G, Gvirsman SD, et al. Changes in rigidity and symptoms among adolescents in psychodynamic psychotherapy. Psychother Res 2011; 21(6):685–97.
92. Deakin EK, Nunes ML. Effectiveness of child psychoanalytic psychotherapy in a clinical outpatient setting. J Child Psychother 2009;35(3):290–301.
93. Scholte EM, van der Ploeg JD. Residential treatment of adolescents with severe behavioural problems. J Adolesc 2006;29(4):641–54.
94. Heinicke CM. Frequency of psychotherapeutic session as a factor affecting the child's developmental status. Psychoanal Study Child 1965;20:42–98.
95. Heinicke CM, Ramsey-Klee DM. Outcome of child psychotherapy as a function of frequency of sessions. J Am Acad Child Psychiatry 1986;25:247–53.
96. Baruch G. Evaluating the outcome of a community-based psychoanalytic psychotherapy service for young people between 12–25 years old: work in progress. Psychoanal Psychother 1995;9(3):243–67.
97. Baruch G, Fearon P, Gerber A. Evaluating the outcome of a community-based psychoanalytic psychotherapy service for young people: one year repeated

follow up. In: Davenhill R, Patrick M, editors. Rethinking clinical audit. London: Routledge; 1998. p. 158–82.

98. Baruch G, Vrouva I. Collecting routine outcome data in a psychotherapy community clinic for young people: findings from an ongoing study. Child Adolesc Ment Health 2010;15(1):30–6.

99. Baruch G, Fearon P. The evaluation of mental health outcome at a community-based psychodynamic psychotherapy service for young people: a 12-month follow-up based on self-report data. Psychol Psychother 2002;75(3):261–78.

100. Target M, Fonagy P. The efficacy of psychoanalysis for children: developmental considerations. J Am Acad Child Adolesc Psychiatry 1994;33:1134–44.

101. Fonagy P, Target M. The efficacy of psychoanalysis for children with disruptive disorders. J Am Acad Child Adolesc Psychiatry 1994;33:45–55.

102. Schachter A, Target M. The adult outcome of child psychoanalysis: the Anna Freud Centre long-term follow-up study. In: Midgley M, Anderson J, Grainger E, et al, editors. Child psychotherapy and research: new approaches, emerging findings. London: Routledge; 2009. p. 145–57.

103. Midgley N, Target M, Smith J. The outcome of child psychoanalysis from the patient's point of view: a qualitative analysis of a long-term follow-up study. Psychol Psychother 2006;79(2):257–69.

104. Midgley N, Target M. Recollections of being in child psychoanalysis: a qualitative study of a long-term follow-up project. Psychoanal Study Child 2005;60:157–77.

105. Cogher L. The use of non-directive play in speech and language therapy. Child Lang Teach Ther 1999;15(1):7–15.

106. Reid S, Alvarez A, Lee A. The Tavistock autism workshop approach. In: Richer J, Coates S, editors. Autism-the search for coherence. London: Jessica Kingsley; 2001. p. 182–92.

107. Wieder S, Greenspan SI. Climbing the symbolic ladder in the DIR model through floor time/interactive play. Autism 2003;7(4):425–35.

108. Alonim H. The Mifne Method—ISRAEL: early intervention in the treatment of autism/PDD: a therapeutic programme for the nuclear family and their child. J Child Adolesc Ment Health 2004;16:39–43.

109. Vorgraft Y, Farbstein I, Spiegel R, et al. Retrospective evaluation of an intensive method of treatment for children with pervasive developmental disorder. Autism 2007;11(5):413–24.

110. Fonagy P, Target M. Predictors of outcome in child psychoanalysis: a retrospective study of 763 cases at the Anna Freud Centre. J Am Psychoanal Assoc 1996; 44:27–77.

111. Target M, Fonagy P. Attachment theory and long-term psychoanalytic outcome: are insecure attachment narratives less accurate?. In: Leuzinger-Bohleber M, Dreher AU, Canestri J, editors. Pluralism and unity? Methods of research in psychoanalysis. London: International Psychoanalytical Association; 2003. p. 149–67.

112. Layne CM, Pynoos RS, Cardenas J. Wounded adolescence: school-based group psychotherapy for adolescents who sustained or witnessed violent injury. In: Shafii M, Shafii SL, editors. School violence: assessment, management, prevention. Washington, DC: American Psychiatric Association; 2001. p. 163–86.

113. Pynoos R, Steinberg A, Wraith R. A developmental model of childhood traumatic stress. In: Cicchetti D, Cohen DJ, editors. Developmental psychopathology, vol. 2. New York: Wiley; 1995. p. 72–95.

114. Saltzman WR, Pynoos RS, Layne CM, et al. Trauma- and grief-focused intervention for adolescents exposed to community violence: results of a school-based screening and group treatment protocol. Group Dynam 2001;5(4):291–303.

115. Layne CM, Pynoos RS, Saltzman WR, et al. Trauma/grief-focused group psychotherapy: school-based postwar intervention with traumatized Bosnian adolescents. Group Dynam 2001;5(4):277–90.
116. Heede T, Runge H, Storebo OJ, et al. Psychodynamic milieu-therapy and changes in personality—what is the connection. J Child Psychother 2009; 35(3):276–89.
117. Wechsler D. Wechsler Intelligence Scale for Children – 3rd Edition (WISC-III₁). Swedish edn. Stockholm: Psykologiförlaget AB; 1998.
118. Exner JE. The Rorschach - a Comprehensive System. 5th edition, Vol. 1. New York: John Wiley & Sons; 2003.
119. Western D. Social Cognition and Object Relations Scale (SCORS) Manual for scoring TAT data, Ph.D. thesis, unpublished manuscript, Ann Arbor, University of Michigan; 1990.
120. Cramer P. The Development of Defence Mechanisms. New York: Springer Verlag; 1991.
121. Eresund P. Psychodynamic psychotherapy for children with disruptive disorders. J Child Psychother 2007;33(2):161–80.
122. Odhammar F, Sudin EC, Jonson M, et al. Children in psychodynamic psychotherapy: changes in global functioning. J Child Psychother 2011;37(3):261–79.
123. Carlberg G, Thorén A, Billström S, et al. Children's expectations and experiences of psychodynamic child psychotherapy. J Child Psychother 2009;35(2): 175–93.
124. Roth A, Fonagy P. What works for whom? A critical review of psychotherapy research. 2nd edition. New York: Guilford Press; 2005.
125. Leichsenring F, Rabung S. Effectiveness of long-term psychodynamic psychotherapy: a meta-analysis. JAMA 2008;300(13):1551–65.
126. Leichsenring F, Rabung S. Long-term psychodynamic psychotherapy in complex mental disorders: update of a meta-analysis. Br J Psychiatry 2011; 199:15–22.
127. Shedler J. The efficacy of psychodynamic psychotherapy. Am Psychol 2010; 65(2):98–109.
128. Westen D, Novotny CM, Thompson-Brenner H. The empirical status of empirically supported psychotherapies: assumptions, findings, and reporting in controlled clinical trials. Psychol Bull 2004;130(4):631–63.
129. Whittington CJ, Kendall T, Fonagy P, et al. Selective serotonin reuptake inhibitors in childhood depression: systematic review of published versus unpublished data. Lancet 2004;363(9418):1341–5.
130. Swanson JM, Arnold LE, Vitiello B, et al. Response to commentary on the multimodal treatment study of ADHD (MTA): mining the meaning of the MTA. J Abnorm Child Psychol 2002;30(4):327–32.
131. Goodyer I, Dubicka B, Wilkinson P, et al. Selective serotonin reuptake inhibitors (SSRIs) and routine specialist care with and without cognitive behaviour therapy in adolescents with major depression: randomised controlled trial. BMJ 2007; 335(7611):142.
132. March J, Silva S, Petrycki S, et al. Fluoxetine, cognitive-behavioral therapy, and their combination for adolescents with depression: treatment for Adolescents with Depression Study (TADS) randomized controlled trial. JAMA 2004;292(7): 807–20.

Dyadic Psychotherapy with Infants and Young Children
Child-Parent Psychotherapy

Erica Willheim, PhD[a,b],*

KEYWORDS

- Child-parent psychotherapy • Dyadic psychotherapy
- Psychodynamic dyadic treatment • Early childhood mental health
- History of parent-infant psychotherapy • Negative attributions
- Child-parent psychotherapy interventions

KEY POINTS

- The history of psychotherapy with very young children and their caregivers has been nearly 75 years in the making with multiple, complementary lines of theoretical inquiry contributing to the present-day field of Infant and Early Childhood Mental Health.
- Infants and very young children exist in a relational context, therefore it is the parent-child relationship that must be the target of therapeutic intervention.
- Intervention with parent-child dyads to mitigate disturbances of infancy and early childhood is supported by a substantial empirical and descriptive literature.
- Child-parent psychotherapy, as a more recent and empirically validated form of dyadic psychotherapy, rests on the foundations of psychodynamic theory and technique, and yet reflects a seamless integration with multiple theoretical perspectives and strategies.

HISTORICAL FOUNDATIONS OF DYADIC PSYCHOTHERAPY

....the history of psychotherapy is, in large part, the story of encounters between existent therapeutic approaches and new clinical populations for whom the existing concepts and techniques were not designed. The specific psychopathology that is clinically addressed is of crucial importance to an understanding of the therapeutic approach that develops. Theories arise with specific clinical phenomena in mind.[1]

[a] Family PEACE Program, Ambulatory Care Network, New York Presbyterian Hospital, Columbia University Medical Center, 99 Fort Washington, New York, NY 10032, USA; [b] Department of Psychiatry, Columbia University College of Physicians & Surgeons, Parent Infant Psychotherapy Training Program, Columbia University Center for Psychoanalytic Training & Research, 1051 Riverside Drive, Unit 63, New York, NY 10032, USA
* 140 West 86th Street, Suite 1-A, NY 10024.
E-mail address: erw9011@nyp.org

Child Adolesc Psychiatric Clin N Am 22 (2013) 215–239
http://dx.doi.org/10.1016/j.chc.2013.01.003
1056-4993/13/$ – see front matter © 2013 Elsevier Inc. All rights reserved.

The history of psychotherapy with very young children and their caregivers has now been nearly 75 years in the making. Multiple, complementary lines of theoretical inquiry have contributed to the field and the clinical interventions now recognized under the heading of Infant and Early Childhood Mental Health. Among the many factors that can be said to have set the stage for the birth of this new form of psychotherapy, one may count: increasing interest in the manner in which early experience shapes adult personality organization; cultural practices and historical events that allowed for the study of early childhood separation from primary caregivers; and shifts in the focus of psychoanalytic practitioners as the field expanded into new settings and was affected by the experience of practitioners.[2]

Attention to the Very Young Child and Caregiver

It was in the late 1930s and 1940s in both England and America that an interest first emerged in the "ill effects on personality development of prolonged institutional care and/or frequent changes of mother-figure during the early years of life."[3] These investigations were groundbreaking in their shift to direct observation of early childhood experience and in the concomitant attention given to the role and importance of the primary caregiver. Such an approach was deeply significant given the backdrop of turn-of-the-century psychoanalytic theory in which (1) information regarding childhood experience was derived from adult retrospection and fantasy, and (2) drive theory held that the primary drive of the infant was oral and independent of the "object," therefore the close relationship with the source of food, namely the mother, was secondary.[3] In other words, an infant orients to the breast and only later to the mother to whom the breast is attached.

In England, where the London Blitz of World War II necessitated mass evacuations of children to the countryside, Anna Freud and Dorothy Burlingham documented their observations that separation from the primary caregiver was subjectively far more disturbing for young children than any other war-related hardship.[4] The culturally normative practice of hospitalizing children with only very strict and sparse "visiting hours" with their parents provided a further natural setting for James Robertson's early 1950s investigations of the impact of separation on very young children.[5] Together with John Bowlby, Robertson would soon describe young children's reactions to prolonged separation from their primary caregiver in 3 progressive stages: protest, despair, and detachment (**Box 1**).[6]

In the United States in the late 1930s David Levy was investigating the treatment of traumatized children, noting the mediating role of the parent in the child's experience of trauma.[7] In addition, the cultural practice of placing abandoned or orphaned children into "foundling homes" provided a novel setting for the observations of psychoanalyst Rene Spitz in the mid-1940s. Spitz documented the extreme physical and

---

Box 1
Progressive stages of young children's response to prolonged separation from primary caregivers

1. Protest

2. Despair

3. Detachment

Data from Robertson J, Bowlby J. Responses of young children to separation from their mothers. Courrier Centre Internationale Enfance 1952;2:131–42.

emotional deterioration shown by these institutionalized infants.[8] He coined the term "anaclitic depression"[9] to describe the poor appetite, weight loss, disturbed sleep, compromised immune status, and social withdrawal he observed in infants suffering maternal deprivation. Similar studies on institutionalized children were later performed by Sally Provence and Rose Lipton at Yale.[10] Two films of the era, Spitz's 1947 *Grief: A Peril In Infancy*[11] and James Robertson's 1952 *A Two-Year-Old Goes to Hospital*[12] provided dramatic illustrations that significant separations from primary caregivers had clearly observable, detrimental effects on young children.

In 1951, sponsored by the World Health Organization, John Bowlby published a highly controversial report entitled "Maternal Care and Mental Health."[13] In this seminal monograph Bowlby reviewed the extant work on the deleterious effects of inadequate maternal care in early childhood, whether from institutionalization or from deprivation of maternal care. He called for changes to accepted practices regarding the care of very young children. This proposition that early real-life experience could determinatively affect later personality development remained hotly contested for some time. As Bowlby would later recall, psychoanalysts "whose theory focused on the role of fantasy in psychopathology to the relative exclusion of the influence of real-life events, remained unconvinced and sometimes very critical."[3] Criticism additionally came from psychologists who objected that the mechanisms whereby early maternal deprivation influenced later personality organization or pathology were insufficiently explained.

Following from the work of Bowlby, Spitz, and Robertson, in the late 1950s and early 1960s American psychologist Harry Harlow used infant rhesus monkeys to conduct a series of experiments on maternal deprivation and social isolation.[14] The results of this work, captured on film, demonstrated that infant rhesus monkeys would feed from a wire mesh "mother" with an attached bottle but, once fed, preferred clinging to and derived comfort from, a wire "mother" covered in soft terrycloth.[15] Significantly, these experiments supported the primacy of the mother-infant relationship apart from oral gratification, although critics at the time maintained that infantile clinging was far more important to monkeys than to humans.

Psychoanalytic Stirrings

Separate from the aforementioned lines of investigation, beginning in the late 1940s, some psychoanalytic circles engaged in increased exploration of the relationships between the mother's own childhood experience, the psychic terrain of the mother as an adult, and the mother's influence on the psychological development of her infant. In the late 1950s Therese Benedek[16] and Grete Bibring[17] wrote for the first time about the psychological relationship between a mother's childhood experiences and her subjective experience of pregnancy and being a parent.[18] Drawing from his work as a pediatrician, British psychoanalyst Donald Winnicott wrote of the centrality of the real mother in the developing psyche of the infant and young child, in contrast to the fantasied mother of concern to contemporaries such as Melanie Klein.[2] Winnicott contributed a wealth of novel theoretical conceptualizations regarding the infant-mother dyad, concepts that are now indelible parts of the infant mental health landscape (eg, the good-enough mother, maternal preoccupation, the mirror-role of the mother, transitional objects, and the holding environment).[19–21] Indeed, it is Winnicott who articulated the frequently cited adage that "There is no such thing as a baby... A baby cannot exist alone, but is essentially part of a relationship."[22] Daniel Stern notes that the "fantasy life of the mother" was also explored by Wilfred Bion in his writings on "maternal reverie."[23–25] Stern suggests that this attention by Winnicott, Bion and others to maternal "reveries, preoccupations, fantasies, and projective identifications (as forms of representations) involving the baby...took on the status of one of the major building blocks for the infant's construction of a sense of identity."[1]

Attachment Theory

In 1969, John Bowlby published *Attachment and Loss*.[26] Synthesizing elements of ethology, object-relations theory, and systems theories, Bowlby proposed that a bio-behavioral system of caregiver-infant interaction had evolved in the service of species survival. Both caregiver and infant are biologically predisposed to engage in behaviors that support the goal of safety and security. For the infant, fear or distress serves to activate the "attachment behavioral system" and motivates proximity-seeking behaviors. Phenotypically, such proximity-seeking behaviors will change as developmental capacities mature over the first year of life, beginning for example with crying, clinging, and smiling and then progressing to approaching the caregiver as mobility is consolidated. Bowlby theorized that based on the caregiver's actual record of providing protection, comfort and safety via the "caregiving behavioral system," the infant would construct an internal working model (IWM) of the self and caregiver in the attachment relationship. It is this IWM that subsequently guides the infant's behavior and expectations of attachment figures, particularly in times of stress and fear.

In the late 1970s the central thesis of attachment theory, that the quality of infant attachment is directly related to the quality of experienced caregiving, was operationalized by Mary Ainsworth and her colleagues[27] in a research paradigm known as the Strange Situation Procedure. Based on the adaptive behavioral responses of 12-month-old infants during a structured series of separations and reunions between infant and primary caregiver, Ainsworth was able to code and classify 3 attachment patterns: "Secure," whereby the infant seeks and derives felt security from proximity/interaction with the attachment figure; "Insecure-Avoidant," whereby the infant avoids proximity seeking/interaction with the attachment figure; and "Insecure-Resistant (Ambivalent)," whereby the infant simultaneously seeks and resists proximity/interaction with the attachment figure (**Box 2**).

Each attachment category reflects a predominant pattern of behavioral strategies linked to the IWM the infant holds of the availability, reliability, and responsivity of

---

Box 2
Infant attachment classifications

Secure (B)

Upon reunion the infant actively seeks and effectively derives felt security from proximity to and interaction with the attachment figure. This is an organized pattern.

Insecure-Avoidant (A)

Upon reunion the infant obviously avoids proximity seeking or interaction with the attachment figure. This is an organized pattern.

Insecure-Resistant (Ambivalent) (C)

Upon reunion the infant simultaneously seeks and resists proximity to and interaction with the attachment figure. This is an organized pattern.

Disorganized-Disoriented (D)

Upon reunion the infant exhibits odd, chaotic, interrupted, mistimed, and incoherent behaviors regarding the attachment figure. This is a disorganized pattern in which all strategies are rendered ineffective and the attachment behavioral system is derailed.

Data from Refs.[27–29]

the attachment figure. This translation of Bowlby's theory into measurable behavioral markers was a watershed achievement that ushered in more than 20 years of intense and robust research on attachment. In addition to the 3 "organized" secure and inse-cure classifications identified by Ainsworth, Main and Solomon[28,29] later added a fourth category termed "Disorganized-Disoriented," relating to the disorganized and incoherent quality of the behavioral pattern shown by some infants with respect to separation and reunion.

The Birth of Parent-infant Psychotherapy

> *Jane begins to cry. It is a hoarse, eerie cry in a baby… On tape we see the baby in her mother's arms screaming hopelessly; she does not turn to her mother for comfort. The mother looks distant, self-absorbed. She makes an absent gesture to comfort the baby, then gives up. She looks away. The screaming continues for 5 dreadful minutes on tape… As we watched this tape later in a staff session, we said to each other incredulously, 'It's as if this mother doesn't hear her baby's cries.' This led us to the key diagnostic question, 'Why doesn't this mother hear her baby's cries?'[30]*

The question posed in this classic passage from the seminal article by Fraiberg, Adelson, and Shapiro, "Ghosts in the Nursery,"[30] signifies the beginning of an entirely new era in the understanding of the parent-infant relationship. Evolving alongside psychoanalytic theories on the role of maternal fantasy in the formation of the infant psyche, Fraiberg and colleagues presented real-time clinical material that vividly illus-trated the manner in which adverse maternal childhood experience could lead to disturbed parent-infant interactions and outright symptomatology in the infant.

Fraiberg proposed that it was the repressed or unacknowledged affects associated with the mother's own negative early childhood experience that were responsible for disturbances in caregiving: "The key to our ghost story appears to lie in the fate of affects in childhood. Our hypothesis is that access to childhood pain becomes a power-ful deterrent against repetition in parenting, while repression and isolation of painful affect provide the psychological requirements for identification with the betrayers and the aggressors."[30] Thus, of the mother who could not hear her baby crying, Fraiberg concluded "her own cries had never been heard," leading to the defensive repression of her experiences of abject neglect, abandonment, and helplessness. Without conscious access to those feelings, the mother internalized and remained unconsciously identified with those who perpetrated her abandonment and, consistent with that identification, she repeated their insensitive pattern of caregiving. This was the first description of what is now referred to as "the intergenerational transmission of trauma."[18]

Stern observes, "This placing of the maternal representation at the core of the parent-infant clinical situation marked the beginning of 'infant psychiatry' of a psycho-analytic inspiration. In a sense, a field was born."[1] Similar clinical evolution regarding the theory and treatment of parent-infant dyads occurred at roughly the same time or soon after in Europe. In Paris it was Serge Lebovici,[31] Leon Kreisler, and Michel Soule,[32] and in Geneva, Bertram Cramer,[33] who developed theoretical schools of psychodynamic parent-infant treatment.[34]

Empirical Foundations of Dyadic Treatment

The proposition that intervening with parent-child dyads is effective in mitigating disturbances of infancy and early childhood is supported by a substantial empirical and descriptive literature. This body of work extends from research conducted at the most micro levels of bidirectional parent-infant interaction,[35,36] to examinations of broader behavioral and dynamic interplay,[37] to clinical interventions.[38,39] The common denominator, however, is the critical importance of caregiver interaction with the infant and the effort to determine which factors drive the quality of that interaction. For the purposes of this review, the focus is narrowed to attachment research as the foundational exemplar of empirical support for dyadic intervention.

Attachment research into the causal relationship between the caregivers' experiences in childhood, their subsequent parenting, and the infant's personality organization emerged with the development of the Adult Attachment Interview (AAI) (George C, Kaplan N, and Main M, University of California Berkeley, unpublished manuscript, 1984). Using a semistructured interview that asked parents about their own childhood relationships with their primary attachment figures, Main and colleagues[40] found that the degree of coherence and integration that characterized parental narratives with respect to attachment could be reliably coded into categories that mirrored those of Ainsworth's infant classifications.

Moreover, when parent-infant pairs were studied, parental attachment classifications were found to be highly correlated with their infant's attachment classification. Secure infant attachment was associated with "Secure/Autonomous" parental attachment, avoidant infant attachment with "Dismissive" parental attachment, resistant infant attachment with "Preoccupied" parental attachment, and disorganized infant attachment with "Unresolved" (with respect to trauma and loss) parental attachment (**Box 3**).[40–42] The implication here was that the quality of the parent's mental representations of self and others in attachment relationships was the mechanism responsible for the intergenerational transmission of attachment quality.[43,44] The quality of the parent's internalized attachment representations was understood to affect the infant's developing IWM of self and others via interactions with the parent arising from those parental representations.

Fonagy and colleagues[45,46] further refined the relationship between adult and infant attachment when they examined an aspect of metacognitive monitoring termed "mentalization": an awareness of and ability to hold in mind meaningful relationships between underlying mental states (feelings, thoughts, intentions) and behavior in the

---

Box 3
Adult attachment correlates of infant attachment classifications

Parental Attachment

Secure/Autonomous

Dismissive

Preoccupied

Unresolved

Infant Attachment

Secure

Avoidant

Resistant/Ambivalent

Disorganized

Data from Main M, Kaplan N, Cassidy JC. Security in infancy, childhood, and adulthood: a move to the level of representation. Monogr Soc Res Child Dev 1985;50(1–2):66–104; and Main M, Goldwyn R. Adult attachment classification system. In: Main M, editor. Behavior and the development of representational models of attachment: 5 methods of assessment. West Nyack (NY): Cambridge University Press; 1995.

self and in others. Rating caregiver AAI narratives on a scale of mentalization (operationalized as reflective functioning [RF]), Fonagy's group found that caregiver RF was highly predictive of infant attachment classification, even exceeding the predictive value of Main's original AAI classifications. High caregiver RF was correlated with secure/autonomous adult attachment and secure infant attachment, whereas low caregiver RF was correlated with insecure adult attachment and insecure infant attachment.

Fonagy and colleagues[47] have suggested that if engagement in RF leads to disturbing negative affect, as might occur if a caregiver reflects on significant childhood experiences of helplessness or distress, RF may be curtailed in an effort to ward off unwelcome and overwhelming affect. Of importance, if a caregivers are involved in such curtailment, or defensive inhibition, they will be unable to perceive, reflect on, and appropriately respond to such states in their infants, leaving infants to manage developmentally unmanageable levels of arousal and anxiety by themselves. Slade and colleagues[48] have advanced this line of inquiry even further by examining caregiver RF with respect to the attachment relationship with the child (rather than with the caregiver's parents) and, indeed, found that it correlated highly with infant attachment status.[49] In addition, researchers working to determine caregiver correlates of disorganized infant attachment have found atypical and dysregulated maternal behaviors to be associated with both trauma and loss in the caregiver's past.[50,51]

Thus, the research into the relationship between caregiver and infant attachment boasts robust empirical evidence that predictive relationships exist between:

1. The caregiver's internal mental representations of attachment relationships as formed in childhood
2. The caregiver's degree of integrated and coherent attachment related mentalization (RF)
3. The manner in which attachment-related representations and affects are behaviorally and affectively enacted in interaction with the infant
4. The infant's IWM, or internalized representation, of self and attachment figure

By extension, we may understand that the caregiver's capacity to self-regulate in the domains of arousal, affect, attention, and behavior will determine his or her ability to assist the infant or very young child in the regulation of the child's own arousal, affect, attention, and behavior.

GENERAL FEATURES OF DYADIC THERAPIES
When is Dyadic Psychotherapy Indicated?

The question often arises, "But why would a baby ever need therapy?" For the sake of simplicity, and diplomacy, we might respond by stating, "sometimes parents need extra help or support" or "some infants or young children present more challenges than others." While not incorrect, most clinical practitioners would agree that these answers do not begin to reflect the actual complexity of situations that benefit from dyadic treatment. Indeed, the question itself is wrong. The essential feature that sets psychodynamic treatment of the young child apart from the treatment of other populations is that infants and very young children singularly exist, develop, and evolve within the relational context.[52] It therefore cannot be "a baby" alone who needs therapy, but rather the baby-in-a-relationship. The unit of treatment, the "identified patient" as it were, is the relationship between the child and parent.[39,53] Alternatively, we may conceptualize the treatment as addressing 3 patients: the parent, the child, and the relationship.[54]

Before discussing clinical situations for which dyadic psychotherapy is appropriate and perhaps necessary to restore a normative developmental trajectory for the child and the caregiver-child relationship, we must affirm that childhood contains a vast number of normative stressors, both internally and externally generated, any one of which may cause transient "symptoms." Some examples might be the 1-year-old who cries bitterly the first few times he is left with a new babysitter, the 2-year-old who seems affectively flat and withdrawn during a 3-day separation from her mother, the 3-year-old who briefly regresses in toilet training following the birth of a new sibling, and the 4-year-old who seems hyperactive and does not sleep well for the first few days and nights in a new home. These types of normative stressors are expectable, even necessary, and typically such reactive symptoms resolve without any professional intervention.

That said, frequently the factor that propels parents to seek professional help, or providers to make a referral, is the young child's overt behavioral presentation. Because very young children have a limited repertoire for expressing distress, the list of early childhood symptoms that may lead to referral commonly includes problems of regulation (sleeping, feeding, eliminating), developmental regression, problems in toileting, inattention, hyperactivity, impulsivity, irritability, excessive or inconsolable crying, defiance, excessive or self-harming tantrums, aggression, hypervigilance, withdrawal, flattened affect, dissociation, somatization, and fearfulness (**Box 4**).[55] These symptoms typically have not remitted over time, are not better accounted for by a medical diagnosis, and are causing subjective distress to the child, primary

---

Box 4
Early childhood symptoms often leading to referral

- Dysregulation (sleeping, feeding, eliminating)
- Developmental regression
- Problems in toileting
- Inattention
- Hyperactivity
- Impulsivity
- Irritability
- Excessive or inconsolable crying
- Defiance
- Excessive or self-harming tantrums
- Aggression
- Hypervigilance
- Withdrawal
- Flattened affect
- Dissociation
- Somatization
- Fearfulness

Data from Schechter DS, Willheim E. The effects of violent experiences on infants and young children. In: Zeanah CH, editor. Handbook of infant mental health. 3rd edition. New York: Guilford Press; 2009. p. 197–213.

caregiver, and often the family system as a whole. As with all psychiatric symptoms, the practitioner will seek the underlying cause of the difficulties, but because of the age of the patient, the cause must be considered within the relational context. What, then, are the factors that may affect the dyadic relationship in such a manner that early childhood symptoms emerge?

Traumatic stress

Examples of traumatic stress that would strongly indicate dyadic psychotherapy intervention include exposure to domestic violence, witnessing community violence, direct physical abuse, direct sexual abuse, severe neglect (see the article by Terr elsewhere in this issue), serious medical illness and instrumentation (see the article by Schechter elsewhere in this issue), and prolonged or repeated separations from primary attachment figures. The term "traumatic" is used here in keeping with the A Criteria for posttraumatic stress disorder (PTSD) found in the *Diagnostic and Statistical Manual of Mental Disorders* (4th edition, text revision) (DSM-IV-TR), which defines trauma as the witnessing or experiencing of events that involve actual or threatened death or serious injury, or a threat to the physical (or psychological) integrity of self or others, with the response involving intense fear, helplessness, or horror.[56] In very young children, 2 additional points require attention. The first is that for the very young child, any threat (or perception of threat) to the primary caregiver is experienced as a potential annihilation of the self. This is one of the most literal examples of what we mean when we speak of the very young child "existing" in the relational context.[55] The second point is that whether the traumatic event occurred to the child alone or to the caregiver and child jointly, it is necessary to treat the dyad. In their model of Relational PTSD, Scheeringa and Zeanah[57] observe that the primary caregiver may either exacerbate or mitigate the child's posttraumatic stress symptoms, and that this is in fact the most important determinant of the child's subsequent adjustment.

A final note here is that dyadic referrals may be made in advance of potentially traumatic life stressors that may present a significant risk for psychiatric or developmental disturbance in the infant or young child. Some examples might be the impending death of a parent from a terminal illness, a significant impending separation from a caregiver such as a parent in the military, or an impending major medical intervention. In such cases, treatment may be used protectively as part of a preventive care strategy.

Constitutional challenges in the child

Significant challenges to the parent-child relationship may result from a child's constitutional challenges. Developmental delays, sensory-motor integration problems, affect regulation problems, prematurity, and autism spectrum disorders do not necessarily, but may, engender problematic reactions in the caregiver. Parental responses such as withdrawal, unrealistic expectations, grief and mourning, overprotection, or hostility can be normative initial reactions but they may also become fixed instead of evolving into a more integrated stance, thereby compromising the optimal development of the individual child and the parent-child relationship. In such situations, dyadic psychotherapeutic intervention is of great benefit.[58]

In this category, mention the paradigm of "goodness of fit" between child and caregiver temperament is also obligatory.[59] Goodness of fit refers to the fit, or lack thereof, between the infant's temperament and the demands of the surrounding environment, including parental temperament. For example, a very energetic, adventurous, and outgoing child might prove challenging for a caregiver who tends to be shy, withdrawn, and cautious. In cases of mismatched dyads, dyadic psychotherapy can often improve the developmental trajectory of the caregiver-child relationship.

Disturbances in caregiving

Any discussion of risk factors for impaired parent-child relationships resulting in early childhood mental health problems must include the following: parental mental illness (eg, schizophrenia, bipolar disorder, personality disorder, major depression, anxiety disorder, PTSD), parental substance abuse, and adolescent motherhood. An additional major risk factor is caregiver history of trauma, particularly interpersonal trauma. Not only can caregiver self-regulation be impaired in such cases, a hallmark symptom of PTSD, but the interpersonal nature of the past trauma very often results in disturbed internal representations held by the caregiver with respect to attachment relationships.[60] These caregivers are the mothers about whom Fraiberg and colleagues[30] wrote so eloquently. Indeed, all caregiving disturbances may pose a significant risk to the parent-child relationship given that:

1. Caregiver self-regulation is compromised and, therefore, the caregiver's capacity to regulate the child is compromised.
2. Caregiver disturbances lend themselves to distortions and misattributions in their perception of the child's feelings, thoughts, and intentions; that is, parental RF is impaired (**Box 5**).

The parent-child relational disturbances that can occur with such caregivers are sometimes colloquially referred to as "attachment disturbances." This term contributes to an unfortunate confusion. Classifications of attachment, as defined by Ainsworth, were never intended as diagnostic categories; they were, and remain,

---

Box 5
Factors contributing to dyadic disturbance and early childhood symptomatology

Traumatic Stressors

- Domestic violence
- Community Violence
- Physical abuse
- Sexual abuse
- Neglect
- Serious medical illness with instrumentation
- Prolonged or repeated separation from primary attachment figure

Constitutional Challenges in the Child

- Developmental delay
- Sensory integration disorder
- Affect regulation disturbance
- Prematurity
- Autism spectrum disorder

Disturbances in Caregiving

- Parental mental illness
- Parental substance abuse
- Adolescent parenthood
- Parental history of trauma

descriptions of infant behavioral patterns reflecting adaptation to the caregiver's track record of providing, or not providing, a "secure base." The single "attachment disorder" that does have defined diagnostic criteria in both the DSM-IV-TR[56] and ICD-10[61] is Reactive Attachment Disorder (RAD).[62]

To describe and codify those psychiatric problems of early childhood and impairments in parent-child relationships for which there are no universally recognized criteria or "codes," leaders in infant mental health have authored the *DC:0-3 Diagnostic Classification of Mental Health and Developmental Disorders of Infancy and Early Childhood* (DC:0-3).[63] Although these diagnoses await empirical validation, they are easily recognizable to the practicing early-childhood clinician. In addition, an alternative model of "attachment disorders" has been proposed to more closely reflect attachment research and clinical practice.[64–66] For example, the term "Secure-Base Distortions" has been suggested to capture abnormalities specific to a preferred attachment relationship that does exist, in contrast to the pathology of nonexistent attachment as defined by RAD. Within Secure-Base Distortions, subtypes of Self-Endangering, Clinging/Inhibited, Vigilance/Hypercompliance, and Role Reversal are intended as descriptions of behavioral adaptations made by the child in an effort to either assure or activate the protective, safe-haven function of the caregiver. For a more comprehensive review of disturbances of attachment, see Schechter and Willheim.[60]

Unique Aspects of Dyadic Psychotherapy

Before focusing on child-parent psychotherapy as a particular evidenced-based exemplar of dyadic psychodynamic treatment, it is pertinent to review several features specific to early childhood dyadic psychotherapy. Zeanah and Boris[66] suggest that there are certain challenges in the assessment of early childhood pathology that are unique to this work because of the young child's natural developmental progression. These investigators outline the following 3 potential "pitfalls" that confront the infant mental health clinician undertaking dyadic therapy.

First, infants and young children are in a constant state of change that is particularly rapid between birth and 2 years, but continues at a fast pace until age 6 years. The brain develops swiftly with attendant marked changes in physiology, cognition, and regulation of affect. Symptoms may therefore morph as development proceeds. At the same time, young children are limited in their repertoire of behaviors, therefore a single behavioral expression may reflect any one of several underlying causes.

Second, during the preverbal period, and even once the child has acquired rudimentary language, the child has a very limited capacity to communicate subjective experience. The clinician necessarily must "infer" the infant's experience. The reporters whom clinicians rely on to give them increased insight into the infant (eg, day-care provider, teacher, babysitter, grandparent, or parent) may be influenced by how well they know the child, in which context they observe the child, or subjective biases they may hold about the child.

Third, there is a constant interplay between the child's rapid development and the ongoing influence of the caregiving environment, often making it a challenge to determine which factor or interaction of factors accounts for the child's symptoms.

Dyadic treatment additionally places unusual pressures on the clinician. From a theoretical perspective, the required range and breadth of competencies are expanded. The clinician, ideally, should have knowledge of: infant and early childhood development, including brain development and developmentally salient anxieties; adult development; psychopathology and diagnostic categories ranging from infancy to adulthood (including the DC:0-3 diagnostic manual[63]); psychodynamic therapy including child-play therapy; attachment theory; trauma theory; and current research regarding parent-child interaction. This is a tall order, and most beginning practitioners will find that they come to the work with perhaps only 1 or 2 of these areas of expertise, but expand their knowledge as the work continues and demands.

From a practice perspective, in contrast to an individual treatment whereby transference and countertransference exist between one patient and one therapist, the dyadic clinician must be attentive to the multiplicity of actual and transferential relationships that simultaneously exist in the treatment room.[1] The clinician must be attuned to the parent's transference to the baby/toddler/preschooler, the parent's transference to the therapist, the toddler's or preschooler's transference to the therapist, and the therapist's own countertransferential responses to parent, child, and the parent-child relationship—noting that both transference and countertransference reactions can be of a positive or negative cast. As in all psychodynamic treatments, the clinician must be on guard for the meaning and treatment impact of these factors.

For the dyadic clinician there can also exist a sensation of excessive or overwhelming sensory, affective, and cognitive stimulation in the treatment room. Working with both parent and child together means having to simultaneously attend to feeling states, behaviors, interactional patterns, play themes and content, and specific trauma material, as they are presented both individually and in interaction.

Finally, perhaps one of the most challenging elements of working with dyads is the practice of not intervening. Just as Fraiberg described the crying of "Jane," Lieberman and Van Horn[67] have presented numerous case vignettes in which the clinician is faced with a crying, distressed infant/toddler/preschooler and a parent who is either nonresponsive or hostile. The clinician struggles with wanting to pick up, hold, calm, and soothe the distressed child. In the moment, the clinician may also struggle with strongly negative feelings toward the parent. The clinician may further struggle to think calmly and clearly in the presence of a highly distressed child. The clinician's challenge in such scenarios is to maintain self-regulation, remain mindful of countertransferential reactions, recall that the infant's best interests may not be well served if it is the clinician who offers comfort, and determine a course of intervention that promotes repair within the dyad. After all, dyadic treatment seeks to reestablish the safety and security of the parent-infant relationship, not the clinician-infant relationship (**Box 6**).

EVIDENCE-BASED DYADIC INTERVENTIONS: CHILD-PARENT PSYCHOTHERAPY

Among the many versions of dyadic treatment that have been developed (eg, Interaction Guidance,[68] Watch, Wait, and Wonder,[69] Parent-Child Interaction Treatment,[70]

Box 6
Unique aspects of dyadic treatment

1. Accurate identification of symptoms in the context of rapid developmental change and a limited repertoire of behaviors

2. Inference of the young child's subjective experience

3. Assessment of symptoms in light of the ongoing interaction between child development and the caregiving environment

4. Mastery of an expanded range and breadth of competencies

5. Management of multiple simultaneous actual and transferential relationships

6. Tolerance of intense sensory, affective, and cognitive stimulation in the treatment room

7. Knowing when to strategically "not intervene"

Clinician-Assisted Videofeedback Exposure Session[71]), the evidence-based intervention that perhaps most exemplifies the integrated use of psychodynamic psychotherapy is child-parent psychotherapy (CPP).[72,73] Because the original literature regarding the theory and clinical application of this intervention is easily accessible for the interested clinician (see References), this article attempts only to summarize the main features of this treatment, with special attention to the role of psychodynamic conceptualization and intervention.

Evidence of Efficacy

The research data that support the efficacy of CPP come from randomized controlled trials across several populations. Research samples have included anxiously attached toddlers of poor Latina mothers with a history of trauma,[74] toddlers of depressed mothers,[75,76] maltreated preschoolers within the child welfare system,[77,78] and preschoolers exposed to domestic violence.[79,80] Taken as a whole, these studies have demonstrated that CPP intervention results in reductions in both maternal and child posttraumatic stress symptoms, decreased child diagnosis of traumatic stress disorder, improvements in the mother-child relationship and child quality of attachment, positive shifts in child attributions regarding self, mother, and relationships, as well as improved child cognitive functioning.[73]

The anchor study most frequently cited as empirical validation for CPP as an evidenced-based treatment model is the 2005 randomized controlled study conducted by Lieberman and colleagues.[79] A sample of 75 mother-preschooler (ages 3 to 6 years) dyads exposed to domestic violence were randomly assigned to two conditions, CPP treatment or case management, with standard community intervention (referral for individual parent treatment). The CPP condition consisted of weekly dyadic sessions for 1 year. Repeated-measures analysis (analysis of variance) demonstrated significant reductions in child trauma symptomatology, child diagnosis of PTSD, and child behavioral problems for children in the CPP condition in comparison with control children. The investigators further found that although maternal functioning had not been a primary target of treatment, maternal avoidance symptoms were significantly reduced along with strong trends in the reduction of global psychiatric distress and PTSD diagnosis for mothers in the CPP condition, compared with control mothers. At 6-month follow-up, CPP-condition preschoolers continued to exhibit significantly fewer behavioral problems, and CPP-condition mothers showed significantly lower scores in global psychiatric distress, suggesting that mothers receiving CPP treatment continued to improve even after treatment ended.[80]

Noting that the age range of this research sample extends up to 6 years, it is important to include the recent framework offered by Lieberman and Van Horn[67] that CPP should be understood as an overarching construct that encompasses the age-specific labels of infant-parent psychotherapy,[81,82] toddler-parent psychotherapy,[76,83] and preschooler-parent psychotherapy.[77] CPP has been manualized since 2005 in the ZERO TO THREE publication, *Don't Hit My Mommy*[84]; however, clinicians are not considered to be certified practitioners until they have received formal CPP training and supervision. Finally, it is important to explicitly state that although CPP is widely known and disseminated by the National Child Traumatic Stress Network as an evidence-based treatment specifically for trauma-exposed children and their caregivers, it is applicable across the continuum of early childhood disorders.

CPP in Practice

Key components of CPP have their origin in infant-parent psychotherapy as developed by Fraiberg and colleagues.[30,81,85] The underlying psychoanalytic conceptualization of intergenerational trauma transmission and the intervention techniques of developmental guidance, concrete assistance, and insight-oriented interpretation used by Fraiberg and her group continue to be cornerstones of CPP. As research and theory have advanced over time, additional paradigms have been integrated into the theory and practice of CPP.[73] Theoretical contributions have come from the "dual lenses" of attachment theory and trauma theory,[86] developmental psychology, psychoanalytic theory, and developmental psychopathology. Intervention contributions derive from social work, social learning theory, and cognitive-behavioral therapy. Most recently, CPP has incorporated a new conceptual paradigm known as "angels in the nursery,"[87] which seeks to recall (or create) benevolent internal models of positive, responsive, and nurturing care.

As a child-centered treatment, CPP prioritizes the goal of a healthy, normal developmental trajectory across all domains. As a relationship-based treatment that locates the mental health of the young child within the relationship with the primary caregiver, the goal of CPP is to strengthen and support that relationship. Embedded in these overarching goals are multiple discrete objectives. CPP seeks to support the attainment of individual affect regulation and integration, resolution of trauma-related symptomatology, and reestablishment of trust in bodily sensations that have been impaired by trauma exposure. Between caregiver and child, CPP works to build the relational qualities of mutuality, reciprocity, communication, and understanding/empathy. CPP fosters security of attachment, the reestablishment of the caregiver as a source of protection and safety, and caregiver-child mutually constructed meanings as opposed to individually held misperceptions about self and other. Additional areas of attention are child cognitive growth, positive conflict-resolution skills, and accurate reality testing (**Box 7**).

CPP Interventions

This section briefly reviews the intervention modalities used in CPP as delineated by Lieberman and Van Horn in the CPP literature. The category of Insight-Oriented

---

Box 7
Goals of CPP

Global Goals of CPP

- Encouraging normal development: engagement with present activities and future goals
- Strengthening and supporting the parent-child relationship
- Maintaining regular levels of affective arousal
- Establishing trust in bodily sensations
- Achieving reciprocity in intimate relationships
- Resolution of trauma-related symptomatology

Trauma-Related Goals of CPP

- Increased capacity to respond realistically to threat
- Differentiation between reliving and remembering
- Normalization of the traumatic response
- Placing the traumatic experience in perspective
- Coconstruction of a mutually meaningful trauma narrative

Interpretation is left for last, so that the use of psychodynamic elements in CPP treatment may be emphasized and expanded upon.

Promoting developmental progress through play, physical contact, and language

This category of intervention relies on the normative pathways of play, physical contact, and putting feelings into words. In treatment, however, these arenas uniquely serve to help metabolize difficult and overwhelming feeling states in a manner that supports individual affect regulation as well as the development of empathic and positive communications between parent and child.

The clinician supports putting feelings into words by at times speaking for the child or speaking for the parent, translating the actions or behaviors of parent or child into a language of feelings that may be heard and understood by the other. Although the technique of putting feelings into words may sound simple, it is probably not an exaggeration to say that this is one of the most powerful and yet delicate intervention techniques in the CPP tool kit. Whether it is an articulation of the feeling state of a toddler ("mommy, that noise scared me and I wanted to be close to you where I feel safe"). the feeling state of a parent ("mommy is crying because it makes her sad when she thinks about how scared you both were during the fight with daddy"), or an articulation of the feelings underlying a ruptured interaction ("you wanted to put in the last piece of the puzzle all by yourself so you got upset when mommy did it, and mommy got upset because she thought she was helping you and didn't understand why you threw the puzzle on the floor"), the translational function of the clinician cannot be underestimated in enhancing mutuality and empathy.

The function of play is at least twofold. The treatment session is an opportunity for parent and child to engage in mutually enjoyable, conflict-free interaction, thus promoting positive communication as well as setting the stage for the more complicated work of cocreating narratives around problematic issues. In addition, however, play is the medium through which children communicate their feelings, expectations, wishes, fears, and anxieties. The clinician again serves as translator, helping the parent to make meaning out of the child's play, supporting the parent should traumatic play themes activate difficult parental feelings or memories, and translating back to the child what the parent may be experiencing.

Promoting physical contact in the form of playful interaction or affection may seem unnecessary but, in some dyads, this basic form of comfort and security is not present. The clinician may need to use a variety of intervention strategies to facilitate warm physical touch between parent and child.

Offering unstructured reflective developmental guidance

Following from Fraiberg, this intervention seeks to make the underlying motivations, feelings, and thoughts of the child understandable to the parent. This aspect is particularly critical when negative parental attributions have obscured the true meanings and intentions of the child's behavior. Parents may be offered basic information on normative child development such as age-specific motor, cognitive, or affective capacities of young children, or information about how their child sees and understands adult behavior and relationships. When appropriate, parents may need guidance about expectable early childhood responses to traumatic experience.

A small sample of this type of guidance includes the following. "Young children imitate their parents' behavior because they want to be like them and assume that their parents' behavior is a model to emulate." "Separation distress is an expression of the child's fear of losing the parent." "Young children use the word 'no' to establish and practice their autonomy." "Memory starts at birth; babies and young children remember experiences before they can speak about them." More concrete guidance may take the form of educating the parent on age-appropriate capabilities, behaviors, or expected milestones.

Normalizing, reframing, educating, modeling empathy, and supporting appropriate limit setting are all components of developmental guidance. The "unstructured" quality of the guidance refers to the fact that these insights are not offered in a set or sequenced manner as they might be in the curriculum of a parenting class; rather, the timing and application of such comments depends entirely on what is happening in the room, in the moment. The "reflective" quality of the guidance is that, in all cases, the goal is to increase the parent's reflective capacity to accurately infer the motivations, intentions, feelings, and thoughts of the child.[45,88] When successful, a parent who has typically been unable to think about her children when activated by traumatic reminders, is able to think about how both she and the child are feeling and, therefore, speak and behave in a manner consistent with that understanding.[54]

Modeling appropriate protective behavior

This intervention is particularly salient when either parent or child, or both, have been so chronically exposed to danger (eg, abuse, domestic violence, community violence) that the thresholds for what activates self-protective behavior in the child and child-protective behavior in the parent is disproportionately high or seemingly nonexistent. Therefore, when a child is engaged in behavior that is dangerous either to himself, others, the parent, or the playroom, and attempts to activate the parent to engage in protective behavior have been unsuccessful, the clinician may mobilize to protect the child by stopping the behavior. This action serves to communicate to the child, and often to the parent as well, that everyone will be kept safe in the treatment and that reestablishing the provision of safety and protection are important goals of the treatment.

Providing emotional support

Lieberman and Van Horn cite psychotherapy research concerning commonalities across all effective therapies[89,90] that support the importance of the therapeutic stance. The therapeutic stance conveys the emotional availability of the clinician and the clinician's willingness to enter into alliance with the patient to achieve the treatment goals. CPP has the additional aim of modeling a posture of respect for each person's unique experience. Particularly for populations that are chronically disenfranchised, this offering of emotional support and validation of the individual's experience can carry with it a powerful message of worth and dignity.

Addressing traumatic reminders

The addressing of traumatic material is a central feature of CPP, and although this fact distinguishes it from other dyadic treatments, it highlights goals that CPP has in common with all treatment modalities for trauma. In the case of traumatic exposure, both the parent and child must be helped to address the symptoms of physiologic arousal, reexperiencing, and avoidance/numbing that typify posttraumatic stress reactions. Physiologic hyperarousal (hypervigilance) can lead to overestimations of threat in the environment resulting in diminished functioning, whereas numbing can lead to underestimations of threat placing child or parent at risk for revictimization. Reestablishing realistic responses to threat and adaptive coping strategies for dealing with threat are thus critical components of trauma work in CPP.

Reexperiencing is problematic in that the parent or child may not be equipped to remember without affectively reliving traumatic incidents. CPP seeks to establish safety in the present, and to enable parent and child to differentiate between remembered experience and present moment feeling state. In addition, as in all trauma treatments, CPP works to normalize traumatic responses through psychoeducation about typical trauma reactions and to help patients gain perspective by integrating their traumatic experience into a larger, holistic view of themselves.

To achieve these goals, the clinician will use a host of strategies, including exercises and activities that increase physiologic relaxation and may be used as coping skills when dysregulation arises. However, central to trauma work in CPP is the facilitation of a coconstructed parent-child "trauma narrative" that directly addresses the traumatic event through play, language, or art. In cases where the parent and child have been jointly exposed, this work may require modifications depending on the parent's capacity to observe and tolerate the child's trauma reenactment play. Similarly, the child's capacity to see the parent visibly upset about the traumatic experience must be gauged by the therapist in the clinical setting. In situations such as these, as well as many others, CPP allows for flexible approaches such as: splitting a session between parent and child; having additional parallel individual sessions with the parent; or using adjunctive phone conversations with the parent until the dyad is ready to engage in joint narrative construction.

Offering crisis intervention, case management, and concrete assistance

Fraiberg taught that when a family is faced with concrete stressors (eg, housing needs, hunger, lack of language proficiency, unemployment, lack of health insurance), preoccupation with these problems of living may preclude any successful engagement in mental health treatment, regardless of how much it may be needed. The solution modeled by Fraiberg's group was to actively engage in helping the family to resolve these real-life challenges. CPP treatment therefore may include interfacing with any number of different agencies, service providers, schools, and legal representatives in the role of advocate, consultant, mediator, or referral source, depending on the issue at hand. In addition, Lieberman and Van Horn remind us that in matters of crisis intervention, the highest priority is always the safety of the family. Given that families referred for CPP treatment have often recently suffered a traumatic event, this guidance is particularly important. In situations of domestic violence, for example, safety must be reestablished before any substantive trauma work can occur.

Insight-oriented interpretation

As noted in the first part of this article, one of Fraiberg's critical contributions to the treatment of young children and their parents was the conceptualization that repressed childhood affects and identification with the malevolent caregiver of the past could determine parental perceptions and behaviors toward the child in the present. Bringing these disowned affects into consciousness serves to, in essence, free the parent from past "ghosts" and thereby free the baby from its role as the object of repetition and reenactment. Using dynamic interpretation, the therapist works to bring the repudiated affects of the past into present awareness. The parent is then supported in connecting these feelings to their interaction with the child. This movement back and forth, linking past and present, is a hallmark of psychodynamic technique and CPP intervention.

To better grasp the use of dynamic interpretation in CPP, it may be instructive to examine a more classically psychoanalytic explanation of the interplay between parent and child, that of the infant as "transference object." Lieberman and colleagues[82] explain: "The transferential component obscures the baby's selfhood for the parents, so that their perceptions of the baby's personality and behavior are colored and distorted by their own experiences." In essence, a parent cannot feel or respond to the infant's actual developmental capacities, emotional needs, underlying motivations, and feeling states. Rather, parental projections, displacements, and other psychic defense mechanisms and maneuvers obscure the real infant. The following vignette illustrates this "obscuring" of the baby, albeit with a slightly older child.

> *A mother and her 3-year-old son have come to the therapist's office for their weekly session. The mother, who suffers chronic and debilitating anxiety deriving from a history of childhood abuse, has had great difficulty engaging in simple play with her child. In this session, and it seems to be a breakthrough, she sits with the child standing directly in front of her and gently tickles him. Each time she tickles him he squeals with delight and wriggles out of reach. He then returns to his spot standing in front of her signaling that he wants her to "do it again." By the fourth iteration of this game, the child is so excited that instead of backing away, he collapses straight down onto the floor laughing with delight. The mother's face immediately looks worried and alarmed. She turns to the therapist and says, "You see? He's scared. He doesn't want to play this game."*

In this example, we see that the mother's internal experience of chronic fear and withdrawal is projected onto her child. She cannot see his true response of enjoyment at this positively toned interaction with her. The therapist might postulate that in addition to this mother's preoccupation with her own internal state of anxiety, she may have become uncomfortable with how well the play was going and defensively excluded the child's pleasurable affect. One line of inquiry might therefore focus on her own early experiences of play to recover why her child's happiness may have become intolerable in the moment. The therapist might respond, "You are feeling that he does not want to play because he became frightened. I can see why you would want to stop the game, to protect him from feeling afraid. You know, what has happened here makes me wonder about any memories you might have of playing with your own parents?"

If, for example, the mother disclosed that her parents had never played with her and that her primary experience of them was fearful, the following interpretation might be offered: "How hard it must have been to always feel afraid and to never experience the joy of simple play with them, of feeling close to them. Because of your experience as a child, it must be very difficult to imagine that your own child could ever experience playing with you as something wonderful and warm and safe." In this manner, disowned affects from the past, that is, sadness and mourning over the lack of parental warmth and moreover generalized fear/anxiety in their presence, might be brought into present awareness. With the mother freed from having to repress these difficult attachment related affects, the child might also be freed from the projection that he is fearful and cannot experience interaction with his mother as safe and pleasurable.

Parental projections and distortions can be normative and, indeed, beneficial to the baby ("s/he's the best baby in the whole world"); they can also be relatively benign ("with those lungs, s/he will be an opera singer"). The cases seen by CPP clinicians, however, are those in which these attributions have become problematic or dangerous to the child's developing sense of self. For example, the child is inflexibly seen as malevolent or manipulative, or excessively needy or aggressive, or unduly powerful, or perhaps unworthy of care at all. Lieberman[91,92] has written about the manner in which negative maternal attributions come to shape and form the child's identity. Deriving from the analytical concept of projective identification,[93] Lieberman has postulated that the parent defensively projects a role, quality, or feeling state onto the child that reflects her own IWMs of attachment or unconscious fantasies (fears, wishes) about the child. The child is then pressured to comply with this projection via the parent's "selective attunement" to states and behaviors that are compatible with that fixed belief about the child. After sufficient time and repetition of this "behaving in ways consistent with the maternal projection," the child ultimately internalizes the projection, which then forms the child's sense of self. The following vignette may help to illustrate this rather complicated process.

During assessment a mother describes to the clinician that her son "nearly punched a hole in my uterus" during pregnancy. She continues, explaining that the now nearly 4-year-old child has been "violent ever since the day he was born" and willfully hurts others, often "smiling or laughing" afterward. She relates her perception of the child's behavior as an objective truth. When asked what generally causes the child to behave aggressively, she responds "nothing, there's no reason, he's just like that." Asked who the child reminds her of, she responds that he is just like her father (a violent alcoholic) who seemed to "enjoy" frightening her and her siblings.

When the clinician meets the child, she is struck by the discrepancy between the mother's description and the child's appearance. Instead of looking like the devil incarnate, he is an attractive little boy, slight of build with a broad smile and "angelic" curly hair. He easily begins exploring the playroom. As he finds each new toy, he plays appropriately with it and several times looks to his mother, seemingly in order to share his excitement, but his mother is not looking at him, she is animatedly telling the therapist about recent problems at her job. After 10 long minutes of playing on his own, the child picks up a toy fire truck, turns in the direction of his mother, and pauses with it poised above his head. His mother abruptly breaks off from her conversation with the therapist and looks at the child. She squints her eyes, purses her lips, and mutters under her breath "you better not." Their eyes lock for a moment and then the child turns slightly away from his mother and throws the fire truck, hard, across the room. As it crashes to the floor, the child turns back to his mother with an odd frozen half smile on his face that the therapist recognizes as a sign of anxious trepidation as to the mother's next move. The mother looks at the therapist and says "I told you he was violent! Nobody ever believes me until they see it for themselves."

In this example, we observe that the mother's repeated, and very nearly exclusive, attunement to "aggressive" behaviors leaves the child with no choice but to behave in a manner compatible with this attribution if he wishes to be seen or known by her at all. The very natural anxiety response that the child then displays following his "bad behavior," expecting a punitive response from his mother, is filtered by the mother through the lens of her attribution, concluding that the child is "laughing and smiling" because he enjoys being violent, as in her childhood she perceived her violent father to enjoy terrorizing her family. As the child continues to develop, repeated experiences of only being known when he is exhibiting aggression will further consolidate the formation of his sense of self as aggressive, and he will increasingly behave in consonance with this identity (**Box 8**).

Ports of Entry

This concept, first introduced by Stern,[1] refers to the question of where and how to intervene in the parent-child relationship to effect change. In CPP, entry points are understood to be a behavior, interaction, feeling state, or attribution that is chosen as the "immediate object of clinical attention."[82] In CPP the choice of which "port" to enter is determined by what is happening in the moment, and the clinician's judgment

---

Box 8
CPP interventions

- Promoting developmental progress through play, physical contact, and language
- Offering unstructured reflective developmental guidance
- Modeling appropriate protective behavior
- Providing emotional support
- Addressing traumatic reminders
- Offering crisis intervention, case management, and concrete assistance
- Insight-oriented interpretation

---

of what will be most effective in that moment; it is not a singular overall treatment strategy nor a single focus of clinical attention throughout the whole of a given session.

In CPP treatments, possible ports include the individual behavior of the child or parent, interactive exchanges between the parent and child, mental representations held by the child of self or of parent, mental representations held by the parent of self or of child, the relationship between the parent and therapist, the relationship between the child and therapist, or the parent-child-therapist relationship. The space allotted in the present article is insufficient to properly illustrate the complexities of choosing ports of entry and appropriate interventions within those ports. For rich and elegant case illustrations of CPP technique in action, the interested practitioner is referred to the extant CPP literature.[67,72,73,82,84,94]

SUMMARY

The present standing of dyadic psychotherapy as a respected treatment intervention for very young children and their caregivers is attributable to a long list of eminent theorists, clinicians, and researchers, as well as the parents and children with whom they have worked. This review briefly traces the historical roots of dyadic therapy from burgeoning interest in early determinants of personality organization, through expanding psychoanalytic and child development paradigms, to the groundbreaking practical and theoretical contributions of Selma Fraiberg. Within a relatively brief time span, the pace of understanding and integration of multiple constructs in early childhood mental health intervention has been robust and impressive. One of the vital outcomes of this journey has been the deceptively simple notion that very young children exist in a relational context and, therefore, it is the relationship that must be the target of therapeutic intervention.

Child-parent psychotherapy, as a more recent and empirically validated form of dyadic psychotherapy, rests on the foundations of psychodynamic theory and technique and yet reflects a seamless integration with multiple theoretical perspectives and strategies. For this reason, practitioners of CPP are perhaps most effective, regardless of which intervention modalities they may use, when their conceptual formulation of the treatment dyad incorporates a solidly dynamic understanding of the parent-child relationship.

REFERENCES

1. Stern DN. The motherhood constellation. A unified view of parent-infant psychotherapy. New York: Basic Books; 1995. p. 1–40.

2. Wright K. Face and Façade—the mother's face as the baby's mirror. In: Raphael-Leff J, editor. Parent-infant psychodynamics, wild things, mirrors, ghosts. London: Anna Freud Centre; 2008. p. 5–17.

3. Bowlby J. The origins of attachment theory. In: Secure Base A, editor. Parent-child attachment and healthy human development. New York: Basic Books; 1988. p. 20–38.

4. Freud A, Burlingham DT. War and children. New York: Medical War Books; 1943.

5. Robertson J. Some responses of young children to loss of maternal care. Nurs Times 1953;18:382–6.

6. Robertson J, Bowlby J. Responses of young children to separation from their mothers. Courrier Centre Internationale Enfance 1952;2:131–42.

7. Levy DM. Release therapy. Am J Orthop 1939;9(4):713–36.

8. Spitz RA. Hospitalism: an inquiry into the genesis of psychiatric conditions in early childhood. Psychoanal Study Child 1945;1:53–73.

9. Spitz RA. Anaclitic depression. Psychoanal Study Child 1946;2:313–42.

10. Provence S, Lipton RC. Infants in institutions. New York: International Universities Press; 1962.

11. Spitz RA. Grief: a peril in infancy (Film). Akron (OH): University of Akron Psychology Archives; 1947.

12. Robertson J. A two-year-old goes to hospital (Film). London, New York: Tavistock Child Development Research Unit, New York University Film Library; 1952.

13. Bowlby J. Maternal care and mental health. Geneva (Switzerland), London, New York: World Health Organization, Her Majesty's Stationery Office, Columbia University Press; 1951.

14. Harlow HF, Harlow MK. The affectional systems. In: Schrier AM, Harlow HF, Stollnitz F, editors. Behaviour of nonhuman primates, vol. 2. New York: Academic Press; 1965. p. 287–334.

15. Harlow HF, Zimmermann RR. Affectional responses in the infant monkey. Science 1959;120:421–3.

16. Benedek T. Parenthood as a developmental phase. J Am Psychoanal Assoc 1959;7:389–417.

17. Bibring GL, Dwyer TF, Huntington DS, et al. A study of the psychological processes in pregnancy and of the earliest mother-child relationship. Psychoanal Study Child 1961;9:9–24.

18. Slade A, Cohen LJ. The process of parenting and the remembrance of things past. Infant Ment Health J 1996;17(3):217–38.

19. Winnicott DW. Collected papers, through paediatrics to psychoanalysis. London: Tavistock Publications; 1958.

20. Winnicott DW. The maturational processes and the facilitating environment. London: The Hogarth Press and the Institute of Psycho-Analysis; 1965.

21. Winnicott DW. Playing and reality. London: Routledge; 1971.

22. Winnicott DW. Further thoughts on babies as persons. In: The child, the family, and the outside world. Harmondsworth (United Kingdom): Penguin Books; 1964. p. 88.

23. Bion WR. Learning from experience. London: Tavistock; 1962.

24. Bion WR. Elements of psycho-analysis. London: Heinemann; 1963.

25. Bion WR. Transformations: change from learning to growth. London: Tavistock; 1965.

26. Bowlby J. Attachment and loss: Vol. I: attachment. New York: Basic Books; 1969–1982.

27. Ainsworth MD, Blehar MC, Waters E, et al. Patterns of attachment: a psychological study of the strange situation. Hillsdale (NJ): Erlbaum; 1978.

28. Main M, Solomon J. Discovery of an insecure-disorganized/disoriented pattern. In: Brazelton TB, Yogman M, editors. Affective development in infancy. Norwood (NJ): Ablex Publishing; 1986. p. 95–124.

29. Main M, Solomon J. Procedures for identifying infants as disorganized/disoriented during the Ainsworth strange situation. In: Greenberg MT, Cicchetti D, Cummings EM, editors. Attachment in the preschool years: theory, research, and intervention. Chicago: University of Chicago Press; 1990. p. 121–60.

30. Fraiberg S, Adelson E, Shapiro V. Ghosts in the nursery: a psychoanalytic approach to the problems of impaired infant-mother relationships. J Am Acad Child Psychiatry 1975;14(3):387–421.

31. Lebovici S. La contribution de la psychanalyse des enfants a la connaissance et a l'action sur les jeunes enfants et les familles deprimes. Congres de la psychanalyse d'enfants. Londres, 1975.

32. Kreisler L, Fain M, Soule M. L'enfant et son corps. Paris: Presses Universitaires de France; 1974.

33. Cramer B. Interventions therapeutiques breves avec parents et enfants. Psychiatrie de l'Enfant 1974;17(1):53–118.

34. Espasa FP. Parent-infant psychotherapy, the transition to parenthood and parental narcissism: implications for treatment. J Child Psychother 2004;30: 155–71.

35. Tronick EZ, Cohn JF. Infant-mother face-to-face interaction: age and gender differences in coordination and the occurrence of miscoordination. Child Dev 1989;60(1):85–92.

36. Beebe B, Jaffe J, Markese S, et al. The origins of 12-month attachment: a micro-analysis of 4-month mother-infant interaction. Attach Hum Dev 2010;12(1–2): 3–141.

37. Brazelton TB, Cramer BG. The earliest relationship. New York: Addison Wesley Publishing; 1990.

38. Stern-Bruschweiler N, Stern DN. A model for conceptualizing the role of the mother's representational world in various mother-infant therapies. Infant Ment Health J 1989;10(3):142–56.

39. Lieberman AF, Pawl JH. Infant parent psychotherapy. In: Zeanah CH, editor. Handbook of infant mental health. New York: Guilford Press; 1993. p. 427–42.

40. Main M, Kaplan N, Cassidy JC. Security in infancy, childhood, and adulthood: a move to the level of representation. Monogr Soc Res Child Dev 1985;50(1–2): 66–104.

41. Main M, Goldwyn R. Adult attachment classification system. In: Main M, editor. Behavior and the development of representational models of attachment: five methods of assessment. West Nyack (NY): Cambridge University Press; 1995.

42. van IJzendoorn MH. Adult attachment representations, parental responsiveness, and infant attachment: a meta-analysis on the predictive validity of the adult attachment interview. Psychol Bull 1995;117(3):387–403.

43. Bretherton I. Communication patterns, internal working models, and the intergenerational transmission of attachment relationships. Infant Ment Health J 1990;11(3):237–52.

44. Crittenden PM. Internal representational models of attachment relationships. Infant Ment Health J 1990;11:259–77.

45. Fonagy P, Steele M, Steele H, et al. The capacity for understanding mental states: the reflective self in parent and child and its significance for security of attachment. Infant Ment Health J 1991;12(3):201–18.

46. Fonagy P, Steele M, Moran G, et al. Measuring the ghost in the nursery: an empirical study of the relation between parents' mental representations of childhood experiences and their infants' security of attachment. J Am Psychoanal Assoc 1993;41(4):957–89.

47. Fonagy P, Steele M, Steele H, et al. The theory and practice of resilience. J Child Psychol Psychiatry 1994;35(2):231–57.

48. Slade A, Grienenberger J, Bernbach E, et al. Maternal reflective functioning, attachment, and the transmission gap: a preliminary study. Attach Hum Dev 2005;7(3):283–98.

49. Zeanah CH, Benoit D, Hirschberg L, et al. Mothers' representations of their infants are concordant with infant attachment classifications. Developmental Issues in Psychiatry and Psychology 1994;1:9–18.

50. Lyons-Ruth K, Bronfman E, Parsons E. Atypical attachment in infancy and early childhood among children at developmental risk. IV. Maternal frightened, frightening, or atypical behavior and disorganized infant attachment patterns. Monogr Soc Res Child Dev 1999;64(3):67–96.

51. Schuengel C, Bakermans-Kranenburg MJ, Van Ijzendoorn MH. Frightening maternal behavior linking unresolved loss and disorganized infant attachment. J Consult Clin Psychol 1999;67(1):54–63.

52. Zeanah CH, Zeanah PD. The scope of infant mental health. In: Zeanah CH, editor. Handbook of infant mental health. 3rd edition. New York: Guilford Press; 2009. p. 5–21.

53. Pawl JH, Lieberman AF. Infant-parent psychotherapy. In: Greenspan S, Wieder S, Osofsky J, editors. Handbook of child and adolescent psychiatry. New York: Wiley; 1997. p. 339–51.

54. Schechter DS, Willheim E. When parenting becomes unthinkable: intervening with traumatized parents and their toddlers. J Am Acad Child Adolesc Psychiatry 2009;48:249–54.

55. Schechter DS, Willheim E. The effects of violent experiences on infants and young children. In: Zeanah CH, editor. Handbook of infant mental health. 3rd edition. New York: Guilford Press; 2009. p. 197–213.

56. APA. Diagnostic and statistical manual of mental disorders. text revision (DSM-IV-TR). 4th edition. Washington, DC: American Psychiatric Association; 2000.

57. Scheeringa MS, Zeanah CH. A relational perspective on PTSD in early childhood. J Trauma Stress 2001;14(4):799–815.

58. Foley GM, Hochman JD, editors. Mental health in early intervention: achieving unity in principles and practice. Baltimore (MD): Brookes Publishing; 2006.

59. Chess S, Thomas A. Goodness of fit: clinical applications for infancy through adult life. Philadelphia. Bruner/Mazel; 1999.

60. Schechter DS, Willheim E. Disturbances of attachment and parental psychopathology in early childhood. Child Adolesc Psychiatr Clin N Am 2009;18:665–86.

61. International classifications of diseases, 10th revision (ICD-10). Geneva (Switzerland): World Health Organization; 1992.

62. Boris NW, Zeanah CH. The work group on quality issues. Practice parameter for the assessment and treatment of children and adolescents with reactive attachment disorder of infancy and early childhood. J Am Acad Child Adolesc Psychiatry 2005;44(11):1206–19.

63. Zero To Three/National Center for Clinical Infant Programs. DC:0–3. Diagnostic classification of mental health and developmental disorders of infancy and early childhood. Rev. edition. Washington, DC: Zero to Three Press; 2005.

64. Lieberman AF, Pawl JH. Disorders of attachment and secure-base behavior in the second year of life. In: Greenberg ET, Cicchetti D, Cummings EM, editors.

Attachment in the preschool years: theory, research, and interventions. Chicago: University of Chicago Press; 1990. p. 375–97.

65. Lieberman AF, Zeanah CH. Disorders of attachment in infancy. Child Adolesc Psychiatr Clin N Am 1995;4:571–687.

66. Zeanah CH, Boris NW. Disturbances and disorders of attachment in early childhood. In: Zeanah CH, editor. Handbook of infant mental health. 2nd edition. New York: Guilford Press; 2000. p. 353–68.

67. Lieberman AF, Van Horn P. Psychotherapy with infants and young children: repairing the effects of stress and trauma on early attachment. New York: Guilford Press; 2008.

68. McDonough SC. Promoting positive early parent-infant relationships through interaction guidance. Child Adolesc Psychiatr Clin N Am 1995;4:661–72.

69. Cohen NJ, Muir E, Lojkasek M, et al. Watch, wait, and wonder. Testing the effectiveness of a new approach to mother-infant psychotherapy. Infant Ment Health J 1999;20:429–51.

70. Eyberg SM, Robinson EA. Parent-child interaction training: effects on family functioning. J Clin Child Psychol 1982;11(2):130–7.

71. Schechter DS, Myers MM, Brunelli SA, et al. Traumatized mothers can change their minds about their toddlers: understanding how a novel use of video-feedback supports positive change of maternal attributions. Infant Ment Health J 2006;27(5):429–47.

72. Lieberman AF. Child-parent psychotherapy: a relationship-based approach to the treatment of mental health disorders in infancy and early childhood. In: Sameroff AJ, McDonough SC, Rosenblum KL, editors. Treating parent-infant relationship problems: strategies for intervention. New York: Guilford Press; 2004. p. 97–122.

73. Lieberman AF, Van Horn P. Child-parent psychotherapy: a developmental approach to mental health treatment in infancy and early childhood. In: Zeanah CH, editor. Handbook of infant mental health. 3rd edition. New York: Guildford Press; 2009. p. 439–49.

74. Lieberman AF, Weston D, Pawl JH. Preventive intervention and outcome with anxiously attached dyads. Child Dev 1991;62:199–209.

75. Cicchetti D, Rogosch FA, Toth SL. The efficacy of toddler-parent psychotherapy for fostering cognitive development in offspring of depressed mothers. J Abnorm Child Psychol 2000;28:135–48.

76. Cicchetti D, Toth SL, Rogosch FA. The efficacy of toddler-parent psychotherapy to increase attachment security in offspring of depressed mothers. Attach Hum Dev 1999;1:34–66.

77. Toth SL, Maughan A, Manly JT, et al. The relative efficacy of two interventions in altering maltreated preschool children's representations models: implications for attachment theory. Dev Psychopathol 2002;14:877–908.

78. Toth SL, Rogosch FA, Manly JT, et al. The efficacy of toddler-parent psychotherapy to reorganize attachment in the young offspring of mothers with major depressive disorder: a randomized preventive trial. J Consult Clin Psychol 2006;74:1006–16.

79. Lieberman AF, Van Horn P, Gosh Ippen C. Towards evidence-based treatment: child-parent psychotherapy with preschoolers exposed to marital violence. J Am Acad Child Adolesc Psychiatry 2005;44:1241–8.

80. Lieberman AF, Ghosh Ippen C, Van Horn P. Child-parent psychotherapy: six month follow-up of a randomized control trial. J Am Acad Child Adolesc Psychiatry 2006;45:913–8.

81. Fraiberg SH. Clinical studies in infant mental health: the first year of life. New York: Basic Books; 1980.

82. Lieberman AF, Silverman R, Pawl JH. Infant-parent psychotherapy: core concepts and current approaches. In: Zeanah CH, editor. Handbook of infant mental health. 2nd edition. New York: Guildford Press; 2000. p. 472–84.

83. Lieberman AF. Infant-parent psychotherapy with toddlers. Dev Psychopathol 1992;4:559–75.

84. Lieberman AF, Van Horn P. Don't hit my mommy: a manual for child-parent psychotherapy with young witnesses of family violence. Washington, DC: Zero to Three Press; 2005.

85. Fraiberg L, editor. Selected writings of Selma Fraiberg. Columbus (OH): Ohio State University Press; 1987.

86. Lieberman AF. Traumatic stress and quality of attachment: reality and internalization disorders of infant mental health. Infant Ment Health J 2004;25:336–51.

87. Lieberman AF, Padron E, Van Horn P, et al. Angels in the nursery: intergenerational transmission of beneficial parental influences. Infant Ment Health J 2005; 26(6):504–20.

88. Fonagy P, Gergely G, Jurist E, et al. Attachment and reflective function: their role in self-organization. In: Fonagy P, Gergely G, Jurist E, et al, editors. Affect regulation, mentalization, and the development of the self. New York: Other Press; 2002. p. 23–64.

89. Luborsky L. Principles of psychoanalytic psychotherapy: a manual for supportive-expressive treatment. New York: Basic Books; 1984.

90. Wallerstein R. Forty-two lives in treatment: a study of psychoanalysis and psychotherapy. New York: Guilford Press; 1986.

91. Lieberman AF. Negative maternal attributions: effects on toddlers' sense of self. Psychoanal Inq 1999;19(5):737–56.

92. Silverman RC, Lieberman AF. Negative maternal attributions, projective identification and the intergenerational transmission of violent relational patterns. Psychoanalytic Dialogues 1999;9:161–86.

93. Ogden T. Projective identification and psychotherapeutic technique. New York: Jason Aronson; 1982.

94. Lieberman AF, Compton NC, Van Horn P, et al. Losing a parent to death in the early years: guidelines for the treatment of traumatic bereavement in infancy and early childhood. Washington, DC: Zero to Three Press; 2003.

Family Intervention as a Developmental Psychodynamic Therapy

Allan M. Josephson, MD

KEYWORDS

• Psychodynamic • Family intervention/therapy • Development

KEY POINTS

- In this article, the term "family" refers to those who have regular interaction with its children and assume the responsibility of meeting their developmental and emotional needs. It implies biological, affective, and legal bonds occurring together or separately.
- This article integrates current findings and practices in developmental theory, family therapy and practice, and psychodynamic theory and practice.
- If a clinician is to understand the inner life of the child, the clinician must understand the family: good family therapy is good developmental psychodynamic therapy.
- The emerging field of developmental psychopathology is conducive to a developmental psychodynamic family therapy. It is a perspective that includes multiple levels of analysis, from the molecular to the cultural, and views mental disorders not as traits or states that reside within the child, but rather the result of a continual interplay between individual (developmental) and extraindividual (family) contexts.
- A case formulation that identifies the relationship between family functioning and the child's mental life naturally leads to an integration of therapies in many clinical interventions.

OVERVIEW

The term family therapy may have outlived its usefulness, in part, because for many it still conjures up the notion of all family members being present for each session. Recent literature has proposed a change of terms from family therapy to family intervention, reflecting the direction of several decades of clinical work.[1,2]

Family intervention is defined as a coordinated set of clinical practices that alters family interaction, family environment, and parental executive functioning and, in doing so, optimizes the development of all family members. The intervention is a collaborative effort with parents and child that maximizes family strengths (ie, protective factors) and minimizes family vulnerabilities (ie, family risk factors) associated with the onset and evolution of child and adolescent psychiatric disorders. These risk factors are

Division of Child and Adolescent Psychiatry, Bingham Clinic, School of Medicine, University of Louisville, 200 East Chestnut Street, Louisville, KY 40202, USA
E-mail address: allan.josephson@louisville.edu

Child Adolesc Psychiatric Clin N Am 22 (2013) 241–260
http://dx.doi.org/10.1016/j.chc.2012.12.006
1056-4993/13/$ – see front matter © 2013 Elsevier Inc. All rights reserved.

not only associated with disorders but also impede overall psychological development, and include a range of family interactions from neglect and rejection to overinvolvement and intrusiveness. In addition to interventions with patient and family, family interventions address the overall family context and external environment outside the consulting room (eg, resolving custody conflicts).

Most importantly, for the theme of this article, family intervention directly influences the developing mind by shaping and modifying a child's inner models through altering ongoing family interactions. There is a reciprocal relationship between life experience and the mental life of individuals: what goes on between individuals affects what goes on within individuals.

The revolutionary idea of the family as system as the sole theory guiding family work has now given way to a multiplicity of ways that clinicians work with families. Some of the terms used to encompass this trend include family intervention science, family treatment, family-based treatment, family-centered treatment, relational processes and disorders, family psychiatry, and family skills enhancement.[1] The term family intervention is more descriptive of current approaches in that the clinician does not solely use a specific school of therapy, but rather endeavors to involve the family in the treatment of each child. The clinician asks "how, and in what way, will I involve the family?" Formal family systems therapy is one specific, intensive type of intervention, but families can be involved in treatment in less direct ways.

This article focuses on the ways whereby family treatment uses developmental and psychodynamic concepts. It reviews how intrapsychic positions are generated and modified through family interaction, and discusses implications for family treatment. This presentation does not propose a new "school" of family treatment, but rather integrates current findings and practices in developmental theory, family therapy and practice, and psychodynamic theory and practice.

Family interventions share characteristics with other psychotherapeutic treatments. Individual therapy concepts, such as developing an alliance, working through conflicts, and dealing with resistance, are helpful in understanding effective family interventions. Family interventions also include behavioral elements, which are often powerfully influenced by psychodynamic factors in the family.

When intervening with families in contemporary psychiatry, a relevant question emerges: "what is a family?" This question, unheard of in a previous generation, often leads to vigorous discussion and, at times, debate among clinicians. In this article, the term family refers to those who have regular interaction with its children and assume the responsibility of meeting their developmental and emotional needs. It implies biological, affective, and legal bonds occurring together or separately. The term parent refers to the individuals who make decisions on the behalf of children. The terms child, and children, refer to any individual younger than 18 years, meaning the use of "child" always refers to child and adolescent. A full range of contemporary changes in family structure is the topic of numerous reviews, discussion of which is beyond the scope of this article.[3]

ANTECEDENT HISTORY

In the middle of the last century, emerging from the child guidance clinics of the early 1900s, the pioneers of family therapy began experimenting with interviewing families. These leaders identified that many individual treatments for children were unduly influenced by families who had difficulty adjusting to changes in their children associated with individual therapies and hospitalizations.[4] John Bowlby wrote in 1949: "I decided to confront the main actors with the problem as I saw it" in describing his decision to do family interviews. He found them so useful that they became routine for his work, although the primary emphasis remained with individual treatment.[5]

The revolutionary idea of the "family as a system" ushered in a dramatic era of change in thinking about the family. Arising from emerging systems thinking in biology,[6] the family system was seen as the unit of treatment. Various schools of family therapy evolved from this theoretical perspective, and the excitement engendered was not unlike that seen when psychoanalysis served as the progenitor of various schools of individual psychotherapies.

The systems concept held sway for a generation, leading to the current status of family intervention as a rapprochement and integration of individual and systemic approaches. This integration sees individual problems and family conflict as interrelated. Previous acrimony between the proponents of individual and family therapy has waned, if not disappeared.[7] As Malone has eloquently stated, "the internal and external are seen as inseparable and intrapsychic and interactional forces, and the interventions related to them, are viewed as interrelated and interdependent."[8] Some have argued that integration is a high standard and that there are few models of family treatment that fully integrate concepts.[9] More commonly, it seems many clinicians practice an eclecticism that pragmatically uses elements of various treatment approaches in a particular case.

From the perspective of child and adolescent psychiatry, development appears to be the strongest unifying, integrating principle in psychodynamic psychotherapy.[10–12] If this is true, it underscores the importance of the family as it is the first and most enduring context for development. If a clinician is to understand the inner life of the child, the clinician must understand the family, as it initiates, and maintains, individual psychodynamics. Consequently, good family therapy is good developmental psychodynamic therapy.

CONCEPTUAL ISSUES

Most clinical syndromes have intrapsychic and interactional components. A young girl with anorexia nervosa refuses to eat food for complex psychological reasons, often related to autonomy and sense of self. Yet this refusal also mobilizes family attempts to get her to eat. An adolescent who engages in self-cutting harm behavior is dealing with intense affects but also implicitly calls for response from others. The child who runs away from home does so for reasons of internal distress, but many times communicates a desire to be found. In a thorough formulation, these clinical syndromes must be conceptualized from the standpoint of the psychodynamic and the interactional, with interventions addressing both components.

This article attempts to integrate systemic and psychodynamic thinking underlying these two perspectives.

The emerging field of developmental psychopathology is conducive to a developmental psychodynamic family therapy. It is a perspective that includes multiple levels of analysis, from the molecular to the cultural. Mental disorders are not traits or states that reside within the child, but rather are the result of a continual interplay between individual (developmental) and extraindividual (family) contexts.[13–15] In this view, risk factors increase a child's chances of developing a psychiatric disorder, and protective factors (ie, resilience) minimize the impact of these risk factors. The perspective of developmental psychopathology goes beyond the disease model of general psychiatry and beyond the systems model toward enriching a developmental, family understanding of patients. Family developmental influences are seen in the internalization of the regulation of affect and behavior, mastery of developmental tasks, and social cognitive/narrative development (shaping the mind).[16] Numerous studies highlight the importance of parenting effectiveness and family stability in children's overall adaptation.[17,18]

The relationship between individual therapy and family therapy requires closer inspection. An evolving notion sees environmental family events as not merely psychosocial stressors, but as direct shaping influences on child and adolescent mental processes.

Clinical example of individual behavior shaped by family experience

Eric, a 10-year-old, fourth grade student, was brought for psychiatric evaluation. The referring request asked the clinician to "adjust the medications for his bipolar disorder." In gathering history, the psychiatrist heard that in art class earlier that day, Eric had picked up a Lego toy and threw it at his teacher. The block struck her on the head, leading to a laceration and the need for an evaluation of Eric's impulsive, aggressive outburst. The stimulus for his act was the teacher's inadvertently knocking Eric's ceramic tiger, which he had just created, off a table to the floor, shattering it. In explaining his behavior, Eric said "the teacher knocked my tiger onto the floor and broke it; she did it on purpose."

Eric perceived this accidental act as malevolent. His developmental history included several years of foster homes necessitated by abusive care given by his aggressive, single father. Teachers and peers saw Eric possessing of a tentative, fearful, mildly paranoid view of the world. Rather than the symptoms of a major mental illness with a need for pharmacologic adjustment, his behavior had meaning in an individual, developmental context, a meaning shaped by his family experience.

Over the last several decades, there has been a rich and evolving literature describing this link: how family interaction becomes part of the mind. Inner working models, described by Bowlby,[19–22] are shaped by family interaction and reflect experiences of attachment. Stern has described mental representations as "an amalgam of remembered history"[23(p9)] of family interaction, including how one interprets the events of family interaction. Historically, family therapy approaches that have attempted the integration of psychodynamic and developmental issues include object relations family therapy,[24–26] intergenerational family therapy,[27] and contextual family therapy.[28] On the other hand, individual theories, such as proposed by Kohut, elegantly describe the evolution of mental life related to the real-life experience with parents.[29,30] In 1991 Fonagy developed the concept of mentalization as the "capacity to conceive of conscious and unconscious mental states in oneself and others."[31(p641)] Grounded in notions of developmental psychopathology, the mind develops primarily from the "outside in…infants finding their mind in the mind of the caregiver."[32(p9)] In their discussion of how mentalizing relates to family therapy, Allen and colleagues[32] draw on the classic work of Fraiberg and colleagues,[33(p388)] who identified how the developing child's mind is burdened with the "oppressive past of his parents." Rutter has commented that "experiences have to undergo cognitive and affective processing so that what happens to individuals influences their mental concepts and models of themselves and their environments."[34(p5)] Vygotsky summarizes how the external becomes internal in this way: "An interpersonal process is transformed into an intrapersonal one. Every function in the child's cultural development appears twice: first on the social level, and later on the individual level; first between people (interpsychological), and then inside the child (intrapsychological)."[35(p57)]

In this article, the intrapsychological is indicated by the interchangeable terms of internal working models, inner models, mental representations, inner world, and mind. Some of the diverse clinical and research literature that identifies how family interaction shapes the child's inner world and becomes part of the self is summarized in **Table 1**.

The developmental psychodynamic approach to family work informs how family processes and interactions regulate a child's development and the child's mastery of developmental tasks, and shapes the child's mind.[36,37] This shaping of the mind is a template for the child's further interactions. In effect the traumatized child believes "I am in the kind of world where I will be hurt" and the indulged child believes "I am in the kind of world where I am special and will be adored by others." These cognitive representations trigger intrapsychic conflict and affect when real-life experience is not congruent with them. The reciprocal relationship between family interaction and the development of a child's inner world provides a rational basis for an integration of individual and family therapy.[8]

The following describes a sequential unfolding of the family developmental psychodynamic process, and is summarized in **Box 1**. The parent brings his or her inner working models to the marriage/relationship. These models are shaped by experiences of the past and strongly influence partner choice. This choice of marital partner leads to the formation of family through the birth of children and determines how the couple begins to parent. In many ways, children and the developmental stages through which they progress are nature's projective device. The behaviors that unfold in development elicit responses from parents deeply influenced by their own family of origin experiences and their own inner world. For example, a dependent woman often chooses a controlling man, and in their evolution as parents the mother runs the risk of being overly responsive in acquiescing to children's demands while the father runs the risk of being harsh and unempathic, not perceiving children's needs. In health, individual differences enrich the parental partnership, whereas in psychopathology, these differences interact in counterproductive ways.

Subsequent family interactions begin to shape the child's inner world and subsequent behavior.

Table 1
Family life experience and mental life

Type of Therapy	Mental Life	References
Cognitive therapy	Dysfunctional cognitions have developmental origins	63
Infant psychiatry/psychology	Infants develop mental representations from caregiver interactions (social referencing)	19–21,64–67
Family therapy	Family members form mental representations of family relationships	68
Child development research	Cognitive perspectives (eg, low self-worth) are generated by nature of relationships with parents	69,70
Psychoanalysis	Intrapsychic conflict has relational origins	24–26,29,30
Child psychiatry	Social experience becomes phenotype/part of the organism	71,72
Developmental psychopathology	Reciprocal effects of genes and environment	38,73,74

Data from Josephson A. Reinventing family therapy: teaching family intervention as a new treatment modality. Acad Psychiatry 2008;32:405–13.

> **Box 1**
> **The evolution of family psychodynamic development**
>
> - The parent brings own inner models to the marriage/relationship.
> - These models are shaped from past experience.
> - These models influence choice of partner.
> - Parenting is influenced by these inner models.
> - Family interactional experience, guided by parents, shapes the inner models of children.
> - Children become adults and use these models, modified through relationship experiences, as templates for their parenting.

With a mother who is overly solicitous, the child begins to see the world as a place "where my demands will be immediately met," and a subtle entitlement ensues. A harsh, emotionally unavailable father begins to elicit a mildly paranoid response, in which "others are there to hurt me, and nothing good will happen when I get close to others." These parental interactions begin to shape the internalized object relations of the children, affect their behaviors, and need to be addressed in clinical treatment. In sum, psychodynamic, developmental, and systemic principles all influence the psychodynamic position of the child.

The case of Karen (**Box 2**) illustrates how these factors are interrelated in treatment of a patient with anorexia nervosa.

PREPARING FOR FAMILY INTERVENTION

The diagnostic case formulation process must drive the psychodynamically informed family intervention. Before conducting therapy, the child and adolescent psychiatrist must assess how families protect, pose risk, and shape the mind. Family interactions profoundly influence the development of attachment, internalized object relations, individual identity, and the regulation of impulses. **Table 2** summarizes the elements of a comprehensive psychiatric formulation that facilitates individual and family work.

Because families are always influential in the clinical encounter, family intervention is not one choice of a modality among many options that the clinician chooses to use or not, but a key to managing all cases. Psychodynamically oriented clinicians find their work dramatically enhanced by observing family processes and appreciating the impact they have on a child's mind. Family events are not merely psychosocial stressors, but are directed by the parents' inner worlds and shape the child's inner world.

In developing family treatment plans, anything impeding the child's development or shaping a deviant inner world is a target for intervention. Family treatment is a developmental psychodynamic therapy that educates parents in behavior-management techniques, alters interactional patterns through formal family intervention therapy, and addresses distortions of the child's inner world. Any 3 of these areas may be impeding emotional development, and they often act in concert.

It should be noted that this article's focus on developmental psychodynamics should not be construed as dismissing the importance of biology. Rutter's work is perhaps the best example of a thoughtful consideration of how genes affect the trajectory of development, and how experience shapes cognitive processes and may influence brain development.[38]

Determining whether the family problems are in need of support and education, or exploration and an expectation of change is a crucial part of the formulation. The disease model of much of contemporary psychiatry typically emphasizes

Box 2
Clinical example of family interactions shaping child behavior

Karen (K.J.), a 14-year-old with anorexia nervosa, lived with her mother, stepfather, and 12-year-old brother. Her mother had previously been married and had 2 daughters, aged 16 and 18, from that marriage. Karen entered outpatient therapy after a 10-day hospitalization had stabilized her weight, gaining back 10 pounds of a 20-pound weight loss. An outpatient course of family therapy was recommended.

As therapy began, it was clear that Karen's mother, Mrs. J., was behaviorally and emotionally overinvolved with her daughter. She frequently observed Karen's eating and exercising, and described their relationship as "being best friends." Mrs. J. stated that "I will often find myself holding her hand when we're walking in the mall. I know this is something I shouldn't do at her age, but I can't help myself." As the pattern of mother and daughter closeness emerged, Karen commented, "I just want to be there for my mother…she needs me." Karen's father was gone frequently in relation to business concerns, and did not attend to her mother's emotional needs when he was physically present. Karen appeared to try to compensate for her mother's loneliness.

Mrs. J.'s closeness with Karen helped "make up for all the problems I had with the other two girls," who were conduct-disordered, substance-abusing youth. Family therapy efforts addressed family structure by getting father and mother to communicate more, have Karen be more independent for eating choices, as well as other choices, and have father more involved with son Jared, who appeared mildly depressed. After several family therapy sessions, the mother requested to be seen alone.

In individual session, mother poignantly described her growing awareness of an intense, life-long emotional dependence on Karen. She revealed an awareness of its current developmental inappropriateness as she described her lonely marriage and her compensation for that by finding Karen "always there for me." In a remarkable statement, the mother related that Karen had been important to her "from the moment I conceived her." She stated "Karen was the baby I wanted more than anything else in the world," and continued that her devotion to her daughter outweighed any other feeling for others, including her son and her husband. Mother revealed her own troubled background in which she had a distant relationship with her single mother, and had found out belatedly that she had been adopted. Though innately intelligent, she was not encouraged toward further academic pursuits. Her father had been absent from her life. She described a premature marriage to a man to whom she was ill suited.

In individual therapy, Karen revealed a dependency and helplessness in relationships with others. She appeared interpersonally ineffective with her friends, and wanted them to initiate relationships, as her mother had with her. She appeared perplexed when they, from her perspective, avoided her, and she began to develop a mild suspiciousness toward them. "They're trying to hurt me; they made it difficult when I returned to school from the hospital." It appeared she expected the same special relationship that she had with her mother. This appeared to be based on an internal working model of relationships in which Karen was the center of others' affections.

Individual work with Karen further revealed her to be entitled and passive. Clinical efforts were directed to help her understand her passivity and her overly close relationship with her mother. As mother was directed toward seeking emotional support from her husband, this intervention revealed a fault in the marriage, years in the making. Mrs. J had always paid the bills, but had conveniently "forgot" to pay the regular monthly car payment. Father was shocked when a bank manager came to their home to state that the car was being repossessed. He was enraged at his wife's lack of forthcoming regarding the budget, and a serious marital crisis lead to a course of couple's therapy.

In therapy, the couple began to look at the roots of their poor communication, father's controlling behavior, and mother's passive/aggressive hostility toward him. The parents began to see how their behavior and emotional needs had set in motion several family interactions. They came to see that not only was Karen in need, but their son Jared was silently suffering from depression-related feelings of inadequacy, as much attention had been focused on Karen. Jared had few friends and was failing in school.

> Family developmental psychodynamic principles evolved from mother's dysthymia and lack of self-confidence. Her emotional overinvestment in the life of her child was related to these individual factors and in part related to the lack of relationship she had with her husband. This overinvestment was crucial in shaping Karen's belief that others thought about her, and were as concerned about her, as much as her mother. This inner model was a direct result of family interaction, and was addressed by interrupting the family interactions that gave rise to it, and then working with Karen individually to address the psychological derivatives of this family interaction.

psychoeducation. These principles include assisting the family in recognizing onset of illness, understanding relapse, describing the effects and side effects of medications, and supporting family strengths as it deals with significant mental illness. Of course, this is an approach that should not be used in family situations whereby the family must be challenged and expected to change how members relate to one another and improve parenting practices.

The first approach, recognizing the strength of the family, educates and empathically supports the family. The second approach, identifying areas of problem, explores issues and empathically challenges a family.

There are specific areas of inquiry that can help the clinician decide when to explore family problems and expect change, and when to educate the family and offer support (**Box 3**).[39]

The data on which to base a formulation include an assessment of family structure, communication patterns, and family regulation of the child's affect and behavior, individual parent functioning, marital functioning, and the stages of family life cycle. These data must be gathered through history taking and observation of family interaction.[39,40]

Family structure refers to hierarchy and power relationships and the invisible boundaries within families. Family communication refers to the clarity and directness of communication and whether the content of communication is congruent with accompanying affect. Family regulation[41] connotes how the family regulates development and behavior.[37] This regulation, performed externally by the family, ultimately becomes an internal regulatory process within the child and is a crucial developmental achievement.[16] The difference in the assessment of individual parents, marital functioning, and family life-cycle history when conducted as part of the evaluation of a child's disorder is that the gathered data are always directed toward treating the child's problems. **Box 4** offers areas of inquiry helpful in a child-focused assessment.[39]

INDICATIONS FOR FAMILY TREATMENT

Although families should be involved with all psychiatric treatments, there are specific indications for a focused family intervention.

1. The clinical presentation is an interactional problem. Problems such as physical and sexual abuse, aggression directed toward a parent, a child running away from home, eating disorder, or separation anxiety all present as interactional problems. Given that almost any childhood behavior problem is interactional and disruptive behavior is the most common problem faced by child psychiatrists, the indications for family interventions are frequent.
2. Parental psychopathology precludes effective parenting. Many times parenting strategies are not effective owing to the problems of parents, including disorders such as substance abuse, aggressive behavior, or personality psychopathology.

Table 2
Toward developing an interactive psychodynamic formulation

Current Picture of Individual Characteristics of the Child

Biological (capacities)	1. General health status
	2. Medical disorder
	3. Temperament (style)
	4. Genetic vulnerability
	5. Perceptual motor disorder
	6. Intelligence
	7. Information processing (eg, attentional process, peripheral sensory, neuropsychological)
	8. Uneven development (eg, precocious sexuality, delayed speech)
Psychological (motivations)	1. Mastery of age-related psychosocial tasks
	a. Trust, quality of attachment
	b. Autonomy, separation from others
	c. Peers, differentiation of relationships, conscience formation, empathy toward others
	d. Achievement, sense of competence, self-esteem formation
	e. Identity, sexual competence
	2. What current mental structures (perceptions, mental representations) are associated with problems in development?
	3. What family interactional experiences have predisposed the child to:
	a. The mastery of developmental tasks or impeded such mastery
	b. Develop adaptive mental structures or maladaptive mental structures
	4. Have family factors perpetuated problems or strengths?
	5. Have family factors influenced defensive behaviors or coping abilities? (eg, regulatory capacities)
	6. Are there specific parent-related dynamics (eg, superego lacunae, self-pathology) affecting the child's development?

Environmental Stressors

Social (environmental demands and expectations)	1. Family factors (acute): divorce, custody battle, family geographic moves, unemployment, and poverty
	2. Interpersonal: peer difficulties
	3. Educational: demands outstripping ability
	4. Developmental: new expectations, traumatic experiences
	5. Cultural disruption (acute): war, environmental disaster
	6. Cultural expectation (chronic): pressure to conform behavior to societal norms

This table offers a summary of factors relevant to most clinical presentations in child and adolescent psychiatry. The template is structured to illustrate characteristics of the child (1) in interaction with environmental stressors (2). The following definition serves as the construct for the interactive template. "Goodness of fit results when the properties of the *environment* and its expectations and demands are in accord with the organism's own *capacities, motivations,* and *style* of behaving."

Data from Thomas A, Chess S. The dynamics of psychological development. New York: Brunner Mazel; 1980. *From* Josephson A. Reinventing family therapy: teaching family intervention as a new treatment modality. Acad Psychiatry 2008;32:405–13; with permission.

Box 3
Determining the approach to the family

Is the family contributing to the problem, requiring an expectation of change; or is it responding to a problem, requiring education and support? Exploring the following areas will help answer the question and suggest a clinical approach to the family:

- Family understanding of developmental norms
- Influence of parental psychiatric disorder
- Quality of parental commitment to the child
- Parental achievement apart from child rearing
- The developmental task mastery of other family members
- Assessment of heritability of the child's disorder
- Level of parents' mutual support of each other
- Relationship of the child's behavior to environmental change

Box 4
Guide to clinical interview

Individual Parent History

- History of developmental years
- Seminal events (eg, sexual abuse)
- Persistent chronic exposure to difficult events
- Presence of a mental disorder and effect on parenting
- Personality strengths/weaknesses/disorders
- Parents' level of insight
- Difficulty with a specific developmental stage (eg, autonomy)

Couple Relationship History

- What attracted them to each other
- Chronologic history of the relationship
- Early relationship expectations
- Effects of previous marriages and children on current relationship
- Legal status of parents' relationship
- Current areas of satisfaction/dissatisfaction: vocation, sexual, financial, parenting

Family as a Unit

- Management of various developmental stages
- Unanticipated/unique challenges (eg, job loss; illness)
- Socioeconomic status
- Religious/spiritual/cultural perspectives
- Seminal events (eg, family moves)
- Relationship to larger community
- Current challenges

A family focus is indicated when there is a mismatch between parental personality style and child temperament.

3. Psychiatric disorders with identified family contributions. Research in developmental psychopathology and family treatment outcome studies demonstrate that there are family concomitants of many disorders which are becoming more clearly becoming defined.[42]

4. Psychiatric disorders requiring psychoeducation. It is recognized that disorders such as major depression, schizophrenia, and attention-deficit disorder have strong biological loadings. Education about the disorders and guiding the family's response to its family member is an important intervention. Even though family processes are not seen as directly etiologically important in some of these illnesses, relapses have been documented to occur in the absence of family intervention.[43]

MAKING THE INTERVENTION: HOW FAMILY THERAPY WORKS

In each clinical case, the issue is not should one intervene with families, but how to do so, when to do so, how to sequence the intervention with other disorders, and which intervention for which disorder. Interventions with families range from brief history-gathering episodes and parent education to extensive intensive individual and family explorations. It is important that clinicians formulate a case accurately because this is the foundation for all treatment.

In developing the formulation, the clinician asks "what is impeding the child's development and what is shaping the child's inner world in a problematic way?", then the addresses these factors. For example, the research literature recently demonstrated that treating maternal depression can lead to remission of a child's psychopathology.[44] In such a case, to help the child one needs to treat the parental depression. This precept is true with any problematic family behavior, such as overprotectiveness or lack of attachment, or individual problem, such as learning disorder.

While meeting with the entire family remains a key component of working with families, the following is a typical sequence of a family therapy that explores problems and maps out the potential for family change through several types of interventions. This section describes the clinical process of making family interventions, with specific attention to the sequencing and coordinating of the interventions. This model may be overwhelming for the beginner but reflects the reality of how family work best unfolds. Stern has summarized this model for working with infants and very young children, but it applies equally to adolescents:

> Regardless of the therapist's persuasion, the therapy is simultaneously an individual psychotherapy (with the primary caregiver), a couples therapy (with the husband and wife), and a family therapy (with the triad), either all at the same time or in sequence.[23(p16)]

Each of these phases does not occur in every treatment, nor do they necessarily occur in the sequence listed, but in more complex, intensive treatments all may be required.[45] The interventions described may be provided by one, or several, therapists. The following sequences target points of intervention along this continuum. The overriding principle of this sequence is that family experience becomes internalized, thus determining how parents parent and how children come to view the world.

Stabilize a Crisis and Address Immediate Needs

Most families come to the clinic wanting to leave with something that can be done for their child. The presenting problem can require urgent attention. Crises may involve environmental interventions, such as removing a child from the home, most commonly by hospitalization. Although not always indicated, pharmacotherapy is increasingly offered as an immediate intervention by many clinicians, fueled by the expectations of contemporary parents.[46] In all nonemergent initial contacts, parents need their anxieties addressed by a treatment plan: a clear description of the nature of the child's problem, what can be done about it, and the family's role in the process.

Parent Management Training

This intervention, supported by a growing outcome literature,[47,48] is not traditionally seen as family therapy. Yet parents are the "executives" of the family, and change must start with them. Many parents, through lack of experience or their own emotional issues, do not know the fundamentals of child development. Furthermore, they often need to be informed of factors related to the onset of disorder, the course of disorder, and what the family needs to do to effectively manage it. This parent education phase is important in disorders with significant biological aspects, such as disorders of attention and learning.

Given the commonality of disruptive behavior problems, parents need a working knowledge of behavior management principles. In milder problems, education and parent management are often all that are necessary. In cases of more serious psychopathology, parental vulnerabilities often preclude the effective implementation of behavior management strategies. For example, a mother's depression and dependency often make limit setting difficult, or a father's anger and aggression may undo the effective limit-setting efforts of the mother. When such events are observed, it can lead to a broadening of therapy. The clinician formulates what needs to change in the family, and empathically holds the family accountable to change while appreciating its difficulty. A next step should be seeing the family together.

Intervention in Family Process

This intervention most closely resembles traditional family therapy. All family members living in the household are invited to attend, and the clinician guides the family in altering problematic interactions between family members. Common interventions include: shoring up parental support of each other when a child is disrespectful to one parent; encouraging parents' authoritative, deliberate limit setting in lieu of a friendly, deferential response; identifying how one parent may undermine the other in limit-setting efforts and facilitating an engagement with a child when there may be evidence of a parent being unempathic to a child's distress. Empathically intervening in various family processes can significantly affect family functioning.

For a generation, family systems therapy emphasized various techniques and described such techniques in a voluminous literature.[49–51] Interventions using techniques such as reframing problems and circular questioning can be particularly useful in uncovering the dynamics of interpersonal and intrapsychic dynamics of specific family members.[52] Often, however, these types of interventions are met with resistance. Systems theory suggests that family homeostasis is the desired state, yet careful study of the individuals in the family often reveals they have their own reasons for resisting change.[53] For example, in setting a limit on a child and experiencing the child's natural resistance, the parent may experience fears of being abandoned by the child. Understanding such fears may require an individual intervention with a parent. When altering family interaction is successful (eg, parents are more effective in setting limits or more engaged with their child), the internalized world of the child shaped by previous dysfunctional interactions may require individual intervention.

Individual Intervention

Change in family interaction is resisted owing to the inner world of parents, which would have to be altered if family interactions were to change. By keeping the parent's internal working models constant, family interactions perform a defensive, protective function for the parent. As in Karen's case, in letting a child move toward independence a parent may experience a previously masked insecurity and a subsequent depressive response. Parental psychopathology may be impeding a child's development to the extent that it needs to be treated in order for the child to stabilize. Enhancing parental self-esteem, coupled with altering family relationships and parent education, is an example of a coordinated intervention. It is always important for the child clinician to remember when intervening with a parent how this work is related to the needs of the identified child patient.

When family interaction work is successful, what remains is a child whose inner world has been shaped as a result of pathologic interactions. A child who has been persistently indulged likely will have a sense of entitlement, and this is where family intervention as developmental psychodynamic therapy has its greatest power. A child's inner world stems from family interactions, but as development unfolds the child has a life independent from those interactions. The family interactions require an intervention with the family, and the inner world requires a specific intervention with the child's intrapsychic dynamics.

Marital/Couple Interventions

Given that the parents' decisions set the stage for many family interactions, this intervention flows from family interventions that are resisted or ineffective. Driven by their internal working models, parents may unwittingly continue to facilitate dysfunctional interactions between themselves, powerfully affecting their children. One parent may have a helpful parenting perspective, but may be undermined by the other, only to have these roles shift in another context. Working on communication styles and parenting can be a prelude for couples to be seen alone to explore their individual perspectives on parenting and identify individual parental vulnerabilities.

Dealing with Siblings

It is not uncommon for family work, initially focused on an identified patient, to indicate that there is another child needing intervention. This child is subjected to the same family dynamics, but may have responded differently because of individual variables (eg, biological differences in attention and learning, birth order, gender, stepsibling status). In addition to gaining attention to their own needs, siblings can often provide a unique perspective of the problems of their sibling, helping parents see things in a different light. Siblings may not be actively involved in regular sessions; however, an initial assessment and other intermittent contacts can flesh out the clinician's understanding of the family.

In sum, the order of these interventions is flexible, and they may not all be needed in each situation. In certain situations, one therapist can sequentially provide all therapies; in others multiple therapists will need to be involved, for pragmatic if not theoretical reasons. The issue of the number of therapists and their relationship with each other remains one of some contention, but perhaps less so than in a previous generation. The reader is referred elsewhere for a more complete discussion.[54,55]

The following case of Blaine (**Box 5**) demonstrates flexible sequencing of interventions from early stabilization and parent management training to family systems, couple, and individual work: the continuum of developmental dynamic family therapy.

Box 5
Clinical example of continuum of developmental dynamic family therapy

Blaine was a 10-year 10-month–old fifth grade student seen for a second psychiatric opinion. At the time of psychiatric consultation, the parents (Michael and Janet) saw Blaine as not being able to control his behavior; his mother believed he was "suffering." He was of average intelligence and had not failed any classes. He and his sister Laura, 2 years younger, were biracial children adopted at the time of birth by Caucasian parents. The adoptive parents had been married for 32 years; mother was 53 years old, and father was 55 years old. Blaine had been in treatment for more than 1 year with little progress, and his parents were frustrated, as well as fearful, about the effects of his "bipolar disorder." Treatment consisted solely of psychopharmacology, with little therapeutic effect, and one major side effect, a 25-pound weight gain.

Blaine's primary symptoms were moodiness, fears, and rages "when he doesn't get his way." When angry he would slam doors, curse, and yell for periods of time, as long as 1 hour in duration. Managing his rages, related to homework expectations, was difficult and emotionally draining for the parents, as it would often take 3 hours to get the homework done. On one occasion, Blaine grabbed his mother by her neck in a conflict regarding lack of homework completion. He couldn't finish assignments unless his mother was there, and even then he would neglect her requests. In exasperation, she then would ask his father to help, who would encourage, cajole, and then, in anger, challenge Blaine to get his homework done. When pushed in this way, Blaine would often threaten to kill himself. He stated "I don't want to do my schoolwork....Mr T. (his teacher) makes me write 5 pages of homework, and it stresses me out." During the homework sessions, Blaine would frequently verbally assault his mother, calling her stupid, ugly, crazy, and a liar, including vulgar epithets.

Therapy began with attempts to help parents stabilize Blaine's current behavior. This meant ensuring Blaine's safety, and that of his parents, by doing careful interviews to assess the veracity and credibility of his verbal threats to kill himself and his parents. The parents were given instruction on how to find emergency care, although they never needed to use such care. The first course of therapy emphasized parent management techniques to facilitate homework completion. The parents were encouraged in their firmness, and a positive reward system was implemented to facilitate task completion. This intervention was modestly successful, but was met with resistance. Predictably, Blaine's resistance was active while his parents' resistance was passive. They stated: "He doesn't handle well what he doesn't want to do. He is the master of delay. He's always been this way since 8 years of age." The latter comment was said with hopeless resignation at the time of consultation. The family noted that he "explodes under pressure, saying things like 'I can't go on like this; I want to die; I'm too tired to do the work'." Mother said "it is breaking my heart to see him like that." Father noted that "Blaine does a lot better when not a lot is demanded of him."

The success of behavioral interventions was limited because of Blaine's distress when parents put pressure on him to complete the most basic developmental tasks (eg, taking a shower). In such instances, he made verbal threats: "How do you think you will like it, when the house is burned down? Or when you are not around?" His younger sister began to act out, as she observed Blaine's behavior. The pleasant couple wanted Blaine to complete homework uneventfully and when his distress mounted, it immobilized them. The behavioral management was difficult to implement because of family psychodynamic factors, which required a family intervention alongside a couple intervention.

In couple work, it was revealed that mother had always wanted children, but father had not. They had been married 22 years before they finally adopted. When the children were younger, Michael adored the children. Yet as they grew older he withdrew from active family life, spending much of his time on the computer, leaving most of the parenting tasks to his wife. Father wanted to be Blaine's friend, making discipline next to impossible. He appeared influenced by his own developmental history of "little discipline, lots of play, and no schedule." The therapy emphasized the need for Michael to support his wife more, and to expect his wife to be less active as the primary limit setter.

One critical incident occurred in family therapy. Blaine physically confronted his parents after they limited his activities with an electronic game. In that session, Blaine's mother tearfully pleaded for help from her husband. As if to take on her father's role, Blaine's younger sister crossed the room and hugged her crying mother. Father verbalized that his son didn't seem to get the concept of limits and wondered why Blaine expressed no concern toward his mother. As therapy progressed and mother continued to insist that she needed support, her husband Michael became mobilized and was more supportive of her. In the couple work, Janet stated "Mike doesn't want to deal with confrontation and the stress that inevitably results from it." Mother saw that "ninety per cent of Blaine's anger has to do with stopping something that is fun, and doing something that he doesn't want to do." The therapist attempted to assist Mike in seeing the normalcy of such behavior.

As family therapy progressed, and the couple began to be more intentional in working together, and effectively addressed Laura's developing noncompliance. Yet Blaine continued to be angry and curse at his mother with provocative statements: "I hate you, I hope you rot in hell, I'll never be your son, because you're an *&$%# idiot."

In couples work, the parents grappled with the issue of diagnosis. The term "bipolar" scared them, because of its immutable, lifelong biological implications and their fears of suicide as a complication. Psychoeducation helped explain what medications can and cannot do. In this work, father stated that "the diagnosis of bipolar changed how we viewed the problem. We believed he couldn't control it. It was chemical." Blaine himself stated that he was no longer responsible for the way he acted. Mother stated "We took the view that we needed to help him control things by finding the right medicine." They acknowledged that the change in therapeutic approach was helpful to them. They told the therapist that "you listened to us more, and you gave us hope. Particularly, you made us stop and look at the real parenting differences between us, and how they were related to Blaine's behavior problem. This made us conscious of things that we were not aware of before and we knew we needed to change. You got us moving in the right direction."

In couples work, mother was able to ventilate, stating "I'm the more parenting person. Mike is the fun parent. This made me angry, because it left me as the only person to get things done." The therapist pursued the goal of getting mother less involved, and father more involved, using improved couple communication. Janet said, "Mike doesn't like the imposition of a schedule," and the therapist was able to point out that children need schedules. Janet pointed out that "Mike doesn't deal with conflict," while the therapist pointed out that active parenting naturally involves conflict and demands solving it.

In individual work, Mike was able to see the influence of his own background "My father wasn't around when I was growing up, and I vowed that I was going to be around more. I wasn't going to make the same mistake. I think his absence affected me. I now wish I'd been closer to my father; I might have learned more." The therapist pointed out that "you corrected but you overcorrected." Mike agreed, noting that "I have wanted to be a friend to my son, and not a parent.... I see it now again in my relationship with Laura. She is trying to control me by getting to my soft spot."

The therapist challenged Michael; with the question, "When children threaten to harm a kind, caring mother, what does this mean?" He responded: "It means the child is too comfortable with not enough limits." Chagrined, Michael came to see how he had enabled his son's tyrannical, verbally abusive behavior toward his mother. He came to understand that his joking approach led Blaine to believe most of his behavioral indiscretions "weren't that big a deal." He also came to see that a medical model, that his son's behavior was a "chemical problem," can lead to pursuing medication changes at the cost of not expecting enough from his son and himself. Unwittingly, Mike came to see that a sole focus on medication minimizes hope in the change process and devalues what families can do to change.

Finally, family work emphasized Blaine's younger sibling and her developing behavior disorder. The parent's identified Laura's noncompliance and challenging of parents to be similar to Blaine's behavior but felt reassured that with their new self-knowledge of their family's, and their own, dynamics they would have solutions to her behavioral challenges.

Individual work with Blaine was beginning to show potential after 2 years, coincident with his advancing age. Earlier in treatment, he was focused on blaming parents for his predicament, his entitlement fueled by his father's indulgence. With Blaine's self-reflection starting with statements such as his wondering, "Why don't I have friends?," the therapist began to plan for individual psychotherapeutic work with Blaine.

Managing the Process

Therapeutic progress with a family may not occur for several reasons: minimal father involvement; a poorly defined role for siblings; inaccurate case formulation; poor communication with an influential biological parent not living with the child; and clinician countertransference issues. There are few contraindications to family interventions apart from those that may facilitate, or escalate, the potential for violence, and those related to boundary violations, such as including family members who have no legal or interpersonal relationship with the child.

Ethical Issues and Confidentiality

For many clinicians, seeing a family raises ethical problems. The simplest of questions focuses the main challenge: "Who is the patient?" Although therapy is initially planned for the identified patient, as family interventions proceed the concerns and problems of other members may become a focus for treatment. When the clinician empathically explores one family member's perspective, he or she may be seen as alienating the patient or another family member. Healthier families understand this apparent unfairness as part of the process of therapy. Families who are influenced by psychopathology are less likely to understand this type of intervention. In such cases the clinician makes a deliberate attempt to relate to all family members, and make the point that in time each person's perspective will be heard. With integrated treatment becoming more common, these concerns may be less prominent than in the past.[55]

Dealing with resistance and difficult families mobilizes special types of countertransference. All clinicians have their own family experiences, and they must guard against their personal situations intruding on the therapeutic process.

RESEARCH

Over the last several decades, there has been a growing literature on evidence-based treatments for child and adolescent psychiatric disorders, increasingly demonstrating the effectiveness of family treatments.[56] Manualized, structured approaches to family treatment have been helpful across disorders, as well as for specific disorders.

Family intervention studies have developed during the past decade, with greater use of randomized controlled trials. Problems and challenges in this research remain, and include: attending to culturally informed family processes; limited attention to comorbid psychiatric disorders; limited long-term follow-up protocols; limited replication of study findings related to different treatment approaches; studies not considering mechanisms of change; and limited attention given to disorders as they occur in real-world settings.

The clinical relevance of studies focusing on a sole diagnostic grouping remains unclear, because day-to-day clinical practice frequently involves complex disorders in youth with more than one condition. Research addressing common processes that cut across disorders may be more applicable to day-to-day practice. Such common therapeutic factors in effective family therapy include: building parenting competence and sustaining hope; motivated families; collaborative goal setting; an empathic treatment alliance; trust in the therapist's acumen; and recognition that therapeutic change is occurring.[57] Furthermore, family treatments are increasingly integrated and, as such, many studies involve more than one approach, such as cognitive behavioral family therapy.

The disorders for which there is significant support for the efficacy of family treatments include conduct disorders, substance abuse, eating disorders, separation anxiety, and psychosomatic disorders.[42,56,58] Even if there is not a specific study to indicate the efficacy of a family intervention, the case can be made that when family intervention facilitates child development, it is a rational course to pursue.

SPECIAL SITUATIONS

There are elements of clinical work that may not typically be seen as a family intervention or developmental psychodynamic family therapy but are crucial in developing family stability. These aspects include: helping parents negotiate community support systems, such as in-home care for developmentally disabled children; supporting parents' efforts in procuring appropriate educational services; and communicating with the legal system.[59]

Aspects of race, culture, gender, sexual orientation, and worldview are important in all families.[60,61] These aspects require specific understanding and often exploration. As the influence of the traditional family wanes, how patients develop their idea of family is influenced by these various factors. Special problems such as divorce, custody, legal issues, and violence are increasingly prominent in contemporary society.[62] These issues and others can complicate any family intervention with a developmental psychodynamic focus.

Finally, many clinicians find that monitoring the long-term course of a child's development typically occurs with more difficult disorders. When the therapist is consistently available to the family, he often discerns another child with clinical needs, and the family becomes and enduring "patient." There are often early, middle, and late phases in the treatment of one child, but treatment can extend when the alliance with the clinician is effective. In these instances, the clinician has the benefit of understanding even more clearly the developmental, family relationships that have shaped the mind.

SUMMARY

Family intervention directly influences the developing mind by shaping and modifying a child's internal working models through altering ongoing family interactions. There is a reciprocal relationship between life experience and the mental life of individuals: what goes on between individuals affects what goes on within individuals. If a clinician is going to understand the inner life of the child, the clinician must understand the family, as it initiates, and maintains, individual psychodynamics. Consequently, good family therapy is good developmental psychodynamic therapy.

REFERENCES

1. Josephson A. Reinventing family therapy: teaching family intervention as a new treatment modality. Acad Psychiatry 2008;32:405–13.
2. Sargent J. Family interventions. In: Shaw R, DeMaso D, editors. Textbook of psychiatric psychosomatic medicine. Washington, DC: APPI; 2010. p. 439–48.
3. Sargent J. Variations in family composition: implications for family therapy. Child Adolesc Psychiatr Clin N Am 2001;10:577–99.
4. Broderick C, Schrader S. The history of professional marriage and family therapy. In: Gurman A, Kniskern D, editors. Handbook of family therapy. New York: Brunner/Mazel; 1991.
5. Bowlby J. The study and reduction of group tension in the family. Hum Relat 1949;2:123–8.
6. Von Bertalanffy L. General system theory: foundations, development, applications. New York: George Braziller; 1968.

7. McDermott J, Char W. The undeclared war between child and family therapy. J Am Acad Child Adolesc Psychiatry 1974;13:422–36.
8. Malone C. Child and adolescent psychiatry and family therapy: an overview. Child Adolesc Psychiatr Clin N Am 2001;10:395–413.
9. Lebow J. Clinical theory and practice integrative family therapy: the integrative revolution in couple and family therapy. Fam Process 1997;36:1–17.
10. Munir K, Beardslee W. Developmental psychiatry: is there any other kind? Harv Rev Psychiatry 1999;6(5):250–62.
11. Wachtel E, Wachtel P. Family dynamics in individual psychotherapy: a guide to clinical strategies. New York: Guilford; 1986.
12. Eisenberg L. Development as a unifying concept in psychiatry. Br J Psychiatry 1977;131:225–37.
13. Cicchetti D, Cohen D, editors. Developmental psychopathology: risk, disorder, and adaptation, vol. 3. New York: Wiley & Sons, Inc; 2006.
14. Kim-Cohen J. Resilience and developmental psychopathology. Child Adolesc Psychiatr Clin N Am 2007;16:271–83.
15. Carrey N, Ungar M, editors. Resilience. Child Adolesc Psychiatr Clin N Am 2007;16:2.
16. Committee on integrating the science of early childhood development. Acquiring self-regulation. In: Shonkoff J, Phillips D, editors. From neurons to neighborhoods: the science of early childhood development. 2nd edition. Washington, DC: National Academy Press; 2001. p. 93–123.
17. Luthar S. Resilience in development: a synthesis of research across five decades. In: Cicchetti D, Cohen D, editors. Developmental psychopathology. 2nd edition. Hoboken (NJ): Wiley & Sons; 2006. p. 739–95.
18. Smith G. Therapist reflections: resilience concepts and findings: implications for family therapy. J Fam Ther 1999;21:154–8.
19. Bowlby J. Attachment and loss, vol. 1. In: Attachment. New York: Basic Books; 1969.
20. Bowlby J. Attachment and loss, vol. 2. In: Separation. New York: Basic Books; 1973.
21. Bowlby J. Attachment and loss, vol. 3. In: Loss, sadness and depression. New York: Basic Books; 1980a.
22. Pietromonaco P, Barrett L. The internal working models concept: what do we really know about the self in relation to others? Rev Gen Psychol 2000;4: 155–75.
23. Stern D. The motherhood constellation: a unified view of parent-infant psychotherapy. New York: Basic Books; 1995.
24. Scharff J, editor. Foundations of object relations family therapy. Northvale (NJ): Jason Aronson; 1989.
25. Slipp S. The technique and practice of object relations family therapy. NJ: Jason Aronson, Inc.; 1988.
26. Slipp S. Object relations: a dynamic bridge between individual and family treatment. New York: Jason Aronson, Inc.; 1984.
27. Bowen M. Family therapy in clinical practice. New York: Jason Aronson; 1978.
28. Boszormenyi-Nagy I. Foundations of contextual therapy. The collected papers of Ivan Boszormenyi-Nagy. New York: Brunner/Mazel; 1987.
29. Baker H, Baker M. Heinz Kohut's self psychology: an overview. Am J Psychiatry 1987;144:1–9.
30. Kohut H. Analysis of the self. New York: International Universities Press; 1971.
31. Fonagy P. Thinking about thinking: some clinical and theoretical considerations in the treatment of a borderline patient. Int J Psychoanal 1991;72:639–56.

32. Allen J, Fonagy P, Bateman A. Mentalizing in clinical practice. Washington, DC: American Psychiatric Publishing, Inc.; 2008.
33. Fraiberg S, Adelson E, Shapiro V. Ghosts in the nursery: a psychoanalytic approach to the problems of impaired infant-mother relationships. J Am Acad Child Psychiatry 1975;14:387–421.
34. Rutter M. How the environment affects mental health. Br J Psychiatry 2005;186: 4–6.
35. Vygotsky L. Mind in society: the development of higher psychological processes. Cambridge (MA): Harvard University Press; 1978.
36. Josephson A, Moncher F. Family treatment. 16. In: Noshpitz J, editor. Handbook of child and adolescent psychiatry, vol. 6. New York: John Wiley and Sons; 1998. p. 294–312.
37. Josephson A, Moncher F. Observation, interview and mental status assessment (OIM): family unit and subunits. 62. In: Noshpitz J, editor. Handbook of child and adolescent psychiatry, vol. 5. New York: John Wiley and Sons; 1998. p. 393–414.
38. Rutter M. Environmentally mediated risks for psychopathology: research strategies and findings. J Am Acad Child Adolesc Psychiatry 2005;44:3–15.
39. Principal Author. American Academy of Child and Adolescent Psychiatry Work Group on Quality Issues, Josephson AM. Practice parameter for the assessment of the family J Am Acad Child Adolesc Psychiatry 2007;46:922–37
40. Josephson A, Moncher F. Family history. 48. In: Noshpitz J, editor. Handbook of child and adolescent psychiatry, vol. 5. New York: John Wiley and Sons; 1998. p. 284–96.
41. Anders T. Clinical syndromes, relationship disturbances, and their assessment. In: Sameroff A, Emde R, editors. Relationship disturbances in early childhood: a developmental approach. New York: Basic Books; 1989.
42. Diamond G, Josephson A. Family-based treatment research: a 10-year update. J Am Acad Child Adolesc Psychiatry 2005;44:872–87.
43. Diamond G, Serano A, Dicky M, et al. Empirical support for family therapy. J Am Acad Child Adolesc Psychiatry 1996;35:6–16.
44. Weissman M, Pilowsky D, Wickramaratne P, et al. Remissions in maternal depression and child psychopathology. JAMA 2006;295:1389–97.
45. Josephson A. The clinical process of sequencing therapies: when, what, how. Scientific Proceedings of the Annual Meeting of the American Academy of Child and Adolescent Psychiatry. Washington, DC: American Academy of Child and Adolescent Psychiatry; 2001. p. 14.
46. Sprenger D, Josephson A. Integration of pharmacotherapy and family therapy in the treatment of children and adolescents. J Am Acad Child Adolesc Psychiatry 1998;37(8):887–9.
47. Kazdin A. Practitioner review: psychosocial treatments for conduct disorder in children. J Child Psychol Psychiatry 1997;38:161–78.
48. Mabe P, Turner M, Josephson A. Parent management training. Child Adolesc Psychiatr Clin N Am 2001;10:451–64.
49. Minuchin S, Fishman H. Family therapy techniques. Cambridge (MS): Harvard University Press; 2004.
50. Haley J, Hoffman L. Techniques of family therapy. New York: Basic Books, Inc.; 1967.
51. Walsh W, McGraw J. Essentials of family therapy: a structured summary of nine approaches. 2nd edition. Denver (CO): Love Publishing Company; 2002.
52. Tomm K. Interventive interviewing: part II, reflexive questioning as a means to enable self-healing. Fam Process 1987;26:167–83.

53. Nichols M. The self in the system: expanding the limits of family therapy. New York: Brunner/Mazel; 1987.
54. Josephson A, Serrano A. The integration of individual therapy and family therapy in the treatment of child and adolescent psychiatric disorders. Child Adolesc Psychiatr Clin N Am 2001;10:431–50.
55. Glick I, Berman E, Clarkin J, et al. Ethical and professional issues in family therapy. In: Marital and family therapy. 4th edition. New York: American Psychiatric Press, Inc.; 2000. p. 683–99.
56. Kaslow N, Robbins Broth M, Oyeshiku Smith C, et al. Family-based interventions for child and adolescent disorders. J Marital Fam Ther 2012;38:82–100.
57. Sprenkle D. Intervention research in couple and family therapy: a methodological and substantive review and an introduction to the special issue. J Marital Fam Ther 2012;38(1):3–29.
58. Henggeler S, Sheidow A. Empirically supported family-based treatments for conduct disorder and delinquency in adolescents. J Marital Fam Ther 2012;38: 30–58.
59. Combrinck-Graham L. Children in families in communities. Child Adolesc Psychiatr Clin N Am 2001;10:613–24.
60. Josephson A, Dell M. Religion and spirituality in child and adolescent psychiatry: a new frontier. Child Adolesc Psychiatr Clin N Am 2004;13(1):1–15.
61. Josephson A, Peteet J, editors. Handbook of spirituality and worldview in clinical practice. Washington, DC: American Psychiatric Publishing, Inc.; 2004.
62. Keitner G, Heru A, Glick I. Clinical manual of couples and family therapy. Washington, DC: American Psychiatric Publishing, Inc.; 2010.
63. Beck A. Cognitive therapy and the emotional disorders. New York: International Universities Press; 1976.
64. Zeanah C, Zeanah P. Intergenerational transmission of maltreatment: insights or attachment theory and research. Psychiatry 1989;52:177–96.
65. Stern D. The interpersonal world of the infant. New York: Basic Books; 1985.
66. Siegel D. The developing mind: toward a neurobiology of interpersonal experience. New York: Guilford Press; 1999.
67. Klinnert M, Emde RN, Butterfield P, et al. Social referencing the infant's use of emotional signals from a friendly adult with mother present. Dev Psychol 1986; 22:427–32.
68. Reiss D. The represented and practicing family: contrasting visions of family continuity. In: Sameroff A, Emde R, editors. Relationship disturbances in early childhood: a developmental approach. New York: Basic Books; 1989. p. 191–220.
69. Garber J, Flynn C. Predictors of depressive cognitions in young adolescents. Cognit Ther Res 2001;25:353–76.
70. Grienenberger J, Kelly K, Slade A. Maternal reflective functioning, mother-infant affective communication, and infant attachment: exploring the link between mental states and observed caregiving behavior in the intergenerational transmission of attachment. Attach Hum Dev 2005;7(3):299–311.
71. Eisenberg L. Nature, niche, and nurture: the role of social experience in transforming genotype into phenotype. Acad Psychiatry 1998;22:213–22.
72. Eisenberg L. The social construction of the human brain. Am J Psychiatry 1995; 152:1563–75.
73. Rutter M. The interplay of nature, nurture, and developmental influences: the challenge ahead for mental health. Arch Gen Psychiatry 2002;59:996–1000.
74. Rutter M. Nature, nurture, and development from evangelism through science toward policy and practice. Child Dev 2002c;73:1–21.

Play Technique in Psychodynamic Psychotherapy

Judith A. Yanof, MD[a,b,*]

KEYWORDS

- Play • Play therapy • Psychodynamic psychotherapy • Metaphor

KEY POINTS

- Imaginary play is often the best way children have of communicating their affects, internal states, fantasies, and complicated conceptual understandings of themselves and the world.
- The opposite of play is not work but reality; and in pretend, children are considerably freer to express conflicted or forbidden aspects of their feelings and their stories.
- We must always be cautious about reading play material as having a one-to-one correspondence with what the child has actually seen, done, or experienced.
- One of the best ways to enter the child's world is to speak to the child from within the frame of the play displacement. Interpreting the unconscious meaning of the play material directly, may shut down the play process.
- Rather than finding the meaning of a particular piece of play, it is often the ability of the therapist to help the child to continue to elaborate different meanings that is the most useful therapeutic technique.
- Today we think of the play as a process that is coconstructed between patient and therapist, and think of the therapist as a participant in the process as well as an observer.

Every child at play behaves like a creative writer, in that he creates a world of his own, or, rather, rearranges the things of his world in a new way which pleases him.
(Freud, 1908).[1]

INTRODUCTION

Play in its broadest sense refers to a wide variety of activities that are universal in human beings of all ages and in many juvenile animal species.[2] This article, however, uses the term "play" to refer to a particular kind of play: imaginary or pretend play. Pretend play has its own developmental trajectory,[2–4] occurs naturally in young children, and is an important factor in their cognitive and social development. Imaginary

[a] Boston Psychoanalytic Society and Institute, 169 Herrrick Road, Newton Centre, Boston, MA 02459, USA; [b] Psychiatry, Harvard Medical School, 25 Shattuck Street, Boston, MA 02115, USA
* 25 Somerset Road, West Newton, MA 02465.
E-mail address: jyanof@erols.com

Child Adolesc Psychiatric Clin N Am 22 (2013) 261–282
http://dx.doi.org/10.1016/j.chc.2012.12.002
1056-4993/13/$ – see front matter © 2013 Elsevier Inc. All rights reserved.

play reaches its peak during the years of early childhood, approximately from age 3 to 7 years. Clinicians who work with children have long used the child's natural capacity to engage in imaginative play as a means of gaining access to the child's inner world, a "royal road to the unconscious." Such is the kind of symbolic play referred to when talking about "play therapy" or "play technique."

Developmental researchers have also studied pretend play for many years in a separate context. Investigators have been interested in play from the perspective of learning about children's cognitive development, organizational level, and their ability to understand another's subjectivity.[5,6] Both psychoanalytic and developmental perspectives may be used in an integrated way to understand how pretend play can unfold and be therapeutic in a clinical setting.[5]

Although play in normal development may have a critical period,[2] in the therapist's playroom, pretend play can be therapeutically effective not only with young children but with children of all ages. This success is often achieved by increasing the frequency of therapy sessions per week and by using the techniques of pretend play in combination with the use of more structured games, music, drawing, and other creative materials. The therapist must actively engage the child in play and scaffold the play when necessary.

WHY PLAY?

Play is privileged as a clinical technique in working psychodynamically with children because it is often the best way children have of communicating internal states, fantasies, affects, and complicated conceptual understandings of themselves and their relationship to the world. Play is also privileged because many believe it is therapeutic in its own right, helping the child to gain developmental capacities that have lagged behind. In development the capacity to play is part of a complicated developmental process. Its emergence has a pivotal place among several developing capacities in the young child, including an explosion of language, the emergence of symbolic functioning, reality testing, triadic relating, and the development of a theory of mind.

Play is Pretend

One of the most important defining characteristics of imaginary play is that it is not real.[1,7] The opposite of play is not work; it is reality.[7] Engaging in pretend play invites an intense affective participation and collaboration with a child in an enterprise that is safe and permissible precisely because it is pretend. Because it is pretend, children are considerably freer to express conflicted or forbidden aspects of themselves and their stories. Children at play are not the monsters, bad guys, or dinosaurs that destroy the world; nor are they the small, helpless creatures that are being attacked[8,9]; they are taking on a role, which can be abandoned or exchanged at will. Important wishes can be expressed without contending with consequences, either from the side of reality or from the side of the superego.[7] The capacity to play can facilitate an exploratory and deepening therapeutic process because it allows access to parts of the self that are not consciously available, parts that are consciously disavowed or repudiated.

There is paradox in playing. Although play is at once "as if" and "not real," it simultaneously involves an intense emotional engagement with the therapist that feels, and is, affectively alive and "authentic."[8,9] There are also similar aspects of this kind of paradox and oscillation in adult psychoanalysis and psychotherapy, especially when working with the complex state of transference or when using free association.[10]

Children who are fully engaged in play, whether inside or outside of therapy, enter a modified ego state or state of consciousness in which attention, perceptions, and thought processes are altered and are redirected primarily to internal experience and fantasy.[2] When things are going well in therapy, the child and therapist can be in both worlds at once, the real world and the world of the imagination, and can fluidly move back and forth. There are always moments, however, when the paradox collapses, when what is enacted becomes "too real" for either the child or the therapist. In these moments the frame of the play collapses, and the parties have to regroup and renegotiate. In these moments the frame of play has failed to contain the affective struggle of the participants.

Play Consists of Actions and Words

One reason that play is such an effective therapeutic technical tool is that children, especially young children, do not use language in the sophisticated ways adults do. Children often communicate with their whole bodies in action rather than in words. If they feel shame, they will hide. If they feel needy, they will use up all the paper supplies in the playroom. Children will tell you how close they want to be to you by moving closer or further away in physical space. Strong affects, in particular, are not easy for children to articulate in words. In fact the therapist's ability, like the parents', to help children name feelings and put their impulses into words is a major contribution in enabling children to eventually contain their feelings, self-regulate, and delay action and impulses. Play in the clinical setting has a similar self-regulating function.

Even when a young child is eager to communicate in words, words may not be the best means of expressing abstract concepts such as emotions. If you ask a young child how she feels, she will often respond with a stereotyped answer such as "I feel happy" or "I feel sad." If you want to get a more nuanced response, you must ask the child a question like, "what happened then?" Such a question will structure the response in the form of a narrative.[11] Pretend play relies on a narrative structure, and it is often the detail of the story that will convey the emotional subtext. When a 3-year-old patient, Jonathan, repeatedly threw the boy doll in the trash basket, it was clear that he was expressing his sense that he could, would, or should be thrown away, and that he felt worthless and bad, like garbage. He could never have expressed this in words.

Play is Metaphorical

It is also important to note that play, like language, uses conceptual metaphor. Lakoff and Johnson[12–14] and other cognitive linguists have revolutionized our thinking by redefining "metaphor," not as a figure of speech but as a fundamental mode of human thought. These linguists believe that metaphor is a nonconscious (different from the dynamic unconscious) way of thinking used by human beings to categorize their experience. Modell,[15] like Lakoff and Johnson, defines metaphor as a "mapping or transfer of meaning across dissimilar domains." The transfer goes from a domain in which there is much concrete knowledge to a domain that is abstract, complex, and much more difficult to define. Lakoff and Johnson[12] use the example "love is a journey" to explain conceptual metaphor in language. In this example, love is a concept that is intrinsically difficult to define and, therefore, is almost always defined in terms of something else; in this case it is compared with a journey, something very concrete. When one says about a love relationship that it "is on the rocks" or that "we can't turn back now," the listener knows immediately what is meant, because of the implicit conceptual metaphor that is part of our everyday thought process. Imaginary play uses conceptual metaphor, just as language does, to categorize experience. In fact, Lakoff and Johnson[12] believe that the ability to use conceptual metaphor may be separate from and antecedent to language.

Clinical example of how play communicates complex conceptual material

Ryan, a 5-year-old boy with a great deal of emotional dysregulation, played out the following story during a therapy hour. A family of plasticine people was at home in the living room. "ET" knocked at the door. ET was "from another planet" and was represented by a plasticine figure with 2 heads and a tail that looked "weird." Ryan told me that ET was an orphan, a "baby orphan," who wanted the family to help him. I was directed to play the part of the family. Under Ryan's direction, the family agreed to help ET and gave him food, but ET ate up all of the family's food. He took the family's car, and drove it until it crashed. He ignored the rules. ET spoke a different language and therefore could not understand the family's rules. He could not control himself and destroyed the family's house. Finally, while trying to fly, he fell off a cliff into a deep pit. At this moment, in a kind of frenzy, Ryan tore ET apart, pulling off his legs, arms, hands, tail, and heads, until the extraterrestrial was just a pile of body parts. Ryan began to toss them into the air and scatter them.

In this imaginative, well-constructed play narrative, Ryan was able to express something very important about how he felt. It was a representation of an inner state whereby feelings were "too big" and threatened to get out of control. Ryan certainly could not have expressed this in words alone. As a young child, he did not have the conceptual language to do this. Yet by using several universal conceptual metaphors as part of his play, Ryan communicated metaphorically his sense of feeling alone (an orphan), insignificant (little, a baby), and different (alien). He also conveyed his sense of feeling internally precarious, uncontained, and coming apart. Most poignantly, at the end of the play sequence, Ryan made ET fragment completely, conveying a lack of self-cohesion. Adults might characterize such a state of mind in a very similar way, using verbal metaphors such as "I feel like I am going to pieces," "I'm falling apart," or "my mind has snapped." Again these universal conceptual metaphors compare an abstract state of mind with a concrete physical object that is brittle and can break.[12] Ryan's communication conveys this state of mind metaphorically in play, rather than words, but in a way that is equally accessible.

Play is a Process

Children have various capacities to play. Children, like Ryan, who have a good play capacity find play pleasurable, and feel safe in communicating their feelings and ideas in play to their therapists, particularly if their therapists make a safe play space and respect their defenses and the use of displacement, which is a main feature of play. For children with a good play capacity, the imaginary play has a process that evolves over the course of treatment. The play has a momentum. It is pleasurable. Over time, an increased degree of complexity is expressed. An increased range of affects is tolerated. An increased elaboration of fantasy emerges, liberating what is being represented from the constraints of both reality and superego. Metaphors evolve, change, and transform. New narratives, solutions, and compromise formations emerge. All of these factors can be used as markers of the treatment process, although there may be periods of regression or impasse, as in any therapy.

THE THERAPIST'S INTERVENTIONS
Listening to Play

Play does not have one meaning: it operates at multiple levels.

Play is complex. Like any communication, it can be read and understood on multiple levels. Play can be the child's representation of an experience from the historical past or a representation of a current life experience that he or she is trying to integrate. Play can be an expression of a child's fears and fantasies, or an imagined solution. Play can be a reenactment or a creative representation of an aspect of an important formative relationship, a phenomenon we would commonly label transference. Play can also be the child's imagined account of what is happening in the new, present relationship with the therapist, a contact through which the child always hopes to find a better, more satisfying way to engage.[16] All these different levels of meaning are oscillating in the play material at any given moment. One must always be cautious, however, about reading play material as having a one-to-one correspondence with what the child has actually seen, done, or experienced (**Box 1**).[17]

The therapist is listening at her best when she can recognize and resonate with the many different levels of meaning that are evolving in the shared play space, but this is difficult to do. Some meanings will feel more salient than others; some will be more elusive. However, an appreciation that the play material does not have one concrete meaning, nor does it operate at one level, is an important place for the therapist to begin. Rather than finding one overarching meaning of a particular piece of play, it is often the ability of the therapist to help the child to continue to elaborate different meanings that is the most useful therapeutic technique. It is also helpful to remember that within a given session the different behaviors and play fragments that occur will always have connecting links, even when the continuity is not obvious. There is always a tension between the goals of communicating a particular insight or understanding to the child and keeping the play space open for further elaboration, to continue to make new meanings. Often interpretations, even when right, can reduce the play to one particular level of meaning, the one that is the most obvious in the moment.

Example of Listening on Different Levels

Let us go back to the example. Ryan expressed in a very nuanced way something about his internal state. As his desires and demands escalated, it felt as if neither he nor his environment could contain them. Under the internal sway of such urgent needs for more food (nurturance, comfort) and more stimulation, no one would remain intact. Furthermore, there was no way of resolving this dilemma, because everyone spoke a different language and no one could understand the other.

As the therapist, I (J.A.Y., the author of this article) could have read Ryan's play communication in different ways. I could have recognized his play as a representation of his real world; that is, a story about a home in which limits or containment were missing or inconsistent, a reading that might be more or less accurate. Or I could have understood his story as a representation of the way he saw himself or was perceived by his parents. In such a reading, I might imagine that Ryan envisioned himself as a child who was so "different" that he felt like he was from another planet, a child that no family could rein in or keep safe. Another way of listening to the play

---

Box 1
Play communicates on multiple levels

1. Play can represent an experience from the patient's past

2. Play can represent current life experiences

3. Play can express fears, fantasies, and imagined solutions to conflicts

4. Play can reenact aspects of important formative relationships (transference)

5. Play can represent the patient's representations of the new, present relationship with the therapist

communication was that it reflected something about my relationship with Ryan in the moment. He might have been telling me that he was feeling uncontained and unheld by me because of something I was doing or not doing. Or the play might reveal his wish to "move in" with me so that I could be his new, idealized "adoptive" family. Ryan might have been trying to discover how I would respond to his escalating excitement and unruly behavior, perhaps both recreating the past (transference) and hoping for a different outcome (new object). Finally, the play might have been a representation of Ryan's internal landscape in which "ET" represented one part of himself (the powerful, aggressive, and thrill-seeking part), whereas "the family" represented another part: an internalized set of rules or values, difficult to adhere to when in conflict with the pleasure-seeking or anxiety-laden impulses. These different ways of understanding the play material might all have been relevant; however, they may not have all been equally salient.

The therapist must determine what aspects of the play are most important, and that will determine how she chooses to respond. Play always occurs in a particular context, never in isolation. Therapists listen on the basis of what they know about the child, their experience with the child, and their experience of the family. Therapists listen with an ear to normal developmental crises or impasses; listen to what the play makes them feel, their countertransference; and listen to how the story is being communicated as well as to the content of the story. It is especially helpful to listen with the following question in mind: "why is the child telling me this story at this particular time?" This question inevitably leads to a curiosity about where the therapist is located in the story, as well as what is now happening in the patient's real life. The following questions immediately come to mind: Is something going on in the therapeutic relationship? Have I been away? What happened in our previous session? Did Ryan get into trouble with a teacher or his mom that day? Children are much more likely than adults to have upsetting experiences at home or school spill over into their therapy sessions.

Working Within the Play Displacement

The unconscious content of the play may often be easy for the therapist to understand, especially if the play has a clear narrative arc and is well structured. However, simply interpreting the play as a statement about the child (a child's wish or fantasy, or representation of reality), even if right, might easily shut down the play space, thus running counter to the child's assumption that his play is pretend and is being received by the therapist as such. Children make this assumption for different reasons. Very young children (younger than 5 years) have no clear cognitive recognition that their play and their internal thoughts are related,[4] whereas for older children the displacement of play makes it a protected place. Older children, even when they understand that their own minds and intentions are at work in creating play, use play defensively to keep themselves from experiencing the potential consequences of reality or conscience. Therefore, timing is everything. One interprets directly from the play only when one thinks that the child is already very close to knowing that the content of the play is about himself and when he is not too defended to hear it.

For instance, if I said to Ryan, "you are so angry you feel like breaking your house apart," he might easily feel accused, frightened, or misunderstood. He might temporarily close down the rich play space that he has just created with me. Disrupting the play space is a frequent, inadvertent consequence of going directly for unconscious forbidden wishes, overriding the patient's defenses, and quickly attributing these wishes directly to the child, as in this example. This kind of direct interpretation might well miss the nuance in Ryan's communication as well. For instance, Ryan does not simply want to break down his house, he also wants to be contained by the family because he is afraid of these destructive wishes. He may even want to be punished because he feels guilty about them.

One of the best ways for the therapist to enter the child's world and to communicate is to do this from within the displacement of the play.[18,19] These kinds of interventions respect the frame of the play. The therapist can comment (1) from outside the play about the play as an observer, still using the patient's play metaphor; or (2) from inside the play as one of the characters in the patient's story. The therapist can even create a new character or tell a related story (**Box 2**).

In the first kind of intervention, the therapist uses her own voice to tell the child what she observes in the play, or to ask for an explanation about the play. For example, the therapist can say to Ryan, as an observer from the outside, "the family doesn't seem to have enough food to keep ET from feeling hungry, what should they do?" or "ET has been starving for so long that he cannot get enough food to fill him up." Each of these comments emphasizes a slightly different aspect of the story; each represents an aspect that the therapist might want to develop for the future. What is technically important about this type of intervention is that even though the therapist speaks from outside the play, her comments respect the displacement of the play, its frame. She does not talk about the child directly. It is ET who cannot be filled, not the child. Such a voice can be comforting because the therapist "gets it," helps contain the affective tension, shows interest, or functions as a witness to the child's communication. Such a technique can feel safer to a child who is not ready to have a true play partner.

The therapist can also talk from inside the play, from the point of view of a character. For instance, as the father I could say, "My gosh, ET is still eating and we are running out of food! What should we do?" or "It looks like he hasn't had any food in days! He is starving!" Talking from inside the play as one of the characters is certainly more playful. The therapist is freer to use her own person to play a role; she can inject more affect into the story and can use voices other than her own. The patient has to have the play skills to respond to this "other" voice, which introduces something different. For example, it is not infrequent for the therapist to express, through her character, a part of the child that the child has disavowed and, therefore, remains unrepresented in the narrative. In Ryan's story this was not the case, as he represented both sides of his conflict: ET felt excited and powerfully strong, as well as frightened of being out of control. However, if Ryan had not been able to represent both sides, the therapist might have chosen to represent the unspoken part—the fear, for instance—through an invented play character. The patient would then have the option of taking in or rejecting the therapist's introduced perspective. Ryan might say, "no, he doesn't say that!" This would tell me that he is not at this moment ready to engage with that aspect of himself. As long as the therapist introduces things in pretend, the child can decide if these things are irrelevant, facilitating, too threatening or, in fact,

---

Box 2
Working in the displacement

1. The therapist can comment about the play from outside, as an observer, still using the patient's play metaphor

2. The therapist can comment from inside the play as one of the characters in the patient's story

3. The therapist can comment by creating a new character or by telling a related story

transformative ways of telling his story. This is also how play works in social situations with peers; it is negotiated. Although the child's story must always be salient, the therapist is more than an observer in the play process; she is a participant/observer, meaning that she must be particularly observant about the impact of her interventions.

It used to be a "rule" among analysts conducting play therapy to only take one's cue from the child, and not to elaborate any part of the story unless the patient had given the therapist explicit directions to do so. I have found this "rule" to be overly cautious in children who have a good capacity to play, and inadequate in children who need help in learning to play. This cautionary rule came from a time when child analytical technique was supposed to look like adult analytical technique, and when adult analysis was considered to be an unfolding of something from inside the patient. There was a concern that anything from the analyst would contaminate the field or the process. Today we think of play as a process that is coconstructed between patient and therapist, and think of the therapist as a participant in the process as well as an observer. The therapist's participation helps the child to scaffold and expand the play.

In fact, the play was not simply a one-way communication from Ryan to me about his experience or state of mind. I communicated something to Ryan about how I contained and dealt with my feelings, particularly my difficulty in having impact, because my "rules" could not keep ET or the family safe. However, when Ryan started to pull ET apart and scatter the small plasticine pieces all over the room, I said in the pretend voice of the father with my full adult authority, "pull yourself together, son." Although I stayed in the play metaphor, I also responded in action, by the tone of my voice and by gently covering what was left of the unthrown pieces with my hand. I regulated the play downwards. This scenario was not thought out; it simply happened. Ryan's plea for containment in the story was now responded to by my "real" containment, via an enactment in the playroom.

Turning Passive into Active

One of the most important therapeutic consequences of pretend play in both natural and clinical settings is that it allows the child to have mastery over situations that are experienced passively and that are uncomfortable or traumatic. Freud[1] understood this, as did Waelder,[20] who described how play helps the child rework difficult experiences by metabolizing, mastering, and assimilating them.

Clinical example of listening, working within the displacement, and turning passive into active

A 5-year-old boy came to my office and acted out a particular story. He played the same story every time he came to see me. In a way it was the same story, but it was always a little bit different. In this story he was "Joe," a deep-sea diver, who had to plumb the ocean's depths and check the ocean floor for signs of trouble. The trouble was usually of an environmental nature, a certain species of fish was about to become extinct or was about to take over another's territory. Joe was the ocean's fix-it man. He would start out on my couch, outfitting himself with a diving suit and something suggestive of an oxygen supply. He would then roll himself over the side of the couch, and swim away into dark and deep waters. But the sea was a very dangerous place, and when he left the safety of the boat, Joe had to make his way among man-eating sharks that could bite off his legs, stingrays that could "paralyze his bones," and, above all, he had to avoid the entangling arms of a giant octopus.

I was Mike, Joe's partner, and my job was to stay up on the boat and monitor his comings and goings on a computer screen. The screen allowed me to be aware of all the dangers that were about to befall him, even the ones he had not yet come upon. I could communicate to him by special underwater cell phone and warn him what lay hidden around the bend. In this way,

I could keep him safe. However, sometimes I wasn't paying attention, and my warnings came too late. Or sometimes he wasn't paying attention, and wandered off beyond our signal area. Then he was in deep trouble. He had to fight off vicious creatures alone and bare-handed. Joe was a skilled and powerful fighter, though, so in the end he always escaped just in the nick of time. Then he would text, "pull me up!" and I would reel him in like a big fish. He would flop down in the boat, breathless from his adventure, and sleep. I would have to tuck him in. Sometimes he would dream about the ocean.

As you can see, Joe's play was very well constructed and coherent for a 5-year-old, an indication that he had a well-developed play capacity and many ego strengths. Knowing something about his history made his play particularly meaningful. In real life "Joe" was an only child. In fact, he was a long-awaited child, as his parents had difficulty conceiving after many miscarriages. From infancy on, he had some very potent allergies. As a toddler he had suddenly become life-threateningly ill when he was inadvertently exposed to one of these allergens. He had to rely on the vigilance of his parents to keep him safe, and they had to be unusually attentive. He became very anxious when they were not around, and they also worried about his venturing forth into the world without them, although they also wanted him to be strong and independent.

In his play, Joe created a wonderful metaphor for his psychic experience. He created an ocean world that had many of the characteristics of his real world. In his ocean world, there were many perilous things that were "ordinary" for the ocean but that had to be avoided by him. There were also many things that were not working the way they should be working, and needed fixing. He knew that he needed to venture forth on his own, but this was very dangerous. In his play, he created a meaningful way of communicating his inner experience to me so that he was no longer alone. Through his play he found a way to make his overwhelming feelings a little more tolerable. He also found a way of incrementally metabolizing his experience piecemeal to find new adaptations and solutions. A major mechanism in the play for doing this was to turn passive into active. In his story he wasn't the littlest one in his family; he was Joe, the grown-up fix-it man. He was, big, strong, and powerful; he was not helpless. He was master of his destiny.

The traumatic aspect of this boy's history made this recurring narrative the focus of his treatment for a long time. However, despite the repetitive nature of this game, it never became stereotyped and inert as it might have become for children whose play is more traumatically stuck. New things were always being added to his play, and new metaphors were always being created, with the potential for finding new solutions.

This play, of course, included much more than simply a mechanism of turning passive into active. It provided a way for exploring the complicated nature of his relationships with the adults in his life. Joe was trying to come to grips with his relationship to his parents, as all children of this age are trying to do. The idealized parents were supposed to magically protect Joe from harm and were supposed to foresee every danger, even dangers that he could not see. Joe's parents were not always able to do this, which made them, at times, disappointing to Joe. It also made him and them very anxious because life could be so unpredictable. His parents were still the main focus of his life, and moving away from them seemed especially difficult for both Joe and them because of fears for his survival. He was young and the world felt particularly dangerous. In the transference I was both an idealized and disappointing parent. Joe wanted me on the boat, at a distance, but connected at all times by a computer monitor and an umbilical rope.

The play also provided a metaphoric way of looking at unconscious conflict and fantasy. Going down, according to Lakoff and Johnson,[12] is a universal metaphor for being further away from awareness, consciousness, or wakefulness. The dangers that were present on the ocean floor were evocative of typical developmental conflicts and concerns that a 5-year-old boy might have. Joe wanted to explore what troubled him, but his mind also felt dangerous to him. In many of his pretend "outings," Joe deliberated between 2 specific dangers: swimming near a man-eating shark that could bite off his legs or getting too close to a giant octopus that could grab him, never to let him go. Joe had unconscious conflict about growing up, made somewhat more difficult by his history. Joe adored his mother, but often held on to behaviors that kept him very babyish. By staying his mother's baby and refusing to grow up, he succeeded in getting her attention and at the same time avoided being a competitive threat to his father. However, when Joe remained a baby he did not feel competent and successful in the world, and feared he could get stuck with his mother forever. In Joe's play he had to fight both fears: the fear of retaliation for his wish for an Oedipal victory (the castrating shark) and his fear of his regressive urges (the entangling octopus). Joe used his play in a very productive way to explore these fears and conflicts about growing up. Through his relationship with me in the transference, he played out his urges to be independent, admired, rescued, babied, disappointed, angry, and competitive.

Transference and Countertransference

Different children use the therapist in different ways, according to their predominant needs. All therapeutic relationships carry vestiges of past relationships; we call this transference. At the same time the repeating and reworking of the past comes in the context of a new relationship in which there is the possibility for a different outcome. Because children are always in the midst of an important developmental process while they are in therapy, many believe that their experience with the therapist is internalized in a more influential, comprehensive, and enduring way than it would be if the developmental process were completed.[21,22]

Children inevitably play out and reenact aspects of their primary relationships with their therapists, just as adults do. Being able to recognize when and how transference is occurring is an important aspect of understanding children and their conflicts, and is an important aspect in communicating with them.

Some argue that transference is not as prevalent in children as in adults because the therapist also has an important role as a "new object" or a "developmental object."[21–26] Because the child is in the midst of development, it is surmised that the therapist is used by the child to fill current developmental needs. Others argue that if the therapist does not take a moral position with the child and does not act as a substitute parent or an educator, but instead maintains neutrality and analyzes the interactions that arise between patient and therapist, one can work in the transference with children in a similar way to the way that one does with adults.[27–29] Although transference is always present, transference reactions are more likely to cohere and consolidate when the therapist is seeing the child more intensively.

Children often do not understand the concept of transference in the way that adults do; that is, they do not understand its "as if" nature.[30] When children feel something about the therapist, they feel it in the present moment and it seems very "real" to them, and often very "big." Rarely do they understand that the strength of their feelings exists because the therapeutic relationship has triggered something from their past or from their current family lives. Because it is difficult for children to comprehend the paradoxic nature of transference, it makes sense to address what is happening between child and therapist in the present and to understand it in the moment.

Often transferences are manifest in the play itself, as they were with Ryan and Joe. Ryan's fear that he would be seen as uncontrollable by his family and Joe's difficulty titrating dependence and independence were important aspects of their relationships with their parents, and they became important in the play interactions with me. These transference feelings led to ways of relating to me that were expressed, enacted, and "played with" in displacement in the play. I did not directly address how the play related to their real lives, because I believed that we were working on these issues productively in play. Nevertheless, I kept the idea of transference very much in mind as I listened.

Sometimes it *is* important to take up transference directly with a child, especially if strong emotions are interfering with the therapeutic work. When children arouse a great deal of feeling in us because of the aggression, hatred, seduction, or neediness that is directed at us, we can almost always be sure that the child is replaying elements of a primary relationship. Nevertheless, it is difficult not to take these strong feelings personally. Interactions around the frame are a very common place for the arousal of transference feelings directed at the therapist to be found. Children may be frightened of entering, or refuse to leave the session; they may be angry in sessions before or after a vacation, and may not want to come back to therapy. Children may feel envious of the toys we have and may want to destroy them, trash the playroom, or use up all our supplies; they may even attack us physically. If they like us too much, they might experience this as a conflict over loyalty owed to a parent. Parents have strong transference feelings to us as well.

Children are often able to acknowledge their intense feelings in the moment, even though they have no appreciation that their sense of abandonment, jealousy, envy, or disappointment has its origins in some previous relationship. Their feelings are best addressed in terms of what they feel in the present coupled with our understanding of what has immediately precipitated this reaction. "You got upset when I told you that our time was up, and then you threw over the box of markers. Maybe you thought I was saying I didn't want to be with you." There are often clear triggers in the therapist's behavior that have contributed to the rupture between therapist and child, and these can also be acknowledged. The therapist may not have been paying attention, or she may have said something that the child found hurtful.

Because children tend to enact their feelings rather than talk about them, the therapist will have to set clear limits to make the play space safe for herself and the child so that the child does not feel too anxious or guilty about what he has enacted. On the other hand, there is always a balance between keeping behavior safe and nondestructive, and wanting to understand what the child is trying to express in action. Therapy has to be a place where the child can express his feelings, even if they are not very pleasant ones. Often things get better on the outside when the "bad" behavior that brought the child to treatment comes into the sessions. For instance, although I do not allow children to destroy my toys or hit me, sometimes it happens that they do, which in turn becomes an opportunity for therapeutic understanding.

Particularly obvious manifestations of transference are those behaviors that concern the child patient's reactions to the presence of other children in the office or waiting room. These other patients who share the therapist's time represent siblings, about whom child patients often have strong and particular feelings. One patient of mine was convinced that the things in her special box had been disturbed or stolen by another child when she was away from the office, even though this was not in the least true. She had felt very deprived by the birth of her sibling some years back, whose arrival coincided with the loss of a favorite nanny. In her mind, all the things that she had lost seemed taken by the birth of this sister. We often addressed and elaborated her fears about losing the things in her special box and her fear that

I could not keep them safe, as well as her own wishes to look in everyone else's box. Although her history and jealousy of her sister were known to her, the issue about losing her place with me was a much more viable way to work on the past. Nor would she have necessarily understood that my other patients were "stand-ins" for her sister.

Whenever a child asks about the therapist's age, or where she lives, or if she has children or not, there is always a fantasy lurking in the question. It can often be very helpful to address the child's underlying concern or interest, whether one answers the question directly or not. The therapist might say: "you are very curious about what I am doing when I am not in this office"; or "you are wondering who I am with when I am not seeing you"; or "you are wondering if I am a mother, and what kind of a mother I would be."

Children who Cannot Play

Many children whom we see in evaluation and later in therapy cannot use imaginative play, and this occurs for many different reasons.[31] The capacity to play is an ego capacity that is important to assess when we evaluate a child.

Children who have autism or are on the spectrum for pervasive developmental disorders (PDD) often cannot play pretend, because they cannot play symbolically.[32,33] It is thought that this deficit is complex, but largely biological in nature; these children have great difficulty developing a robust theory of mind. Play techniques have been developed specifically for working with these children, emphasizing a foundation of shared attention and engagement.[34] Although we know that play is universal in human development, we also know that it is highly susceptible to the impact of environmental factors such as trauma, troubled attachment, and even nutrition.[2,35,36] Research shows that children who are securely attached by age 3 years are 3 times more likely to play pretend with their peers than children who are not.[36,37] Children in secure relationships with their caretakers tend to be interested in using toys, playing pretend, and exploring the world because of their primary investment and identification with their parents who introduce these interests to their children, while providing a secure base. Preschool children with disorganized attachment, on the other hand, are more likely to completely inhibit fantasy play or act out chaotic, violent fantasies that have no play resolution.[36,38,39] Children cannot play when they cannot coherently organize their experience.

Children who have suffered severe trauma are another group of children whose play is impaired. The play of traumatized children is often stuck in rigid and repetitive forms that seem to go nowhere. The play may actually be communicating some aspect of the trauma in a concrete way while simultaneously interfering with the development of a creative, coherent narrative. Working with this kind of traumatic play may be arduous, but incremental changes are important signs of progress.

We also see children who have difficulty playing because they have internal conflict and play inhibitions. Sometimes these children can play pretend at home quite well but do not want to play with their therapist because it feels too revealing. For children who are frightened of their feelings and thoughts, the freedom of pretend can feel less safe than a structured board game because internal thoughts and feelings can "pop out" without warning or control.

Clinical example of a child unable to play

I worked with an 8-year-old boy who was inhibited and very anxious about his impulses. David refused all my many attempts at pretend play. He was a chess whiz and only wanted to play chess and defeat me at this game until he felt safer. David eventually became an excellent pretend player, but only after a long time and only when we began to meet multiple times a week. The inroad to pretend play occurred one day when I had been particularly frustrated about losing a chess game to him once again. In a pretend voice, full of real frustration, my king began to complain that he was totally fed up because no one in his kingdom was doing their job to protect him and that he was tired of having so few moves. He always felt "boxed in." Although David usually rejected my use of pretend and playfulness, on this day he answered the king and gave him some important advice that opened up a completely different level of play, the beginning of fantasy play. Perhaps the element of revealing my authentic frustration, alongside David's identification with the king's sentiments and my perseverance over time, brought about a different response.

HOW THE CHILD PLAYS

When a child is a "good player" the therapist has a much easier time finding a way to engage, enjoy, and facilitate the deepening of the play. The therapist has more degrees of freedom in terms of what can be addressed and in what forms it can be addressed. Every child/therapist pair develops their own play process that is unique to the dyad and has their fingerprint on it. With children who have more difficulty playing, the therapist's skill in facilitating the process and engaging in play will be more crucial. Of course, it is not simply play that the therapist is interested in. The use of language, action, particular words, interruptions of play, the expression of affect or lack thereof, somatic events, facial expressions, gestures, and eye contact are all part of what the therapist will use to understand and make meaning with the child. Much of what I have talked about so far is the aspect of the play that is in symbolic, narrative form, but there are also many aspects that are delivered in action and are communicated in nonsymbolic ways.

Play Disruptions

Play disruptions[40] occur when too much anxiety arises from a conflict during play, with the play being interrupted by the child.

Clinical example of disruption of imaginary play

Suki, an 8-year-old girl who had a very ambivalent relationship with her mother, played out the story of a polar bear family with small animal figures. The bears split up to find food. The father and daughter bear went in one direction; the mother and baby in the other. The father and daughter had great success and stuffed themselves, as if at a delicious banquet. The mother and son faced a vanishing food supply, wandered and wandered, and soon began to starve. At this point in the story, Suki got ashen and said "this story could not really happen," and put away the toy animals because playing pretend was "too babyish."

Suki got anxious at the point in the story when her fantasy of Oedipal victory and her aggressive impulses toward mother and baby became "too real" and too threatening. She anxiously stopped the game, reminding herself that it could not really happen. In a similar way, children can interrupt the play by needing to use the bathroom, by insisting on visiting their mothers in the waiting room, or by being unable to continue the narrative arc of the story. Sometimes the play disruption takes the form of shutting down the play, as it did with Suki. At other times the disruption takes the form of enacting the impulse, as when Ryan began to scatter the Lego pieces all over the room or when a child suddenly hits the therapist instead of the mother doll. The play disruption can also involve a somatic discharge such as soiling. Noting what occurred before the play was disrupted is of critical importance to the therapist in understanding the nature of the child's conflict and what got in the way of playing.

The therapist has several options in dealing with play disruption. The therapist can observe it but not address it, or can point out to the child that the disruption happened in response to something that worried her (a form of defense interpretation). If Suki were receptive, the therapist might say something about the impulse that actually made her so anxious: "you began to worry what would happen to the mother bear because she got too close to starving."

The therapist wants to be able to contain the child's fantasies, conflicts, and difficult emotions, and to use play to explore and organize as much about the child's inner affective life as the child can manage. The therapist is not interested in taking a moral position regarding the play, nor interested in "cleaning up" the child's story or giving the child a particular solution to the story. The therapist is interested in why a child is having trouble finding a satisfactory solution. The therapist's job is to help the child structure the story and to expand the narrative, finding the right words to capture what the child is trying to convey.

The therapist's ability to play freely and enjoy play is an important aspect of engaging a child in pretend. Some child therapists are very wary or guilty about "just playing," as if it were not doing the serious work of therapy. Playing is often the best way to deepen the therapeutic engagement. Play can feel intimidating to the therapist, just as it can for the child, because of its open-endedness and because one uses the deepest recesses of one's own experience to participate. Therefore, the therapist has to feel confident in her capacity to contain the internal affective elements aroused in both herself and the child. Of course, there are always moments when the frame of pretend collapses under the weight of the affective struggle, at which point the therapist must move in, reinstitute the frame, and repair the disruption.

Play often stops when impulses break through. Letting the child know that there are ways to tell his story that are safe and won't make him feel too scared or too guilty is an important part of reestablishing the frame for the child. For instance, if a child wants to examine the therapist while playing the doctor game, it is helpful to move the play from the macroscopic sphere to the microscopic sphere.[40] I might say, "show me what you want to do to me on this doll; then you can pretend anything you want." Macroscopic play is likely to be more overstimulating than symbolic play with toys. Macroscopic play is also more limited in what can be permitted to be actualized. One can frequently help a child calm down and become more organized by moving to a more structured form of play.

Clinical example of disruption of real play

One day during an intensive psychotherapy with a very inhibited 6-year-old girl, Heather convinced me to play a game of tag with her in my office. Although I don't usually play tag because the space is small and the game itself involves tagging, a kind of touching, I agreed because of her insistent request, which I heard as a need to show me something. Quite soon after I began to chase her, she grabbed off her shirt in a frenzy of anxiety and excitement. I stopped the game, saying that this game had gotten her too excited. I added, nevertheless, that I really wanted her to find another way for her to tell me the story of the "clothes coming off." With a great deal of scaffolding on my part, she was then able to make some drawings of something she had witnessed that was very overstimulating and frightening to her.

Although this was a tag game and not imaginative play, I have considered this example as similar to a play disruption. Helping the child reestablish the play frame by putting her feelings in the form of a narrative story was helpful to her.

Play Enactments

Play can also be used to enact something with the therapist in a defensive way. It is not that the play does not have communicative value, but that the enactment carries the emotional valence.

Clinical example of play enactment

One patient of mine, a 9-year-old girl, played that she was the queen doll and I was the servant doll every time we met. She would dump out her doll's wardrobe and I would have to tidy up her clothes repeatedly. I had no voice in the play and had to say whatever the queen doll wanted to hear. When I did something that was more rebellious or assertive, I was made to suffer more humiliation or banished to the dungeon.

Certainly one could understand this play as communicating something about my patient's experience of feeling dominated in her family, and as an attempt to counteract this experience by turning the tables, an identification with the aggressor. Nevertheless, as this play enactment continued without change, it began to lose its metaphoric capacity. The sadomasochistic relationship was transferred to the therapeutic relationship, in the guise of play, whereby the nature of what was happening between us was not at all playful.

Therapeutic play at its best involves a situation in which both patient and therapist have a voice and are willing to acknowledge the other person's initiatives. I often talked through my servant doll about how she felt: sad, frustrated, enraged, and full of revenge. I also talked about the ways that my doll did not like being the "lowly servant" and was trying to find ways to elevate her sense of self and self-worth, but I could not find a way to be heard from within the play. Nor could the sadomasochistic impasse be addressed from outside the play because the patient denied that there was "really" anything demeaning going on at all; it was all "pretend." I saw this response from my patient as a further communication: a way she conveyed to me her sense that humiliating things went on in her family that no one could acknowledge or own.

I eventually had to extricate myself from this enactment by refusing to play unless we had different ground rules. Although this did not seem like an optimal solution at the time, it brought the patient's fury at me into the open and we were able to work productively on her envy and hate. It is important to recognize, however, that the many months of playing out the sadomasochistic enactment provided important experience that we had both lived through. This shared experience became a background and a reference point that enabled the work that followed.

HELPING CHILDREN TO PLAY

Winnicott[41] wrote that when children cannot engage in play, it is the task of the therapist to help them to play. Often this is true for the very young child and for the child with an impedance in the capacity to play. The therapist must introduce play and scaffold it, just like the mother of the infant who introduces the peek-a-boo game (a pretend game about separation) and toys to her child as part of the child's development.

The initial engagement of the child patient is important, and engaging a child through play, without a lot of talk, is one of the most successful ways of beginning play therapy. Children are often delighted that the therapist has toys in the office, and children will often begin by playing out their most pressing affective themes. Nevertheless, the therapist often needs to invite the child into the play mode and give him permission to play. In *The Piggle*, Winnicott[42] has a particularly engaging way of initiating play with a very young, inhibited child.[6] Winnicott starts out in a corner of the room away from the child, makes friends by himself with a teddy bear, and asks the young patient to come and show the bear the toys.

I often start to play by telling a story or putting something that has actually happened between the patient and me into a puppet show for the child, using animal puppets with pretend voices. I might try to involve the child by asking what names to give the characters. I often inject something playful about the names of the characters to let the child know that we can depart from reality, revise it, or poke fun at it. I ask the child for input about what should happen next. I try to pick a theme that will be appealing to the child and, as time goes on, I add what the child cannot or will not do for himself. I scaffold the play, helping the child to structure and expand the play.

To shape my interventions I use my own imagination, but whatever I say is informed by everything I know about the child, both consciously and unconsciously: the child's history, family experience, the previous transactions between us, and the child's interests, favorite books, and favorite shows. I aim to stay in the neighborhood of something that will be of interest to the child. Obviously I try to start with less charged themes. This attempt to engage the child in play is a process of trial and error, and the therapist must take her cues from the child about what is working and what is met with negativity, what may be built on, and what is best to abandon for the moment. The play space is a joint imaginary arena that has to be negotiated between patient and therapist.

Equipping a Playroom

Therapists have their own individual preferences for what toys they have, but if the therapist wants to encourage imaginative play, the best toys to have on hand are nonmechanical, noncomputerized toys that can be used open-endedly for symbolic play. Dollhouse figures, dollhouse furniture, small animals, blocks, action figures, cars and trucks, Lego bricks, and plasticine food all lend themselves to creative play. The office should also be well stocked with markers, paper, tape, scissors, whiteboard, and Play-Doh so that drawing, writing stories, constructing, destructing, and repairing can all be easily accomplished.[28] Having said all of this, there are of course many creative and successful ways to introduce pretend play with different toys. It is also important to have a place where the child's projects and drawings can be kept safely in between sessions and out of sight of other patients, because attention to and care for the child's projects promotes a sense of continuity and conveys a sense of value about the therapeutic work. Symbolically this makes a space in the therapist's world (and mind) for the child and the "work" of therapy. I encourage patients to leave their projects in the office, but I never make it a rule. I often make a copy of a child's drawings or stories to keep in the office if the child wants to take them home.

HOW TO TALK TO PARENTS ABOUT PLAY

I believe the therapist must be actively engaged with parents to make the child's treatment work. Therefore I see parents separately, but regularly, whenever I see a child in treatment. Of course, the child is informed that I see the parents regularly. The goal of this adjunctive parent treatment is to help parents to be better parents. I try to be flexible in working at whatever level the parents are able to work in order that this goal is best achieved. This flexibility includes being available to parents in a time of crisis, helping them understand why their children are having trouble, advocating for their child's needs with other psychological helpers and educators, talking to parents about development, and helping them understand the dynamics in the family. I also try to understand who parents are psychologically and to work with them on how their own conflicts get played out with the child, whenever we can work at that deeper level (**Box 3**).

Outside the playroom, I try to remember that the child is a very important member of a family system and is significantly affected by parents' perspectives and behavior, both positive and negative. In parent work, I try to intervene to improve the parent/child relationship. I do this while keeping the child's specific communications to me confidential, and the parents' specific feelings and concerns about their child confidential as well. Although there are complications and difficulties in this ability to relate to both parents and children, I believe this approach has the best chance for therapeutic success. I convey that I am a person who is there to help the family, not just the child. I convey that there is a need for me to keep confidentiality in my relationship with the child, and that this is a matter of how the relationship works best.

Some parents think that their children are supposed to talk in therapy, so I explain that therapy with children is very different from adult therapy. I inform parents that play is often the best way that a child can communicate to me, because children, especially young children, cannot talk about their feelings in the same ways that adults can. Although play is fun and compelling, it is not an avoidance of work; play is actually the work the child is supposed to be doing.

Early in the consultation I often give examples to parents of how I listen to play as a communication and how I use play to work on a problem. I may use an example from play the parent has witnessed with the child, or an example from a common clinical situation that does not breach the child's confidentiality. For example, I explain that if a child is inhibited and afraid to talk about anger, playing about being angry with a crocodile puppet is a helpful, liberating step. I try to describe what I have observed about the child and what meanings I give to these observations. I am also clear about what I do not yet know and what I will be trying to find out. I find that treating the parents as partners in the child's treatment is a helpful way to frame the relationship.

Box 3

Helping parents be better parents

1. Be available to the parents in times of crisis

2. Help parents understand why their child is having difficulties

3. Advocate for the child's needs with other health care providers and educators

4. Talk to parents about child development

5. Help parents understand family dynamics

6. Seek to understand the parent psychologically

7. When possible help parents understand how their own issues get played out with the child

8. Maintain the goal of improving the parent/child relationship

9. Treat the parent as a partner

Preparing a Child for the First Visit

Preparing a child for the first visit is an important part of the process of engaging the child and the parents. My preference is to meet the parents alone initially to get a good understanding of their concerns about the child. It is also important for me to find out how the parents plan to prepare the child for his or her first meeting with me. By eliciting this information from the parents initially, the therapist will obtain a good sense of how the parent is conceptualizing the therapy, as well as what the parent feels is important to communicate or avoid communicating to the child. I usually suggest that things often work best if parents describe the therapist as a doctor or person who helps children with their worries by talking and playing with them. I also suggest that parents address directly why the child is coming to see me. It is always better to lead with something that the child will want assistance with, rather than a behavior the parent wants to extinguish or labels as "naughty." For instance, it is better to say we are seeing the worry doctor because "you are unhappy at school" rather than because "you don't listen to the teacher."

THE THERAPEUTIC ACTION OF PLAY

Psychoanalytic investigators differ among themselves about what accounts for cure in psychoanalytic treatment and psychodynamic therapy. There is now a fascinating debate in adult psychoanalytic theory about the contribution of words and the nonverbal: the place of language in mental life and in therapeutic change.[43–48] This debate has implications for treatment technique. Similarly, in work with children there is debate over what should be decoded from the play, put into words and interpreted directly to the child; what should be verbalized and left as part of the play dialogue, and what should be left unspoken altogether.[8,9]

The increased interest in what is communicated implicitly and nonverbally in psychodynamic therapy is a result of increased data from the neurosciences, infant research, and cognitive psychology. We now know that much of what is transmitted in a room between two people goes on outside of their conscious awareness. We also know that therapeutic change can occur in conscious and nonconscious brain systems, and that these systems can enhance each other, rather than working in an either/or way.[49] Implicit or nonconscious change is possible during play not only because procedural relational systems (implicit relational knowing) can shift,[43] but because in a rich play process symbolic ideas can be "played with" metaphorically, just as they can in language, without necessarily being made explicit through interpretation.[8,9] At the same time, narrative, an important part of the play process, helps organize internal affective states by lifting subsymbolic affective states partially into consciousness.[50]

In the last 2 decades an increasing number of clinicians working with and writing about children have taken the position that helping the child to engage in the play process is just as important as verbalizing the meaning of the play content.[5,8,9,16,17,30,36,51–56] Even when the play content is not explicitly decoded or interpreted, these investigators have been impressed that the play process is therapeutic in its own right and can bring about change. If we think of play as making contributions to development in natural settings, it is not difficult to imagine that helping a child to play in the clinical setting might have important benefits as well.

In development, imaginary play reaches its peak during early childhood (age 3–7 years) and is an important capacity that emerges in confluence with other significant developmental capacities such as the emergence of language, symbolic functioning, self-regulation, reality testing, triadic relating, and theory of mind. Developmental research shows correlations between these emergent capacities rather than causal connections,[2] therefore it is not exactly clear what relationship these capacities have to each other, what the specific function of play is, or how play contributes to development. Nevertheless, there are several compelling hypotheses that have been generated in the psychoanalytic and developmental literature.

Pretending is introduced very early to the infant by the caregiver, and is understood even in its most elementary forms by the infant as something "not real" and something pleasurable; this occurs well before the infant can pretend back. One hypothesis about the function of pretend is that the caregiver organizes and regulates the infant's emotional experience by a process of affect-mirroring whereby the caregiver plays back the infant's emotional states to the infant through facial and vocal expressions that are "marked," exaggerated, or "pretend," not real.[3,57]

Fonagy and colleagues[3] hypothesize that, over time, the infant learns to decouple mental states from reality through the building up of second-order representations communicated by the caregiver's marked responses. These investigators see this very early use of "pretend" as a way of establishing affect regulation and see it as a way the child learns to separate inside from outside, me from not me, and as an important forerunner of mentalization. Mentalization is the human being's unique capacity to understand that there is not a single perspective of the world, but that meaning is personally created and is subjective.

Psychoanalytic investigators have written that playing, apart from its particular content, contributes to mastery,[1,20] integration and repair of disturbing experience,[20] problem solving,[19] regulation and integration of affect,[58] making experience meaningful and coherent,[17,55,58] promoting reality testing and theory of mind,[3,4] developing insightfulness,[59,60] and enhancing the ability to achieve intimacy in relationships through communication and shared meaning.[58] A therapist is a highly skilled play partner. By scaffolding and expanding the child's play, a therapist helps the child to hone a developmental tool that can be used to make sense of important affective themes in life, and that can be used to structure and organize future experience. Play in this sense is not so much about uncovering meaning as discovering meaning.[5]

Unlike reveries and daydreams, play is primarily social. Even when children play alone, as many 2-year-olds do, the play is often about social experiences or requires approval from the sidelines.[5] At ages 5 to 7 years, imaginary play becomes an even more complex social activity that occurs with peers. Children negotiate how they will play together: they have to decide what stories and themes will be played out, who will pretend to be whom, and whose perspective will prevail. This process involves turn-taking, flexibility, an understanding that different people have different ideas, and the willingness to compromise in order to stay engaged and part of the game. Participating in this kind of social play is obviously related to the child's capacity to mentalize and to participate in joint making of meaning. For children in whom these social capacities are impaired or lag behind, the play process enhances these developmental skills.[36]

SUMMARY

Imaginary play is privileged as a clinical technique in working with children, because it is often the child's best way of communicating affects, fantasies, and internal states as well as complex conceptions about the self and the world. Pretend play relies on a narrative structure and, like language, uses conceptual metaphor. It also uses nonsymbolic, action components that communicate meaning. Because imaginary play is pretend, children are freer to express their forbidden and conflicted thoughts in play, removed from the constraints of reality and their conscience. Consequently, one of the best ways for the therapist to enter the child's world is to do so from within the displacement of the play process. Interpreting the unconscious meaning of the play material directly or attributing the feelings or wishes directly to the child may easily shut down the play process, as well as miss some of the nuance. Because play can be read on multiple levels, it is important to be open to the many different levels of meaning on which the play may be operating. We cannot assume a one-to-one correspondence between the child's play and what the child has actually experienced. Rather than finding one overarching meaning of a particular piece of play, it is often the ability of the therapist to help the child to continue to elaborate different meanings that is the most useful therapeutic technique.

There are many children who cannot play for a variety of clinical reasons, and it is the therapist's goal in these cases to teach the child, as far as possible, to use play as a means of self-expression and as a way to create meaning in the presence of another. Many investigators believe that just as play promotes growth in normal development, play in therapy enhances a child's capacities to relate, negotiate shared meaning, and regulate affect, quite apart from the particular symbolic content of the play itself.

REFERENCES

1. Freud S: Beyond the pleasure principle (1908). In: Strachey J, editor and translator. Standard edition, vol. 18. London: Hogarth Press; 1955. p. 1–64.
2. Gilmore K. Pretend play and development in early childhood (with implications for the oedipal phase). J Am Psychoanal Assoc 2011;59(6):1157–81.
3. Fonagy P, Gergely G, Jurist EL, et al. Affect regulation, mentalization, and the development of self. New York: Other Press; 2002.
4. Mayes LC, Cohen DJ. Children's developing theory of mind. J Am Psychoanal Assoc 1996;44:117–42.
5. Slade A, Wolf DP. Children at play. New York: Oxford University Press; 1994.
6. Scarlett WG. Play, cure, and development: perspective on the psychoanalytic treatment of young children. In: Slade A, Wolff DP, editors. Children at play. New York: Oxford University Press; 1994. p. 48–61.
7. Neubauer PB. The many meanings of play: introduction. Psychoanal Study Child 1987;42:3–9.
8. Yanof JA. Technique in child analysis. In: Person ES, Cooper AM, Gabbard GO, editors. Textbook of psychoanalysis. Washington, DC: American Psychiatric Publishing, Inc; 2005. p. 267–80.
9. Yanof JA, Harrison AM. Technique in child analysis. In: Gabbard GO, Litowitz BE, Williams P, editors. Textbook of psychoanalysis. Washington, DC: American Psychiatric Publishing, Inc; 2012. p. 333–48.
10. Modell A. Other times, other realities. Cambridge (MA): Harvard University Press; 1990.
11. Siegel DJ. The developing mind: how relationships and the brain interact to shape who we are. New York: Guildford Press; 1999.
12. Lakoff G, Johnson M. Metaphors we live by. Chicago: University of Chicago Press; 1980.
13. Lakoff G. Women, fire, and dangerous things. Chicago: University of Chicago Press; 1987.
14. Lakoff G, Johnson M. Philosophy in the flesh. New York: Basic Books; 1999.
15. Modell A. Imagination and the meaningful brain. Cambridge (MA): MIT Press; 2003.

16. Ferro A. The bi-personal field: experiences in child analysis. London: Routledge; 1999.
17. Mayes LC, Cohen DJ. Playing and therapeutic action in child analysis. Int J Psychoanal 1993;74:1235–44.
18. Ritvo S. The psychoanalytic process in childhood. Psychoanal Study Child 1978; 33:295–305.
19. Neubauer PB. Playing: technical implications. In: Solnit AJ, Cohen DJ, Neubauer PB, editors. The many meanings of play. New Haven (CT): Yale University Press; 1993. p. 44–53.
20. Waelder A. The psychoanalytic theory of play. Psychoanal Q 1933;2:208–24.
21. Freud A. Normality and pathology in childhood (1965). In: The writings of Anna Freud, vol. 6. New York: International Universities Press; 1974. p. 25–63.
22. Lilleskov RK. Transference and transference neurosis. In: Kanzer M, editor. The unconscious today. New York: International University Press; 1971. p. 400–8.
23. Tyson P. Transference and developmental issues in the analysis of a prelatency child. Psychoanal Study Child 1978;33:213–36.
24. Sandler J, Kennedy H, Tyson R. The technique of child analysis. Cambridge (MA): Harvard University Press; 1980.
25. Abrams S. Differentiation and integration. Psychoanal Study Child 1996;51: 25–34.
26. Abrams S, Solnit AJ. Coordinating developmental and psychoanalytic processes: conceptualizing technique. J Am Psychoanal Assoc 1998;46:85–103.
27. Klein M. The psychoanalysis of children (1932). New York: Delacorte Press/Seymour Lawrence; 1975. p. xv–xvi.
28. Klein M. The psychoanalytic play technique. Am J Orthopsychiatry 1955;25: 223–37.
29. Chused JF. The transference neurosis in child analysis. Psychoanal Study Child 1988;43:51–81.
30. Yanof JA. Language, communication, and transference in child analysis. J Am Psychoanal Assoc 1996;44:79–116.
31. Gilmore K. Play in the psychoanalytic setting: ego capacity, ego state, and vehicle for intersubjective exchange. Psychoanal Study Child 2005;60:213–38.
32. Cicchetti D, Beeghly M, Weiss-Perry B. Symbolic development in Down syndrome and autism. In: Slade A, Wolf D, editors. Children at play. New York: Oxford University Press; 1994. p. 206–37.
33. Cohen DJ, Volkmar FR. Handbook of autism and pervasive developmental disorders. New York: Wiley; 1997.
34. Woidor S, Greenspan SI. Climbing the symbolic ladder in the DIR model through floor time/interactive play. Autism 2003;7:4.
35. Wachs T. Multidimensional correlates of individual variability in play and exploration. New Dir Child Dev 1993;59:43–53.
36. Lyons-Ruth K. Play, precariousness, and the negotiation of shared meaning: a developmental research perspective on child psychotherapy. J Infant Child Adolesc Psychother 2006;5:142–9.
37. Howes C. The collaborative construction of pretend. Albany (NY): State University of New York Press; 1992.
38. Main M, Kaplan N, Cassidy J. Security in infancy, childhood, and adulthood: a move to the level of representation. In: Bretherton I, Waters E, editors. Growing points of attachment theory and research. Monograph for the series of child development, vol. 50 (1–2), serial no. 209. Chicago: University of Chicago Press; 1985. p. 66–104.

39. Solomon J, George C, DeJong A. Children classified as controlling at age six: evidence of disorganized representational strategies and aggression at home and at school. Dev Psychopathol 1995;7:447–63.
40. Erikson E. Studies in interpretation of play I. clinical observations of play disruption in young children. Genet Psychol Monogr 1940;22:557–671.
41. Winnicott D. Playing: a theoretical statement (1971). In: Playing and reality. London: Tavistock; 1986. p. 38–52.
42. Winnicott D. The piggle. New York: International Universities Press; 1977.
43. Stern DN, Sander LW, Nahum JP, et al. Non-interpretive mechanisms in psychoanalytic therapy. Int J Psychoanal 1998;79:903–21.
44. Harrison AM, Tronick E. "The noise monitor": a developmental perspective on verbal and nonverbal meaning-making.in psychoanalysis. J Am Psychoanal Assoc 2011;59:961–82.
45. Rees E. Introduction. J Am Psychoanal Assoc 2012;60(2):227–9.
46. Vivona JM. Is there a nonverbal period of development? J Am Psychoanal Assoc 2012;60(2):231–65.
47. Bucci W. Is there language disconnected from sensory/bodily experience in speech or thought? J Am Psychoanal Assoc 2012;60(2):275–85.
48. Litowitz BE. Why this question: commentary on Vivona. J Am Psychoanal Assoc 2012;60(2):267–74.
49. Gabbard GO, Westen D. Rethinking therapeutic action. Int J Psychoanal 2003; 84:823–41.
50. Bucci W. Pathways of emotional communication. Psychoanal Inq 2001;21:40–70.
51. Winnicott D. Playing and reality. London: Tavistock; 1986.
52. Cohen PM, Solnit AJ. Play and therapeutic action. Psychoanal Study Child 1993; 48:49–63.
53. Solnit AJ, Cohen DJ, Neubauer PB. The many meanings of play. New Haven: Yale University Press; 1993.
54. Neubauer PB. The role of displacement in psychoanalysis. Psychoanal Study Child 1994;49:107–19.
55. Ablon SL. The therapeutic action of play. J Am Acad Child Adolesc Psychiatry 1996;35:545–7.
56. Frankel JB. The play's the thing: how the essential processes of therapy are most clearly seen in child therapy. Psychoanal Dialogues 1998;8(1):149–82.
57. Gergeley G, Watson JS. The social biofeedback theory of parental affect-mirroring. Int J Psychoanal 1996;77:1181–212.
58. Slade A. Making meaning and making believe: their role in the clinical process. In: Slade A, Wolff DP, editors. Children at play. New York: Oxford University Press; 1994. p. 81–107.
59. Sugarman A. A new model for conceptualizing insightfulness in the psychoanalysis of young children. Psychoanal Q 2003;72:325–55.
60. Sugarman A. The use of play to promote insightfulness in the analysis of children suffering from cumulative trauma. Psychoanal Q 2008;77:799–833.

Games Children Play

Board Games in Psychodynamic Psychotherapy

Jill Bellinson, PhD[a,b,c,d,e,f,g,*]

KEYWORDS

- Play therapy • Middle childhood • Psychodynamic psychotherapy
- Psychoanalytic psychotherapy • Board games in psychotherapy
- Psychotherapeutic play

KEY POINTS

- Actions are the language of early childhood; words are the language of adulthood; and structured game play can be the language of the developmental stage in between known as latency or middle childhood.
- The issues we see in board game play in the treatment room, as long as we allow children to use the game creatively rather than insist on the box-top rules, are often precisely the issues that led to the referral for treatment.
- Playing board games, we can observe when and how children bend and break the rules, understanding and interpreting what makes them frustrated or overwhelmed or unable to bear an assault to their self-esteem.
- Children use games during treatment to contain their uncomfortable feelings and unacceptable behaviors, freeing the child to function productively in the real world.

Zach and I are playing Mousetrap. He throws the die, counts his turn, and asks me what the square he has landed on means. He performs the assigned task and hands me the dice. This continues through much of our session, as we build the mousetrap and take our chances gaining and losing ground or pieces of cheese.

Disclosures: Dr Bellinson is on the Board of Directors of Division 39 (Psychoanalysis) of the American Psychological Association and Past-President of the Child and Adolescent Section of the division. She is Associate Editor of the *Journal of Infant, Child, and Adolescent Psychotherapy* and author of *Children's Use of Board Games in Psychotherapy* and numerous articles on psychodynamic and psychoanalytic treatment.

[a] William Alanson White Institute, New York, NY, USA; [b] Adelphi University, New York, NY, USA; [c] Institute for Psychoanalytic Training and Research, New York, NY, USA; [d] New York Institute for Psychotherapy Training, Brooklyn, NY, USA; [e] Metropolitan Institute for Training in Psychoanalytic Psychotherapy, New York, NY, USA; [f] Clinical Psychology Doctoral Program, City University of New York, New York, NY, USA; [g] Clinical Psychology Doctoral Program, Teachers' College, Columbia University, New York, NY, USA
* Private Practice Psychologist and Psychoanalyst, 229 West 71st Street, New York, NY 10023.
E-mail address: bellinsonj@nyc.rr.com

This description suggests the kind of blocked communication and defensive use of time that many therapists believe arise from structured games in the playroom. In the early history of our literature, there were only a handful of articles[1,2] about using board games productively in child therapy, and most of these recommended using games to forge alliances before beginning treatment with children rather than as part of the treatment itself. Supervisors often advised young therapists to keep board games out of the playroom.

DEVELOPMENTAL CONTEXT OF BOARD GAMES

Children do play structured games in their lives; it is their preferred mode of play through most of their school years. Games permit expression and working through[3–6] of many of the developmental tasks of middle childhood, referred to as the latency period in psychoanalytic theory. Children learn to sit still, wait their turn, delay gratification, share with peers, tolerate losing, and find ways to restrain the direct expression of their impulses (**Box 1**). Such are the developmental tasks of latency[7,8] and the demands from society for school-age children. We expect the normal play of latency-age children to show a decrease in dramatic play and an increase in the structure of their games.

Clinical example of developmental progression expressed in board games

Consider the play of Isaiah, at age 6 years:

We sit on the floor to play Memory, in which we turn over cards and try to find their match. This version of the game has circular cards, in the form of Pokeballs on their back side, and Pokemon figures to try to match. We play by the rulebook for a while, turning over 2 cards (or occasionally 3 or 4, when Isaiah needs an extra turn) to search for the right Pokemon figures.

When Isaiah is matchless for a few turns, he begins to imagine battles between the 2 non-matching figures, and he then directs me to participate with him. We each turn over a card, making suitable noises as we reveal our respective Pokemon figures, which then battle using the powers they have on television: "Pikachu, I choose you! Head-butt, now!" we say. "Charizar, lighting bolt! Now!" This is so stimulating that Isaiah regresses, and we have to stand to continue the battle; soon he has us eliminate the cards to become Pokemon figures ourselves, battling with our own imaginary lightning bolts and fireballs. This continues dramatically and expressively for a few minutes, after which Isaiah has us sit on the floor and begin the next round of Memory.

Box 1
Developmental tasks of latency addressed in board games

Developmental tasks of latency addressed in board games include learning to:

- Sit still
- Wait your turn
- Delay gratification
- Share with peers
- Tolerate losing
- Restrain the direct expression of impulses

Isaiah clearly demonstrates a typical developmental progression from using the self as a play figure, through using action figures—here, the cards and their Pokemon drawings—to a fully sublimated game of remembering and matching. Isaiah begins with the most mature behavior, playing the game by the rules, but as he becomes excited he reverses the developmental trajectory. When he cannot maintain the structure and control of the sublimated version, he regresses to action figures; when this, too, becomes overstimulating, he regresses further to an infantile stage at which his own body is his only means of expression. This process allows him to release his bound-up physical energy, which enables him to sit down to a more mature version of play, until his energy builds again, and we repeat the sequence.

At 6 years, Isaiah is too young to be fully rid of magical thinking, but he is working toward it. In a few years, by the time he is 9 or 10, we expect he will no longer need direct motoric expression of his thoughts and feelings. However, he will not yet be able to talk as adolescents and adults do in treatment, and board games may then be his preferred recreational activity. If we are going to provide effective treatment for children during these years, we have to learn to play board games therapeutically.

PLAYING BOARD GAMES PSYCHOTHERAPEUTICALLY

Although the activities of structured games may be developmentally appropriate for latency-aged children, the play itself seems devoid of psychodynamic meaning. What latent content could possibly be revealed in dice-throwing and money-counting? How on earth could we discover anything about children's unconscious when they simply pick up cards and put them down?

Therapeutic Games

There are certainly games designed to be psychotherapeutic[9,10]; these were created to elicit information about the child's life and inner world. Games such as Gardner's[9] Talking, Feeling, Doing Game ask children, and the therapists playing with them, to talk about their thoughts and feelings. The games can be interesting and fun, and a helpful aid, for children trying to talk but in need of prompts.

But most children do not talk; they shrug and grunt, and seem to dread questions and conversations. The language of childhood is action; they express themselves in behavior rather than words, particularly when they are emotionally stimulated by anxiety or other complex feelings. A Talking Game might not seem playful for them; in the words of one 8-year-old who tried it, "why would anyone want to play that game?" In addition, the issues raised are those on the cards drawn at random, and might not pertain to the child playing at all, and might overlook the issues most pressing for the child. Therapists, too, are often uncomfortable with therapeutic games because they, too, are expected to self-disclose in answer to the cards they draw.

Ordinary Games

The alternative to using contrived therapeutic games is to use the ordinary games children play, which on the surface might seem not to be therapeutic at all. I (J.B., the author of this article) use the term "board games" to mean any structured game, regardless of whether it is actually played with a board. Games played with cards, dominoes, marbles, and other material all apply, as long as there are rules one is expected to follow.

I do not discuss electronic games here, although I have done so elsewhere,[11,12] because their use is somewhat different from games in which materials can be directly manipulated by the child. Children do play electronic games, often incessantly, and we should find ways to use them in therapy as well. However, while there are tricks, short-cuts, and "cheats" for electronic games they are not under the direct control of the playing child, so they do not lend themselves to the therapeutic techniques for playing described in this article.

We have to find ways to therapeutically use board games that on the surface do not seem to contain much communicative material—at least, if we follow the rules. The rules call for throwing the dice, counting the squares, and paying the money: all deadly dull activities that are psychodynamically uninteresting. Play according to the rules does indeed lack communication of deeper, psychodynamic material.

CHILDREN IN THERAPY DO NOT FOLLOW THE RULES

The good news is: children in therapy do not follow the rules! Their presenting problem is often just that. Children cannot sit in their seats, do not do what they are told, refuse to share, will not wait their turn, and are easily overwhelmed by their own frustration. These issues are precisely those most evoked by structured games. Moreover, these are the issues we see in board-game play in the treatment room, as long as we allow children to use the game creatively rather than insist on the box-top rules.

If we allow children to play the game as they need to, stretching and bending rules whenever and wherever they need to, following or breaking or creating the structure of the game, they will show us just how they experience their world. Allowing the children to play as they need to makes sense in dramatic play; we would never tell a child how to use dollhouse figures or what to draw with crayons. We need to apply these same therapeutic rules to the way we use board-game play in the treatment room. We can observe when and how children bend and break the rules, understanding and inter-preting what makes them frustrated or overwhelmed or unable to bear an assault to their self-esteem.

In Isaiah's case, for example, we can understand that he was interested in mastering self-control. His interest in a structured game was a sign to me that he was develop-mentally ready to explore rule-following, and, probably, that he wanted help with it. He played by the rules until he could no longer bear the frustration, then showed me his difficulties and his methods of coping. First, he took extra turns. He wanted to continue to follow the rules (taking turns, turning over one card at a time, giving over the turn if a match was not found), but needed a little extra help, like a handicap would be in golf. So he turned over 3 or 4 cards instead of 2, and still relinquished his turn if he did not find a match. When even this was too frustrating, he lost his ability to maintain the structure and regressed to a stage of more active, motoric play. Interestingly this release of energy allowed him to recover his ego strength, regain his self-control, and return to the structured game. I took this to indicate the psychic structure in his life outside the treatment room as well, where he could not maintain the structure of rule-following at school and at home. There, too, he needed motoric release of his pent-up frustrations. There, too, he was capable of recovery on his own if allowed the time and space to do so. I can watch this pattern in dramatic play, and I can also see it in the rhythms of Isaiah's structured game play, as long as I allow him to stretch and bend rules in any way he decides to.

Many therapists focus on keeping children such as Isaiah rule-bound, perhaps worrying about appearing to condone cheating. Such a therapist might admonish him to turn over only 2 cards per turn, sit in his seat, and finish the game, and that ther-apist might obtain compliance from Isaiah. Teachers and parents can often keep chil-dren following their rules as long as they stay with the child and repeatedly remind them. However, that therapist would not have succeeded in helping Isaiah develop the ability to follow the rules independently, and would not have understood anything about Isaiah's reasons for being unable to do so.

My understanding of Isaiah's difficulties was that he was developmentally not yet able to succeed. His attempts to follow rules, even during his struggles, suggested how hard he was trying. His excited dramatic play indicated the level of energy (perhaps anxiety) bound in his attempts to play. His spontaneous return to the game, independent of anything I did or said, revealed his determination and capacity to regain his mature developmental level after a brief regression.

CHOICE OF PLAY

When children come into my office, I follow their lead on what to do and where to do it. The children can choose toys, art materials, or board games, or roam aimlessly around the room, demonstrating their approach to life and to the treatment process itself. This freedom to choose applies to their choice of board games as well. If we allow children to define their own play during their sessions, the game a child picks tells us something about him or herself.

- Does she pick a game appropriate to her age level, or something for much younger or older children? Here we can learn something about how she fits in her own skin, whether she longs to remain a baby or to grow up faster.
- Does he want games of luck or games with some skill involved? This choice shows us, for instance, how he is likely to approach schoolwork: blindly hoping for the best or trying hard to succeed, confident in his skills or preferring to not even use them, believing he is a victim of his unfair teachers or the master of his own fate.
- Does she play the same game over and over, or does she like to explore many different kinds of games; that is, does she cling to the comfort of the tried and true, or is she a risk-taker?
- Does he prefer games with hostile options, such as games in which he can send me back to Start or sentence me to Jail or impose a flat tire on my trip? If so, how comfortable (or flamboyant!) is he with his own aggressive impulses? (**Box 2**)

STYLE OF PLAY

After we consider what games children choose, we can watch the style of their play. Are they active or passive? Dramatic or subdued? Do they tell us the rules or ask us? Do they want to use the rules or make up their own? If they make up their own game, is their new game structured—like Isaiah, who makes an adventure battle when two different Pokemon pieces turn up on the Memory game? Or is it unstructured—like Claire,[4] who uses the Clue board for an imaginary dinner party and ballroom dance? These choices parallel children's approaches to life, so we can interpret the way they

---

Box 2
Features to observe in game choice

- Is the game age appropriate?
- Is it a game of luck or skill?
- Is the same game played over and over again?
- Does the game have hostile options that allow the expression of aggression?

use games as the way they experience other life events, just as we would with dramatic play in a dollhouse or with action figures.

Most informative is the way children show themselves when they break the rules. Some children start immediately, from the first move, as if even beginning to follow a structure is unbearable for them. Many play according to box-top rules for a few turns, but then play creatively when something happens to make them need to break rules. Some children may not be able to stand it when I get ahead by a little, or by a lot. Or it may be too painful to lose a turn, go to jail, or tolerate setbacks. At those moments, when the rules become too constraining, children protect their self-esteem by changing the game. When they do this tells us what kinds of situations put their self-esteem at risk.

Some children worry most about my position: am I lucky, am I ahead, am I gaining on them? Others barely notice my place in the game, and care only whether their own turn is good enough.

How children change the game is also expressive. Do they do it openly, or try to hide it? Some pretend that they aren't changing the game ("it's on the line," "I dropped the dice"), others admit they did ("I don't like that number," "I'm taking a do-over?"). Or is the threat they feel so overwhelming that they cannot continue to play the game at all? If so, do they quietly abandon the game to do something else (some children start game after game, never progressing past their first setback) or do they feel so bad about themselves that they throw the game around the room and lose their ability to stay related to us? And for how long? Can they throw the game, scream, and start over, or do they need to storm out of the treatment room, for a minute or for the rest of the session? (**Box 3**)

We can watch all this unfold in a session, much as we watch a dollhouse drama unfold or follow a painting being created, trying to understand what our child patients are experiencing and what they are trying to tell us about themselves. We can play along, just as we do when our action figures are shooting at each other. And we can interpret what we see: "it's hard for you to stand it when I get ahead"; "it feels too bad when you get sent back to Start"; "you need an extra turn so you don't lose this game"; or, a bit ironically, "isn't that lucky that the dice turned out just like you hoped for!"

Box 3
Observing the child who changes the rules

When does the child change the rules?

- Immediately?
- When something happens in the game the child cannot tolerate?

How does the child change the game?

- Openly or covertly?
- By quitting the game?
- Switching to a different game?
- Switching to a different activity?
- By having a tantrum?

Does the child need to avoid the therapist when the rules change?

A case illustration: style of play

Let us look back at the example given at the beginning of this article, the Mousetrap player, Zach. He plays very close to the box-top rules, most of every game for several sessions. He is young (not yet 6 years) so he takes some time to understand the game, and he prefers the excitement of the 3-dimensional trap we create to the mundane routine of the structured play, as is appropriate to his age. Soon, he asks that we build the whole mousetrap before we begin the game; this turns out to be less satisfying than he expected, because it takes such a long uneventful time to proceed to the end this way, so we return to building as we go. Next, he refuses to land on special squares; this means he never goes back to Start or loses a turn or a piece of cheese, but it also means he never gets extra pieces of cheese, because he does not distinguish beneficial special squares from disadvantageous. This progression is common to many children who play the game: the mousetrap is indeed fun, so they often create the trap faster than the board calls for, and they almost always ask to try it out as every piece is added. Bad-luck squares are avoided by many children in many games.

Zach's next modification is more unique. He lands on the Turn Crank square, where he can place me under the basket and trap me in the mousetrap, thus winning the game. Instead, he leaves me where I am—several squares back from being trapped—and places the mice not in use under the basket. He then traps them with glee, over and over again, and delights as we pretend to make them scream.

This approach to play parallels Zach's approach to life. He cannot bear setbacks of any kind, and when he is threatened with bad news he refuses to hear it. He changes the subject, or runs out of the room, or hits his sister (which also changes the subject), or hides in the bushes. At home, he also shouts, "No! I'm NOT going to do that! NO!" In the office at this early stage of our work, he protects me from his outbursts but he continues to avoid setbacks in every game we play, and he includes me in the avoidance as well:

- In the Mousetrap game he keeps both of us out of the trap, and prefers to trap other anonymous mice instead.
- In Candyland, we remove all the picture cards before we begin to play
- In Don't Wake Daddy, we move around the board—he much faster than I, skipping squares if needed—but neither of us is allowed to push the button that might cause Daddy to wake up.
- Similarly, in dramatic play, we use only the toothless puppets (no sharks or alligators), and we eat only cookies if we want to, whether we've finished our vegetables or not.

These are all metaphoric expressions of Zach's experience in living: he is happy and productive, intelligent and mature, collaborative and cooperative—as long as things go his way. Setbacks and disappointments are unbearable, so he refuses to have them; in the playroom—so far—by removing them from the field, in real life by angry and regressive outbursts. I can see his discomfort rise and fall in the board games just as in dramatic play or in reports from his parents, and I can interpret them and help him with them wherever they arise.

Board games, then, represent just one more mode of expression for understanding a child's psychodynamics. Actions are the language of early childhood; words are the language of adulthood; and structured game play can be the language of the developmental stage in between known as latency or middle childhood.

THERAPIST TECHNIQUES

Once we understand and formulate the psychodynamics communicated by a child's board-game play, how do we use the play? How can it be therapeutic?

First, a word about the way I structure my own play. For children not yet engaging in the structure of the game, I play along with them. So I participate in imaginary battles or dinner parties or candy-eating orgies whether those take place on the floor, in a doll-house, or on a game board. When a child demonstrates that she wants to play a struc-tured form of a game, I play by the box-top rules. I remain a steady, predictable object, a model of polite society. I can be relied on to be bound by the rules no matter how tempting it may be to stretch them to get ahead, and I am benevolent even though I lose every round, every game. When a child tells me "you can play that way, too. "Really," I say, "I know, but I like to play the way the box-top says to." My patient can be reassured that my own boundaries are secure, and his own need to take extra turns, miscount the squares, escape from Jail, and win at all costs will never be challenged.

I am not saying that I do not notice these breaches. I am not always successful, but I do try to see the child's creative play as soon as it begins, and remark on it in some way.

I use several different kinds of comments at these times (**Box 4**).

- Interpretations of awareness:
    "It took a lot of throws to get the number you wanted."
    "You landed on that Extra-Turn square when I thought your number came out on the one before."
    "You seem to get every 'slide' square every turn."
    "You're going to keep picking till you get a 'Sorry'."
- Interpretations of feelings:
    "You didn't like that number."
    "You really want the Princess Lolly card."
    "It hurts so much to have to go backward."
    "You hate it when I have a lucky turn."
- Interpretations of circumstances:
    "You need to be waaaaay ahead of me."
    "You missed it three times, and now you're going to make sure you get it."
    "You're dealing yourself all the good cards so I won't have any chance."
    "One lose-a-turn was OK for you, but two is too many."

Notice that none of these mention winning or losing the game. The end result is likely to be that my patient wins and I lose, but that is still many minutes away. I focus on the immediate situation and my patient's response to it. He was unhappy that I got an extra turn from throwing doubles, so he took two (or four) turns of his own; she did not get a match on her last turn, so she steals a pair of cards from me; he got very close to Home, and could not bear to wait another turn or two. This way, there are dozens of opportunities for interpretations during every board game, long before either of us wins or loses.

Box 4
Kinds of therapist comments on the child's play

- Interpretations of awareness
- Interpretations of feelings
- Interpretations of circumstances
- Interpretations of outcome: winning/losing

Interpretations of outcome:

- Winning
  "You needed to win, and you did."
  "You got it! You took that win!"
  "You beat me, AGAIN."
  "You love it when you win."
- Losing
  "How did I lose, again?"
  "I lose every single time."
  "I never stand a chance when I play with you." (pretend crying)

When I talk about my losing, I try to be sure I remain playful (I try to be sure I FEEL playful!) while I express the experience of feeling like a loser. I assume my patient feels that way often, and my describing the feeling with empathy will show her that I understand what it feels like to be in that situation. I survive the loss and can describe the feeling without anger or retaliation, and I am always open to playing, and losing, again. In this way, I create an environment where my patient can win, can play aggressively, can act out his rage or revenge toward those who win over him, and can take whatever steps he needs to express and work through his feelings safely, even when the structure of the game itself, by the rulebook, implies otherwise.

TREATMENT PROGRESS

What I have found in many years of using board games in this way is that children can work out their difficulties with the structure demanded of them in their lives. The first step in this process is often that they play creatively with me and fairly with their friends. Richard played chess by 'Richard Rules' in my office and box-top rules with his uncle and classmates.[3,4] Frances played "spit" with me—starting before my cards were set up, removing my cards from the pile or placing hers under mine, grabbing the smaller pile at the end of each round—while her relationships with peers became conflict-free. Kal threw game equipment around the room whenever he began to lose, so he could be fairer and neater in school.[4]

In this way, children use games during the treatment to contain their uncomfortable feelings and unacceptable behaviors, freeing them to function productively in life outside.

Later, children try out challenges in their board-game play before they risk anything in their outside life. Adena played Monopoly backward and tried Life without homeowners insurance,[4] frightening gambles for someone who was desperate for security in her life. Frances allowed herself to lose a round, and then a whole game, to see how it felt, within the safety of our therapeutic relationship. Zach tries to push the plunger in Don't Wake Daddy—first letting me do it, while he holds his ears against the scary noise.

Thus, the games serve as a holding environment[13] and fertilize the development of a transference neurosis,[14] bringing symptoms into the treatment room so they can be directed against me as a game opponent, allowing them to be worked through within the game play.

COUNTERTRANSFERENCES

One challenge of playing this way is that it stirs many feelings in the therapist, who must lose over and over again to an opponent who demands special privileges and breaks every rule. Our own competitive impulses can impede our ability to be therapeutic partners for our child patients, and must be monitored and controlled. I find that I usually do not feel very competitive because I don't pay much attention to the game itself; my focus is on how my patient is playing, when and why the play changes, and what his inner experience might be as he plays. I watch for what stirs my patient's need to change the rules, I think about what is unfolding between us as that need rises and falls during a session, and I talk about my patient's feelings and actions as we play. I know I'm going to lose many or most games, not because I allow my patient to win (I wish for my patient to win, when I see her trying to abide by the rules but still needing to win, but I don't alter my own play to purposely lose a round or a game), but because I know my patient needs to be the winner, so she will be bending the rules to guarantee that, and because I am paying attention more to that process than to the outcome of the game I am unlikely to win. Of course, this shift of my attention to the process rather than the winning of the game protects my own self-esteem as I play: I was not really playing to win, so I did not really lose!

As therapists we do have to examine our own countertransferences, and clear the playroom of them whenever possible. If we love a game, or are exceedingly good at it, we should not have it in the room, lest we lose track of our patient's interests and needs in favor of our own. Similarly, if we hate a game, or have a difficult history with it, we should not stock the game on our shelves. A friend whose brothers hostilely trounced her at Monopoly when she was growing up should not have Monopoly in the room.[3,4] I tend to get absorbed in games of physical play, finding it hard to keep my mind on interpretation rather than the play itself, so I do not keep sports equipment in my office.

All this does not mean we will never play those loved or hated games; children bring in whatever they need to, so they will bring their own box or create a game whenever it suits their psychological needs. It remains important for us to be aware of our own feelings and attend to them as they arise in our work. Children in my office create basketball, bringing their own or using my wastebasket and crumpled-up paper, so I play basketball when children want to. Children bring in Stratego, Battleship, and Connect Four, all games I avoid for varying reasons of my own personal preference. I have to be especially careful at such times to scrutinize my own thoughts and feelings, so I can remain focused on my patients' play and experiences rather than my own.

Children's choice of games not available in the playroom is also informative, of course. Are they telling me my games are not good enough? That they need to change rules of play on even such a basic level? The second or third time they bring a game I do not have, are they intentionally stirring those feelings of discomfort in me? I still have to inspect my own countertransference at these times, but I also can interpret the child's participation in the process.

SUMMARY

After children in therapy grow out of the stage of dramatic play, and before they develop the ability to engage in talk therapy, they typically play structured board games. This activity is developmentally appropriate for them, and needs to be a clinically appropriate activity for us as their therapists. If we allow them to play creatively, stretching and bending rules when they feel the need to win or protect their self-esteem, we can learn a great deal about their psyches, thus meeting our goals to gather information about them and help them with their difficulties, and their goals to get help while enjoying the play that comes most naturally to them. These children can show us what is on their minds and how they struggle in life, and we can interpret these issues in structured games just as we can in dramatic play or dream recall. Our child patients can improve their functioning and eliminate their symptoms because we create an attentive holding environment[13] where their problems can unfold. The children show us their difficulties and we interpret their experience, and they work through their impediments to healthy functioning. Children play games, and we all win the therapy.

REFERENCES

1. Loomis EA Jr. The use of checkers in handling certain resistances in child therapy and child analysis. In: Haworth MR, editor. Child psychotherapy. New York: Basic Books; 1964. p. 407–11.
2. Meeks JE. Children who cheat at games. J Am Acad Child Psychiatry 1970;9(1): 157–70.
3. Bellinson J. Shut up and move: children's use of board games in psychotherapy. J Infant Child Adolesc Psychother 2000;1(2):23–41.
4. Bellinson J. Children's use of board games in psychotherapy. Northvale (NJ): Jason Aronson; 2002.
5. Herman J. Treating the cheater: an ego and self psychological approach to working through of the cheating syndrome in the treatment of latency age children. J Infant Child Adolesc Psychother 2000;1(2):59–70.
6. Krimendahl EK. "Did you see that?": a relational perspective on children who cheat in analysis. J Infant Child Adolesc Psychother 2000;1(2):43–58.
7. Peller LE. Libidinal phases, ego development, and play. Psychoanal Study Child 1954;9:178–98.
8. Sarnoff C. Latency. Northvale (NJ): Jason Aronson, Inc; 1976.
9. Gardner RA. The talking, feeling, doing game. Cresskill (NJ): Creative Therapeutics; 1973.
10. Gardner RA. Psychotherapeutic approaches to the resistant child. New York: Jason Aronson, Inc; 1975.
11. Bellinson J. I beat the level: children's use of Gameboy as therapeutic communication. J Infant Child Adolesc Psychother 2005;4(2):198–208.
12. Bellinson J. Introduction to where the wired things are: children and technology in treatment. J Infant Child Adolesc Psychother 2011;10(4):389–91.
13. Winnicott DW. Maturational processes and the facilitating environment: studies in the theory of emotional development. London: Hogarth Press; 1965.
14. Chused JF. The transference neurosis in child analysis. Psychoanal Study Child 1988;43:51–81.

Mentalizing-Based Treatment with Adolescents and Families

Efrain Bleiberg, MD[a,b],*

KEYWORDS

- Mentalizing • Mentalizing-based treatment • Automatic/implicit mentalizing
- Controlled/explicit mentalizing • Attachment • MBT-A • Mentalizing formulation
- Mentalizing loop

[*Search Tags:* Mentalizing antecedents: psychic equivalence, the pretend mode, the teleologic mode, effortful control of attention, Representation of experience, Remoralization, Remediation, Rehabilitation of mentalizing, The spectrum of interventions, The therapist's stance, Emerging BPD]

KEY POINTS

- Mentalizing-based treatment (MBT), an evidence-based treatment model, is rooted in a psychodynamic framework and in attachment theory and research, and offers a bridge to social neuroscience.
- MBT for adolescents (MBT-A) is based on the view that a core problem for many adolescents is a vulnerability to a breakdown of their mentalizing capacity in particular emotional and interpersonal situations, thus placing mentalizing at the center of the treatment process.
- The basic aim of MBT-A is to promote skills that reestablish mentalizing when it is lost and maintain it in the face of the challenges when it is present.
- The MBT-A protocol outlines competencies that therapists must show to promote mentalizing in patients and families.
- MBT-A deemphasizes interpretation of unconscious motivation, promoting, instead, curiosity about the mental states that patients can link to subjectively felt reality and how these mental states motivate and explain behavior in self and others, making relationships more effective and supportive and allowing affects to become more understandable and manageable.

[a] Child and Adolescence Psychiatry, Menninger Department of Psychiatry & Behavioral Sciences, Baylor College of Medicine, One Baylor Plaza, Houston, TX 77030, USA; [b] Psychiatry, Texas Children's Hospital, One Baylor Plaza, Houston, TX 77030, USA
* Child and Adolescence Psychiatry, Menninger Department of Psychiatry & Behavioral Sciences, Baylor College of Medicine, One Baylor Plaza, Houston, TX 77030.
E-mail address: ebleiberg@menninger.edu

Child Adolesc Psychiatric Clin N Am 22 (2013) 295–330
http://dx.doi.org/10.1016/j.chc.2013.01.001   **childpsych.theclinics.com**

INTRODUCTION

A 17-year-old girl participating in a group focused on mentalizing-based treatment (MBT) was being introduced to the notion that mentalizing refers to the ability to attend and to understand the intentional mental states that are the basis of our behavior. As she grasped that she was being invited to pay attention to how we access minds (our own and those of others), she blurted out "Oh, minds … that is a scary place," and then added "and you wouldn't want to go there alone!" (Allen J, personal communication, 2006).

Such a cry from the heart speaks to the challenges of MBT. If minds can be scary, arguably there is no more scary place than the mind of an adolescent, in which a convergence of neurodevelopmental changes and psychosocial and developmental demands compromises the ability to mentalize. MBTs encourage patients to engage in mentalizing in various relationship contexts (the 1-on-1 context of individual psychotherapy; the context of a group of peers in group therapy; or the context of family interactions in family treatment) and to pay attention to:

a. Specific emotional and relational contexts in which mentalizing becomes "so scary" that it breaks down or is defensively inhibited
b. Skills and attitudes needed to restore the ability to mentalize

This article:

1. Reviews the process of mentalizing, its components, and role in self-regulation and attachment.
2. Examines the neurodevelopmental changes affecting the adolescent's capacity to mentalize and the role of such compromised mentalizing in the adolescent's vulnerability to adaptive breakdown and psychopathology, in general, and to emerging personality disorders, in particular.
3. Discusses the principles, objectives, and core features of mentalizing-based treatment and its application to adolescents (MBT-A) and families (MBT-F).

WHAT IS MENTALIZING?

Mentalizing denotes the pervasive human disposition to understand and interpret human behavior (our own and that of others) as based on mental states (ie, thoughts, feelings, needs, desires, even misconceptions and delusions). Such interpretation makes behavior (and people) meaningful, intentional, and predictable.[1,2] Mentalizing is an aspect of social cognition that lies at the core of our humanity, anchoring our subjective sense of self (our sense of agency, continuity, and the unity of our selves) and our ability to engage in reciprocal, sustaining, effective interactions with others.

A focus on subjective experience and intentionality (ie, on the dynamic forces that give direction to human behavior) is, of course, the hallmark of the psychodynamic approach. However, a mentalizing framework emphasizes not what we have in our mind (ie, the content of our thoughts and motivation) but the capacities and processes that we use to access and interpret mental states. In so doing, the concept of mentalizing links a clinical and theoretic framework rooted in the psychodynamic tradition and in attachment theory with neuroscientific efforts to elucidate the brain processes underlying mentalizing capacity[3–5] and with developmental research aiming at documenting the trajectories leading to robust mentalizing or to the specific mentalizing dysfunctions associated with psychopathologic conditions.[1,6] From this perspective, all psychiatric disorders involve dysfunctional mentalizing, linked to disordered self-experience and an impaired capacity to understand and engage with others.

A growing body of brain imaging studies of social cognition[4,5] documents that mentalizing is a dynamic capacity, affected by stress and arousal, particularly in the context of attachment relationships. Furthermore, this dynamic capacity is not a unitary skill or trait but a multifaceted capacity, with its adaptive functionality residing in the flexible balance between various dimensions of processing of experience. Luyten and colleagues identified the following 4 dimensions of mentalizing processing (**Fig. 1**):

1. Automatic/implicit–controlled/explicit
2. Internally focused–externally focused
3. Self-oriented–other-oriented
4. Cognitive–affective

Automatic/Implicit–Controlled/Explicit

The most fundamental dimension of mentalizing is the polarity of automatic/implicit mentalizing versus controlled/explicit mentalizing. Automatic mentalizing[7] is a form of unreflective, fast, parallel processing that is activated by specific cues or signals and requires little effort, attention, awareness, or intention. This form of processing is nonverbal and is encoded as implicit memories, the activation of which generates procedural patterns of physiology, motricity, perception, and affect.

Controlled or explicit mentalizing, on the other hand, involves the sequential, relatively slow process of representing experience. It requires attention, reflection, and effort. Memories of controlled processing are encoded as explicit memories that are potentially accessible to conscious awareness and can be verbalized. Robust, adaptively balanced mentalizing involves flexibly switching from predominantly automatic to more controlled mentalizing and vice versa, a shift that is guided by an awareness of one's own and others' mental states. For example, when playfully interacting with his spouse, a man relies on automatic, intuitive, unreflective feelings and procedural patterns and expectations about self, the other, and self with the other. On noticing that his wife has become unusually silent and emotionally distant, he switches to reflecting and enquiring about what may be wrong and what may be going on in her mind.

Internally Focused–Externally Focused

A second dimension in mentalizing processing, emerging from neuroimaging research,[8] refers to processing that focuses on visible physical features or actions of oneself or others, or processing that relies on imagining one's own or others' internal, not observable, subjective experience.

Self-Oriented Other-Oriented

Mentalizing also involves a balance between a focus on one's own mental states (self-orientation) and a focus on the mental states of others (other-orientation).[9,10]

Implicit/Automatic		Explicit/Controlled
Non-conscious, non-verbal, non-reflective	VS	Conscious – or potentially conscious – verbalizable, reflective
Affective	VS	Cognitive
External	VS	Internal
Self	VS	Other

Fig. 1. Aspects of mentalizing.

Cognitive–Affective

Full mentalization entails the balanced integration of cognition (described as theory-of-mind propositions: eg, "I–believe Johnny–took the cookies") and affect (the embodied or empathizing processing: eg, "I feel bad–you feel hurt–by what I said").[11]

Stress and Arousal Effect on Mentalizing

As mentioned earlier, a key feature that affects the capacity to maintain a flexible, adaptive mentalizing balance is the effect of stress and arousal on each mode of mentalizing. Stress and increased arousal facilitate automatic mentalizing, along with an activation of the attachment system, which, as[12–15] noted, is preprogrammed to be triggered by fear and built-in cues signaling danger to the survival of the self. Controlled mentalizing, on the other hand, is facilitated by arousal up to a certain level of stress (the switch point), at which point, controlled mentalizing becomes inhibited (**Fig. 2**).[16–20]

Neural Systems Related to Mentalizing

Each of the 4 dimensions of mentalizing is related to relatively distinct neural systems. For example, evidence from neuroimaging studies points to 2 different neural systems underlying automatic and controlled mentalizing.[21] Automatic mentalizing has been linked to activation of the amygdala, basal ganglia, ventromedial prefrontal cortex, lateral temporal cortex, dorsal anterior cingulated cortex, and the mirror neuron system. These are phylogenetically older brain circuits that rely heavily on sensory information and procedural matching (feeling the other's feelings or evoking feelings in the other that match our own). Brain circuits implicated in controlled mentalizing include the medial prefrontal cortex, the lateral prefrontal cortex, lateral parietal cortex, medial parietal cortex, medial temporal lobe, and anterior cingulated cortex. These are phylogenetically newer brain circuits that rely on linguistic, categorical, symbolic information that seeks to generate representational or narrative coherence (produce categories or stories that are coherent and make sense) (**Fig. 3**).[22–24]

Patient Mentalizing Ability

A central aspect of the mentalizing-based approach to treatment is the assessment and monitoring of the individual patient's mentalizing abilities in each dimension,

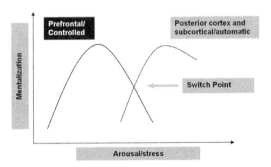

Fig. 2. A biobehavioral switch model of the relationship between stress and controlled versus automatic mentalization (based on Luyten and colleagues, 2012). (*Adapted from* Luytman P, Fonagy P, Lowyck B, et al. Assessment of mentalization. In: Bateman A, Fonagy P, editors. Handbook of mentalizing in mental health practice. Washington, DC: American Psychiatric Publishing; 2012; with permission.)

IMPLICIT/AUTOMATIC	vs	EXPLICIT/CONTROLLED
Amygdala, basal ganglia, ventromedial pre-frontal cortex, dorsal anterior cingulated cortex	vs	Lateral prefrontal cortex, medial prefrontal cortex, lateral parietal cortex, medial parietal cortex, medial temporal lobe, rostral anterior cingulated cortex
Older circuits relying on sensory information (external)	vs	Newer circuits involved in linguistic and symbolic processing (internal)
Perceived, felt, procedural, non-conscious, non-verbal, unreflective	vs	Interpreted verbal conscious (or potentially conscious), verbal and reflective
Fast, requires little effort, focused attention or intention	vs	Slower, sequential, requires attention, intention, and effort
Facilitated by arousal	vs	Inhibited by arousal

Fig. 3. Implicit/automatic versus explicit/controlled.

particularly in the specific attachment contexts in which mentalizing impairments are manifested. Therefore, the mentalizing-based evaluation yields a specific mentalizing profile, as is discussed later. Adolescents, particularly those with an emerging border-line personality disorder (BPD), often present a mentalizing profile characterized by a predominance of unreflective, rigid, automatic assumptions, held with unjustified certainty about the internal states of mind of self or others, overly focused on external features of self and others, and emphasizing overwhelming affective states. This profile is evident in the context of the stress associated with attachment, which can be rapidly hyperactivated, a context in which they engage in excessive and typically inaccurate efforts to interpret other people's mental states (hypermentalizing).

For example, a young girl of 16 years, on noticing that her therapist has shifted his gaze to check how much time is left in the session, explodes, stating that "I know you cannot stand my neediness." When relating the incident in a group session she "cannot stop thinking" that her peers find her "disgusting, fat, needy, and a jerk."

The therapeutic interventions of a mentalizing-based approach aim to restore or promote more balanced mentalizing in the specific contexts of attachment and stress in which the balance is lost, tailoring the interventions to the mentalizing capabilities that the patient shows at that moment.

HOW DOES MENTALIZING ARISE? THE DEVELOPMENTAL ANTECEDENTS OF MENTALIZING

The development of mentalizing is inextricably linked to the extent to which the human infant is preadapted, that is, biologically prepared for "social fitedness,"[25] a disposition for social affiliation that drives the social-cognitive capacities undergirding human interactions.[26]

Attachment System

The attachment system, as pointed out,[12–15] is activated by fear, that is, by built-in cues that have been associated by evolution with threats to the safety and survival of the self. The stress associated with such cues, such as hunger, cold, or a loud noise, activates a procedural pattern of physiology, motricity, affect, and vocalization that has evolved to seek the availability of caretakers[13,14] and the experience of "felt security" or "safe haven."[27] This pattern is associated with the downregulation of the state of stress that results from the caretaker's responding with a matching, reciprocal, protective, regulating response to the infant's distress and emotional signals.[28] This pattern of interaction generates an "internal working model"[13,14] of the self as effective and of others as responsive, a model underlying the secure pattern of attachment. Downregulation of stress, in turn, activates exploration and learning and the infants' confident, procedural expectation that they are effective in evoking protective, regulating responses from available and responsive caretakers.

As infancy research shows, normal infants are exquisitely disposed and remarkably capable of orienting themselves toward other humans[26,29,30] and to recognize and seek out to establish a contingent (cause-effect) relationship between their emotional signal (eg, the baby's cry) and the social outcome of that signal.[31] For example, when a parent responds to the baby's crying by saying "Oh, honey, you are sooo hungry" and then proceeds to soothe, comfort, and feed the baby, the baby is disposed to establish that the parent's response is contingent on (is caused) by their crying.

Psychic Equivalence

This disposition to seek out a contingent, procedural match is a driver of the first pre-mentalistic mode of processing: psychic equivalence. In psychic equivalence, infants seek to evoke a match in another human being of their procedural internal state of affect and physiologic activation. This precursor of mentalizing includes the activation of a frontoparietal mirror neuron system that is involved in understanding in an automatic, implicit, bodily sense the emotions and action of others and in evoking in others a bodily understanding of our emotions and actions.[32,33] This disposition generates a conviction in one's guts that "what I feel and perceive" is the same (is matched) by what others feel and perceive.

This conflation of what is me (what I experience) and what I assume I share with others can be charming, as when a 3-year-old, asked what his mother wants for her birthday, responds without a hint of doubt "A spaceship." It is with the same certainty that the same child just knows that "there is a monster under the bed," despite his parents efforts to reassure him. This certainty points to the equation of "what is in my mind" and "what is real."

A similar isomorphism between mental and real is found in adults who experience a traumatic reminder as real feelings that are relived instead of remembered. The young woman cited earlier, who responds with rage to her therapist's glance at the clock with the conviction that "if I think that he hates being with me and wishes to reject me, then he does hate being with me and is rejecting me," shows the equation of mental and real often experienced by patients with BPD.

The development of controlled/explicit mentalizing requires the particular environmental input provided by an attachment context. As careful observation of mother-infant interactions[29,34,35] shows, average caretakers successfully match the procedural qualities of their infants' signals about one-third of the time, a percentage arguably as good or better than average therapists with their patients. The average caretakers maintain a highly contingent engagement[36] using communicative cues such as eye contact and the exaggerated, marked,[31] and slightly distorted mirroring of the affective qualities of the infant's signals that we refer to as motherese.

These qualities of attachment seem to facilitate several related developmental conditions and achievements:

1. The maintenance of an optimal level of arousal: that is, the Goldilocks point of arousal, which is not overwhelming and does not prompt fight (aggression), freeze (dissociation), or flight (anxiety), nor does it fail to engage.

2. The activation of attention and learning: optimal arousal in the presence of a regulating attachment figure who contingently mirrors (in time and emotional tone) and marks this response activates attention and learning.[37] This activation of learning points to what Csibra and Gergely suggest is an evolutionary adaptation for pedagogy, a built-in disposition to acquire vital social information in the context of attachment. As Csibra and Gergely point out, it seems that the attachment context has evolved to prompt the baby to respond to the message: "pay attention, I am going to show you some vital skills–such as 'do's and don'ts,' language and, as we will see, *mentalizing*–that you must acquire to survive and adapt." An attuned and contingent attachment seems to signal to the infant that it is safe to acquire new information.

3. The acquisition of the effortful control of attention: contingent and marked mirroring seems to facilitate the coming on line of the brain structures underlying the capacity to direct attention voluntarily.[38] The ability to direct attention, in turn, affords infants the realization of perspective, that is, that what they see is not necessarily what others see; instead, that they can direct others' attention toward their own perspective, a developmental milestone (joint attention) normally achieved by 9 months **(Fig. 4)**.[11]

4. The uncoupling of mental and procedural and the representation of experience: the caretaker's contingently mirrored and marked response does not present infants with a facsimile of their own response: parents do not cry back in response to their baby's crying. The contingent and marked response of the caretakers captures key procedural qualities of the infant's internal states, but reflects them in a different behavioral display. Such response, suggests Stern,[26] helps infants uncouple internal, emotional states from overt behavior; that is, it shifts infants' attention to their own and their caretaker's mental states. Furthermore, the displays are marked, that is, exaggerated, slowed down, and involving a great deal of eye-to-eye and high-contingency contact. This marking seems critical to help infants understand that the caretaker's display reflects the caretaker's perspective (their

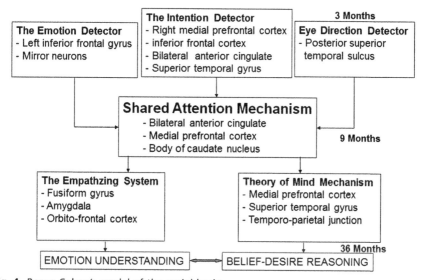

Fig. 4. Baron-Cohen's model of the social brain.

representation) of the infants' own emotional state, rather than expressing the care-taker's own mental states. This process seems crucial to enable infants to inter-nalize the representation of their own experience, a process that brings to life Winnicott's[39] statement that babies find themselves when looking at their mother's face.

Internalizing the reflection (or representation) of their own emotional experience seems to set in motion the capacity to represent internal experience, that is, to process and experience one's thoughts not as what is but as a thought or a feeling that conveys a perspective that can change, be combined with others to form cate-gories (such as 1 category to encompass all the mental images of different care-takers), acquire meaning and symbolic value (1 thought or mental state can stand for others, like a word can describe a whole range of objects or events), and impute to others intentions, thoughts, and emotions that may be different from one's own.[6]

5. The pretend mode and joining automatic/implicit/procedural and controlled/explicit/representational mentalizing: the emergence of representational capacities generates a mode of processing that allows children to play with multiple perspec-tives without experiencing such play for real but, instead, as an experience completely disconnected from the real. Practicing and perfecting symbolic/repre-sentational processing may be one of the key evolutionary functions of play and a reason for its preservation in the development of children in all cultures. Play (the pretend suspension of disbelief) collapses if one asks a child happily pretend-ing to shoot with his "finger-gun" if the finger is really a finger or a gun. Pretend mode does not link up with "for real" until a functional integration of automatic and controlled mentalizing is achieved.

   Such functional integration of the psychic equivalence generated by automatic/procedural/implicit mentalizing and the pretend mode that results from controlled/representational/explicit mentalizing normally takes place between ages 3 and 5 years, leading to full mentalizing. A precursor of this integration is a mode of processing, the teleologic mode, in which mental states can be recog-nized as not necessarily shared but counting only when expressed in observable, overt behavior, a phenomenon common in borderline personality (eg, "I can feel loved only if you hug me").

   Neuroimaging evidence[40] points out that activation of regions of the prefrontal cortex modulates and inhibits the automatic disposition to psychic equivalence and the conflation of experience.

6. Full mentalizing is thus a developmental acquisition involving the automatic, immediate mapping or matching of the self onto the other and the other onto the self followed by a second system consisting of the medial prefrontal cortex and the anterior cingulate cortex, which processes information about the self and others in more controlled abstract and symbolic ways, is accessible to intro-spection and verbalization, and allows for consideration that others have minds with intentions, perspectives, thoughts, and feelings that can be different from ours.[22,41]

In a fundamental way, psychological disorders can be conceptualized as failures of the mind to represent and fully mentalize its own activities, intentions, and contents of self and others, either persistently, as in autism; episodically, as in the manic episode of a bipolar disorder; or in particular states (eg, stress or specific interpersonal or emotional contexts, as in the emerging dramatic personality disorders of adolescence).

NEURODEVELOPMENTAL CHANGES, MENTALIZING, AND EMERGING BORDERLINE PERSONALITY FEATURES IN ADOLESCENCE

Over the last 3 decades, clinicians and researchers[42–45] have noted, with increasing empirical support, that a substantial percentage of adolescents present symptoms of affective dysregulation, impulsivity, and instability in relationships and in self-image that are hardly distinguishable from the symptomatic picture that qualifies for a diagnosis of (BPD) in those older than 18 years.

Such emergence of symptoms of BPD during adolescence should be looked at in the context of adolescents' heightened vulnerability to psychiatric problems and adaptive breakdown. Starting with Offer and Offer's[46] classic study of adolescent boys, tracking the course of adolescence reveals that about one-fourth to one-third of adolescents experience a tumultuous adolescence, marked by a vulnerability to adaptive breakdown, emotional storms, impulsivity and self-harmful behavior, dramatic and rapidly fluctuating mood, pervasive misery, deterioration of coping and adaptive competence, struggles with identity, conflicts with parents, and painful questions about self-esteem.

Epidemiologic studies[47–49] point to a marked increase in the rate of psychiatric disorders in adolescence, showing that both internalizing and externalizing problems increase during adolescence. In the natural history of most psychiatric disorders, including depression, drug abuse and dependency, bipolar disorders, eating disorders, and psychotic disorders, the onset of adolescence plays a significant role in the emergence, organization, or exacerbation of these disorders.

Disruptions in Mentalizing

Growing evidence suggests that disruptions in mentalizing are at the heart of the adolescents' heightened vulnerability to adaptive breakdown and psychopathology, in general, and to borderline signs and symptoms, in particular.

Fonagy and Luyten[50] summarized a large body of neuroscientific research that supported the view that adult patients with BPD seem to have a lower threshold for the fight-or-flight system[51–53] and an associated disposition to deactivate explicit/representational/controlled mentalizing. As discussed, this aspect of mentalizing is mediated by the lateral prefrontal cortex, the medial prefrontal cortex, the medial parietal cortex, and the anterior cingulate cortex. These structures undergo massive reorganization during adolescence, as reviewed in the next section.

Brain Structure Reorganization in Adolescence

Research evidence, cited by Fonagy and Lutyen,[50] documents that, in adults with BPD, emotional arousal leads to hyperactivation of the amygdala and a rapid and specific deactivation of the neural circuits involved in explicit/representational/controlled, internally focused and cognitive aspects of mentalizing. This deactivation leads to a shift to implicit/procedural/automatic, externally focused, affective processing involving the amygdala, basal ganglia, and ventromedial prefrontal cortex. As Siever and Weinstein[54] concluded, in patients with BPD, the areas in the prefrontal cortex that are responsible for social judgment, emotion evaluation, and top-down affect regulation are not used effectively in suppressing or modulating the limbic activity that generates aggression, affect instability, and automatic psychic equivalence processing. These neurobiological markers of BPD bear striking similarities to the normal neurodevelopmental features of the adolescent brain,[55–59] which involve significant brain remodeling and transformation.

This normal transformation of the adolescent brain is evident in the decrease or pruning in gray matter volume, particularly in the brain structures involved in social cognition and mentalizing. Such structures experience steady growth and increased volume up to puberty, then decline markedly. Thus, the trajectory of growth of gray matter in the prefrontal cortex resembles an inverted letter U, reaching its apex of greatest volume and thickness at age 12 years.

As the pruning proceeds during adolescence, enhanced connectivity between gray matter centers is achieved by a steady increase in white matter (myelin) density in the axons linking the gray matter centers that are not undergoing pruning.[60,61]

These findings suggest that adolescence may be a critical stage in the development of mentalizing and social cognition. During adolescence, the capacity to ascribe emotional significance to social cues and to regulate emotional responses and inhibit automatic, defensive reactions in social interactions matures as it is subserved by more rapid, efficient, and specific communication between specialized brain centers.[60,62–64]

Behavioral and neuroimaging studies give evidence of the impact of brain reorganization on the adolescent's mentalizing and social-cognitive capabilities, particularly generating declines in aspects of executive function, response inhibition, effortful control of attention, emotional self-control, and in the overall capacity to functionally integrate and balance implicit/procedural/automatic mentalizing and explicit/representational/controlled mentalizing.[65–68]

For example, social perspective taking is disturbed during adolescence.[69,70] The capacity to decide whether words match the expression of emotion declines in speed and accuracy,[71,72] because adolescents are markedly less able to recruit the frontal and prefrontal cortex when reading the emotions conveyed implicitly and procedurally in a picture of a human face. Conversely, in responding to an explicit/verbal/symbolic inquiry, such as the question of whether it is a good idea to swim with sharks, adolescents are less effective than adults in concluding that it is a bad idea to engage in such risky behavior. Differences in effectiveness correlate with adults' greater activation of the insula and the right fusiform face area in response to the risky probe, suggesting a capacity to assess possible outcomes by linking explicit, controlled, reflective processing with implicit, automatic, procedural processing that gives an embodied sense of the self in danger.[73] Adolescents' brain response, on the other hand, remains largely at the dorsolateral prefrontal cortex, with minimal limbic input that would allow the potential risk to be felt for real rather than as a pretend or purely representational image that fails to bridge from the mental to the real. Sharp[74] gave evidence of hypermentalizing (ie, excessive and largely inaccurate mentalizing) in adolescents who meet criteria for BPD and seem to fail in their attempts to integrate cognition and affect.

Evidence thus points to neurodevelopmental changes in adolescence affecting and likely generating disturbances in the regulation of mood, affect, impulse, and action by explicit, controlled, cognitive mentalizing, a capacity that lags behind developmentally until the maturation of the brain circuits underlying it is completed in the mid 20s (M Zanarini, McLean Hospital and Harvard Medical School, 2003, unpublished data).[55,75,76] The changes of normal adolescence seem exaggerated and significantly amplified in the case of adolescents, whose adaptive breakdown and signs and symptoms meet criteria for BPD, and seem to persist in those adults who continue to show signs and symptoms of BPD, as discussed later.

EMERGING BPD IN ADOLESCENCE

Children reaching adolescence with an enfeebled capacity to mentalize are less able to adaptively negotiate the developmental challenges of adolescence: to integrate a vastly changed body and a reorganized sense of self; to manage increased sexuality and newly acquired procreative capacity, to regulate heightened affective intensity; to deal with a greater capacity for abstraction and symbolization; to meet the pressures of peer-focused norms and expectations and the demands to transition to adult roles and to autonomy, separation, and intimate and committed relationships. The context in which these developmental challenges are negotiated involves the broader culture's structures and values, social- economic pressures and opportunities, family history and current functioning and, crucially, a brain undergoing a massive reorganization that compromises the capacity to recruit perspective taking and top-down regulation when faced with stress, intense affect, and attachment needs. This is a biopsychosocial perfect storm, which arguably creates the conditions for adaptive collapse and the emergence of BPD in vulnerable adolescents. As Baird and colleagues[77] described it, the effect of neurodevelopmental changes in vulnerable adolescents is "like attaching a 330-horsepower motor to a cardboard box." The box in question is the fragile capacity to mentalize, a capacity that is precipitously lost when the 330-horsepower motor of emotional arousal and attachment needs is activated. Psychological defenses, consisting of the active inhibition of mentalizing, arguably are organized in adolescence to deal with the youngster's intense despair and helplessness.

Adolescence seems to be a point in development at which early difficulties in attachment and in the development of mentalizing join with a neurodevelopmental reorganization that weakens mentalizing and mentalizing-mediated affect regulation, impulse control, and the capacity to represent the self and one's relationships. Such convergence takes place at a time rife with psychosocial demands and developmental challenges that thus create the conditions for the symptomatic expression of BPD.

The roots of enfeebled mentalizing can be traced to an interaction between constitutional vulnerabilities[78–83] and exposure to neglect, trauma, and invalidation in early attachment relationships.[84–90]

BPD: Familial and Heritable

Studies of psychiatric patients[88,91] show that BPD is familial, and twin studies[92–94] document that BPD is heritable. The developmental model that best describes the emergence of the mentalizing failures characteristic of BPD is a transactional diatheses-stress model. This model was tested by Belsky and colleagues[95] in a prospective longitudinal study of a birth cohort of 1116 families. This study showed that constitutional factors (eg, anxious or aggressive temperament, or a constitutional disposition to intense and negative affective instability and reactivity and low threshold for activation of impulsive motoric responses) exert an influence on the environment by:

a. Affecting parents' capacity for emotional attunement and mentalization, particularly in parents with similar temperament or traumatic histories
b. Impairing infants' capacity to benefit from the regulating qualities of the attachment relationship

Attachment Disorganization

A complex developmental cascade crucially involves the development of disorganized attachment.[96] The conditions for disorganization of attachment are present when infants' signals of distress and activation of attachment evoke distress and a nonmentalizing response in the caretaker. Caretakers' defensive response of fight-or-flight results in increased distress and dysregulation in the infant, rather than the downregulation of distress brought about by contingent matching. But increased distress also triggers activation of attachment, setting in motion a vicious cycle of distress and attachment begetting more distress and more activation of attachment and less mentalizing in both infant and caretaker. The result is a ready triggering to the hyperactivation of the attachment system manifested in a "rapidly accelerating tempo of intimacy in interpersonal relationships,"[1(p277)] and loss of mentalizing and catastrophic emotional reactions at the prospect of rejection, loss, or misattunement. Such mutual evocation of mentalizing loss increases controlling, coercive, defensive behavior.

Exacerbated stress associated with hyperactivation of attachment primes the brain to more rapidly respond to stress with dissociation of implicit/procedural/automatic mentalizing, and explicit/representational/controlled mentalizing; that is, as **Fig. 5** shows, a lowering of the threshold for dissociation[16,19] of automatic and controlled mentalizing.

Dissociation

In adolescence, these vulnerable youngsters show a disposition to loss of mentalizing and the dissociation of controlled and automatic mentalizing, which is triggered by stress, loss, rejection, or the failure of interactive partners to match the youngsters' state of mind.[97,98] These triggers evoke overwhelming states of hyperarousal, subjective dyscontrol, and an inner sense of falling apart that reflects the loss of the sense of coherence provided by controlled mentalizing.

Adolescents begin to anticipate this potential to mentalizing breakdown and dissociation and defensively seek to actively dissociate before dissociation and loss of control passively happens to them. Thus, they seek to distract or numb themselves with a variety of addictive or addictivelike patterns, such as deliberate self-harm,[99–101] purging, drug use, promiscuity, or escape into a pretend existence made readily available by the Internet. However, addictive, numbing behavior increases attachment disorganization and psychophysiologic dysregulation and excludes youngsters from competence-building avenues, alienating them from mainstream peers, and increasing involvement with deviant peers and maladaptive patterns of coping and affect regulation.[102,103]

Furthermore, dissociative efforts, although they provide a measure of relief and an illusory sense of control, also intensify the youth's disconnection from their own subjectivity and sense of intentionality and self-directedness.[104] Thus, they find themselves increasingly falling into a dark despair that resists the comprehension that is available only when controlled mentalizing gives us access to our subjectivity and the verbal and representational means to communicate our experience. Deprived of

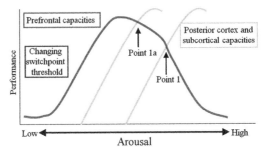

Fig. 5. Mayes' (2000)[129] adaptation of Arnsten's dual arousal systems model: implication of the hyperactivation of attachment. (*Adapted from* Mayes L. A developmental perspective on the regulation of arousal states. Semin Perinatol 2000;24:267–79; with permission.)

access to their own intentionality, they experience their behavior as happening to them, because their actions, compelled by powerful forces of raw affect, lead them to enact automatic responses they witness like someone watching a movie. Disconnected from their own subjectivity, they feel numb.

Dissociation also compromises access to other people's subjective experience and leads to ever greater aloneness, because they feel deprived not only of the presence of another person but also of the mentalizing means with which to achieve a sense of connection and reciprocity with other human beings. Thus, they desperately hypermentalize,[74] reading suspiciously in others' faces an anticipated slight or rebuff.

However, aloneness intensifies distress and hyperactivates attachment, fueling the young persons' need to coercively evoke, through manipulative, nonmentalistic means teleologic (physically observable) matching response from others. This matching provides the concrete assurance of reciprocity that counters feelings of aloneness and self-fragmentation.

Mentalizing Cycle Among Adolescents and Caretakers

Completing the vicious cycle, the youngsters' coercive, manipulating behavior arouses intense emotions in others, including parents, teachers, and clinicians. Parents often feel increasingly out of control, anxious, enraged, paralyzed, and unable to mentalize.[105–107] In response to their own mentalizing breakdown, parents try even more desperately to control their children and squelch their manipulation and misbehavior, a stance that typically reinforces the adolescent's retreat from mentalizing. Thus, in a tragic transactional sequence, the adolescents' attempts to cope with loneliness and loss of control through inhibition of mentalizing and addictive, nonmentalizing, and coercive patterns evoke nonmentalizing and coercion from parents and others. Such transactions result in self-perpetuating and self-reinforcing vicious cycles that leave families feeling stuck, exhausted, and engaged in an arms race of nonmentalizing that reinforces persistent misery and maladjustment (**Fig. 6**).

MENTALIZATION-BASED TREATMENT OF ADOLESCENT BREAKDOWN AND EMERGING BPD (MBT-A)

The implications of this model of adaptive breakdown and emerging BPD in adolescence involve a therapeutic approach focused on promoting the adolescents' and their family's capacity to mentalize in the context of emotional arousal in attachment

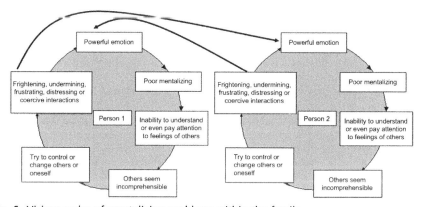

Fig. 6. Vicious cycles of mentalizing problems within the family.

relationships. Focusing on promoting mentalizing while attachment is stimulated provides a conceptual and clinical framework that can structure treatment and organize treatment interventions in a coherent model.

MBT was originally developed by Anthony Bateman and Peter Fonagy[108,109] to treat BPD in adults. Mentalizing Based Treatment – Borderline Personality Disorder (MBT-BPD) is now robustly supported by empirical evidence of effectiveness in the treatment of adults with BPD.[110,111]

From the common trunk of MBT, treatment models with varying degrees of empirical evidence of effectiveness have been developed for families[112]; antisocial personality[113]; at-risk mothers and infants[114–116]; eating disorders[117]; depression[4]; trauma[118]; drug addiction,[119] and, as is discussed in this article, for adolescents (MBT-A).[120–122] The empirical evidence of MBT-A is preliminary, although highly encouraging.[123]

The common element in all MBT protocols is placing mentalizing at the center of the treatment process. MBT is not defined by a structure of specific techniques but by the process of stimulating mentalizing and developing an attachment relationship: to reestablish mentalizing when it is lost and to keep it going when it is present.

To stimulate mentalizing, the mind of the patient (the patient's subjective experience) becomes the focus of treatment. The objective is for patients (and their families) to find out more about how they think and feel about themselves, about others, and about themselves in relationship with others; how their thoughts and feelings give direction and meaning to their behavior; and how distortions in understanding themselves and others lead to maladaptive behavior, even although such behavior is often an effort to maintain some sense of safety, stability, and control and to manage distressing and incomprehensible feelings.

A mentalizing framework with adolescents requires consideration of the vulnerability to mentalizing breakdown in adolescents discussed earlier, in particular in adolescents with BPD. Therefore, a critical principle of MBT-A is to recognize the adolescents' developmental need for a mentalizing scaffolding, normally provided by the adolescents' family, to support and bridge the adolescents' transition to greater mentalizing competence and stability.

However, coercive, nonmentalizing interactions in families of adolescents with BPD maintain, reinforce, and exacerbate nonmentalizing in both teenagers and parents, leading to self-reinforcing vicious cycles and hopeless impasses. In the throes of these vicious cycles, as pointed out earlier, parents feel stuck, helpless, angry, ashamed, and more disposed to punish, criticize, reject, or disengage than to seek to understand, mentalize, offer emphatic support, provide effective limits, and model how to connect thoughts and feelings and manage emotional arousal without turning off mentalizing.

Thus, a basic goal of MBT-A is to assist families in shifting from coercive, nonmentalizing cycles to mentalizing discussions that can result in the realistic hope (or remoralization) associated with a sense of choice and agency, more effective communication, and greater trust.

The notion of coercive cycles, driven by emotional arousal and threats to the safety and continuity of the self and attachments, helps parents appreciate the transactional nature of the problems experienced by their adolescents and their families and defines a crucial goal: enlisting the parents as partners in treatment. Such partnering aims to shift discussions about behaviors that need to be controlled (discussions that resemble a dialogue of the deaf between parents who bemoan their children's out-of-control behavior and the teenagers who bristle and reject their parents' efforts to control them) to mentalizing conversations that enable family members to hear and understand each other's perspective. This shift aims at rekindling the markers of mentalizing: curiosity, respect, empathy, mutuality, and agency in all family members. Empathy, of course, does not preclude limit setting. The attachment processes conducive to mentalizing, as discussed earlier, are built on a foundation of trust engendered by effective, responsive, regulating caregiving, which includes support and containment of stress and of the fight-or-flight automatic, defensive reactions that lead to destructive and self-destructive behavior.

MBT-A is thus framed along the lines of assisting parents in maintaining their own mentalizing first, so that they can support their children's mentalizing, as airline safety instructions direct parents to first place the oxygen mask on their face, before seeking to help their children breathe.

Such an approach involves an invitation to parents to explore the experiences and situations in which they feel buffeted by emotional turmoil and struggle to adopt a mentalizing position and the identifying of the interventions and resources that can support them and their mentalizing capacity.

To help create a common framework with the parents and to help them counter the feelings of shame, guilt, hopelessness, and despair that fuel nonmentalizing cycles, the MBT-A clinicians provide the family with a mentalizing formulation. The formulation is a profile of the adolescent's and the family's mentalizing strengths (a review of the family's caring, empathy, and capacity to offer understanding and support) and vulnerabilities (an account of the particular ways [eg, going into pretend mode or focusing on external behavior and losing sight of what goes on in the mind] and the emotional and interpersonal contexts [eg, when feeling vulnerable and wishing for support and validation or when feeling left out] in which mentalizing fails or is inhibited). Thus, formulation highlights how breaks in mentalizing give rise to coercive behavior and defensive reactions of fight-or-flight that undermine reciprocity and collaboration and the capacity to engage in treatment.

The mentalizing formulation offered to the family also includes profiling the adolescent's neuropsychiatric/addictive vulnerabilities and diagnosis. As suggested earlier, all psychiatric/addictive disorders of adolescence involve a dysfunction of mentalizing, including an impaired capacity to interpret self and others, and maladaptive and nonmentalizing modes of perceiving, feeling, thinking, coping, communicating, and relating to others.

However, the relationship between mentalizing impairment and neuropsychiatric and addictive disorders is bidirectional: mentalizing deficits exacerbate neuropsychiatric/addictive problems by interfering with the capacity to collaborate and use help. Neuropsychiatric/addictive dysfunction affects arousal, attention-control, affect regulation, cognition, and impulse, all of which interfere with the capacity to mentalize.

Thus, a second goal of MBT-A is to assess and provide psychotherapeutic, educational, or pharmacologic remediation for the neuropsychiatric symptoms that emerge either during acute psychobiological decompensation or as trait vulnerabilities representing an enduring diathesis to dysfunction. The specific MBT-A interventions that are discussed later aim to offer opportunities to practice restoring mentalizing, with the goal of setting in motion the rehabilitation of mentalizing.

In summary:

1. MBT-A aims to shift from coercive, nonmentalizing cycles involving adolescents and their families to mentalizing conversations that can promote remoralization, based on rekindled hope and improved sense of agency and understanding.
2. Remoralization is supported by providing the family with a mentalizing formulation that outlines the adolescents' and the family's mentalizing strengths and

vulnerabilities; reviews the stressors affecting the family and the parents' mentalizing; and identifies the neuropsychiatric, addictive dysfunctions affecting (and being affected by) mentalizing vulnerabilities.

3. Remediation of neuropsychiatric/addictive problems with specific psychotherapeutic, educational, and pharmacologic interventions serves as a launching pad for the longer-term rehabilitation of the mentalizing capacities that generate agency, reflection, and connections with others and promote more effective means to manage stress, adversity, and vulnerability.[124–126]

4. The specific MBT-A interventions actively and systematically seek to promote mentalizing, particularly in the emotional and attachment contexts in which it breaks down or is defensively inhibited. Such mentalizing in attachment interventions aims to rehabilitate the capacity to mentalize.

MBT-A was designed for and has been evaluated[74,123,127] in adolescents who meet criteria for BPD, engage in self-harm or experience a significant adaptive breakdown that results in behavior that is dangerous to themselves or others and elicits destructive responses from the environment. However, I suggest that promoting mentalizing in adolescents is the core active ingredient or mechanism of therapeutic action of treatment interventions with adolescents. Thus, MBT-A is proposed as a general framework to organize treatment of adolescents.

Rossouw and Fonagy[120,123] developed a year-long, manualized psychotherapy program involving weekly individual MBT sessions and monthly MBT-F sessions aiming at enhancing the adolescents' and their family's capacity to represent their own and others' thoughts and feelings accurately in emotionally challenging situations. A mentalizing framework was also developed by Bleiberg and Williams as a way of organizing a 3-week to 12-week inpatient and partial-hospital program at the Menninger Clinic.[120] The overall process of MBT-A is outlined in **Fig. 7**.

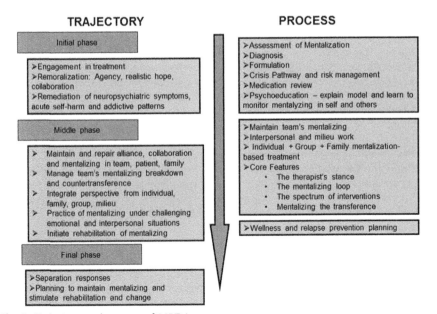

Fig. 7. Trajectory and process of MBT-A.

ASSESSING MENTALIZING TO ORGANIZE MBT-A: THE DIAGNOSTIC FORMULATION OF MENTALIZING STRENGTHS AND VULNERABILITIES

1. The first step in MBT-A is to arrive at a diagnostic formulation that includes the following items: the adolescent's psychiatric diagnosis and symptom severity. This assessment outlines the impact of the psychiatric disorder on mentalizing capacity and the effect of mentalizing problems on the impairments associated with the psychiatric disorder
2. The presence of emerging features of personality disorder
3. The adolescent's psychological capacities mediating treatment response, particularly, as is described later, mentalizing strengths and vulnerabilities, and the emotional and interpersonal contexts in which mentalizing problems emerge
4. Family functioning, identifying stressors impinging on the family and the family's mentalizing capacities in relation to emotionally challenging situations

The assessment of mentalizing in the parents, the adolescent, and the family can be accomplished with structured instruments that measure different aspects or dimensions of mentalizing. Without attempting to be exhaustive, **Box 1** outlines a selection of measures that assess aspects of mentalizing in adolescents.

A comprehensive assessment of mentalizing is based also on clinical evaluations in various attachment contexts. The adolescents and their family's involvement in individual, family, and group interventions allows for a naturalistic clinical evaluation of both the young person's and the family's mentalizing strengths and vulnerabilities, particularly in relation to the challenges brought about by individual, group, and family sessions.

An important aspect of the development of a mentalizing formulation is the engagement of the adolescents and the families in the ongoing assessment of their own mentalizing capacities. To facilitate such engagement, MBT-A includes psychoeducational groups, which are referred to as explicit mentalizing educational groups. These groups use discussions and role playing, which seek to bring to life what mentalizing is and how one can tell what good and bad mentalizing looks like; the skills and attitudes involved in mentalizing, such as curiosity, openness, agency, and reflection; the relation of mentalizing and attachment and how mentalizing breaks down under stress and when the sense of self or the connection to significant others is threatened; and how to use treatment to promote mentalizing, particularly in the challenging situations in which it fails or is inhibited.

Adolescents and families are explicitly helped to recognize when their own and other people's mentalizing is working, as reflected in the deployment of the skills and attitudes outlined in **Boxes 2–4** and, when mentalizing is failing, as indicated by

---

Box 1
Measures: adolescents' characteristics

Mentalizing Capacity

- Basic Empathy Scale
- Avoidance and Fusion Questionnaire–Youth
- Movie for Social Cognition
- Reflective Function Questionnaire
- Working Alliance Inventory

An example of an MBT-A formulation

Background

Jason, a 15-year old, presented to our service with a history of outbursts of rage, depression, and self-loathing, drinking to intoxication since age 12 years, and abusing benzodiazepines, opiates, and marijuana on a daily basis. He experienced severe distress when alone in his room, and his distress sometimes led to self-harm. Jason is an only child of a family dominated by conflict and emotional distance. From infancy, he was described as extraordinarily sensitive and prone to react intensely and angrily to frustration or disappointment. Testing at age 12 years revealed a verbal IQ of 150, significantly ahead of his performance IQ of 110. His sophisticated language had made him sound like a grown-up since he was in elementary school but, despite his obvious gifts, he had had such difficulties in school that he had been expelled from 4 schools.

Jason had become increasingly absorbed in pornographic Web sites and felt alienated and unsupported by his parents, of whom he spoke disparagingly. He believed that his father was incapable of understanding anyone's feelings and that his mother was trying to "get inside his head" to control him. On admission, he spoke sadly of his hopelessness, although he proudly described his talent for telling others what they wanted to hear and his conviction that he was able to trick even the most skilled therapists.

Coping skills

Jason's sensitivity and intense reactivity seemed to have left him exposed, from early in life, to having to figure out how to cope with conflict, uncertainty, stress, and angry feelings. He came to believe that his own feelings were overwhelming to others, and that he was so "hard to deal with" and incomprehensible that others ignored or rejected him or tried to control him and "squelch" his feelings. Whenever he feels vulnerable, frustrated, or in need of help and understanding, he quickly feels in danger of losing control over his own feelings and feels ashamed and exposed to rejection or humiliation. He tries hard to distract himself from feeling so vulnerable, lonely, and helpless, and from noticing how others ignore him, reject him, or fail to notice him, on the one hand, or "get" him so completely (get "inside of his mind") that he feels at risk of losing control of his own mind. His solution is to cope by trying to disconnect himself from intense feelings, especially feelings of vulnerability, loneliness, anxiety, and anger, by numbing himself with drugs or engaging in self-harm, by going into a pretend mode of Web-based observation of relationships from the outside, instead of engaging in real ones, and by seeking to trick others and himself with the illusion that he can control his own feelings and the reactions of others.

Personality style

Jason is a sensitive, intelligent and articulate person. However, he expects that others would either ignore him and be totally unaware of his needs and feelings, or that they would be overwhelmed by his needs and feelings and try to control his mind. Both the prospect of being ignored and that his needs will not be noticed, or the expectation that his feelings are overwhelming to others and will lead to loss of control, are profoundly distressing to him and keep him on his guard, because he expects to get hurt and humiliated. He is ready to distance himself from his feelings and holds himself apart from others. This distance leaves him feeling even more alone and disconnected, which only adds to his distress and wishes to form attachments. These wishes to form relationships are the feelings that he finds threatening and overwhelming, because he fears rejection, humiliation, and loss of control. Thus, he explodes with rage to put more distance or tries to numb himself.

Engagement in therapy

Jason is likely to be challenging to engage in therapy. He may wonder if the clinicians are really interested in him or will ignore him and fail to understand his needs. On the other hand, he may worry that if he allows himself to trust the clinicians and show them his feelings, especially when he wishes to feel understood or wishes to get help, that he would end up being humiliated or taken advantage of.

Self-destructive behavior

Jason uses substances to numb himself and put distance from his feelings. He also uses self-harm as a way to manage his feelings. At times, it feels as if the only thing he can do to cope with his feelings and with other people is to explode with rage. These ways of coping are damaging to Jason's health and to his relationships and are likely to keep him stuck in ways of coping that lead to more and more pain and isolation.

Effective mentalizing

Jason often shows a great ability to understand what is in the mind of others. He also tries to understand his own thoughts and feelings. Jason's sensitivity to, for example, how his father is confused about what Jason feels and, on the other hand, how his mother is sensitive to him, and the reactions he has to his understanding of his parents' thoughts and feelings, are painful and stressful and make it difficult for him not to fall into patterns of coping that, although resulting in pain and problems in his relationships, also give him a sense of control and connection.

Mentalizing problems

Jason often comes to points when he feels overwhelmed by his own feelings and his awareness of others people's feelings, particularly the feelings of the people closest to him. He then falls into a pattern in which, on the one hand, he feels completely sure of what other people think and feel, as if he could tell for certain that what he has in his mind is also what is in other people's minds. He usually assumes that others think hateful or negative thoughts about him, that they don't care or that they wish to hurt him, control him, and humiliate him. This assumption leaves him feeling lonely, angry, and overwhelmed. He then believes that the only way he can manage his feelings is to distract himself or numb himself, pretending not to care and even pretending not to feel lonely, angry, and overwhelmed. A related way to put distance from these vulnerable feelings is to turn his feelings into actions, particularly actions involving his own body, as when he self-harms or uses drugs or in actions that cause other people to feel as lonely, angry, and overwhelmed as he feels.

Family mentalizing

Jason's family has been stuck in a dialogue of the deaf, in which everyone feels not heard or understood and have no hope that that anyone else can appreciate their individual perspective, much less accommodate and take into account their needs and feelings.

Jason's parents see Jason's problems differently and often feel blamed by the other parent for Jason's difficulties. When feeling stressed, the parents experience a difficult time, being open to a different perspective, which leads to vicious cycles in which, as Jason becomes more distressed and feels angry and misunderstood, he adopts behaviors that become even more distressing for the parents, who then have a more difficult time understanding Jason. This situation, in turn, leads him to feel more distressed, angry, and misunderstood and so on, until everyone feels hopeless and out of control.

Treatment plan

Jason and his parents have agreed to become involved in a treatment plan that starts with a course of hospitalization. The purpose of the phase is to help shift the vicious cycles described earlier so that both Jason and his parents can regain a sense of control, hope, and connection based on a better ability to understand each other and communicate and collaborate more effectively.

An important goal of the hospital plan is to sort out how Jason can understand and manage his feelings in a way that he can cope with feelings without using self-destructive behaviors that hurt him, his health, and his relationships. These behaviors include abusing substances and making himself numb by harming himself or getting absorbed in pornography. Completing a plan to interrupt these self-harming patterns, managing crises, and staying on track after leaving the hospital are goals of this phase of treatment.

A second goal of the hospitalization is to stabilize symptoms of depression and anxiety, which make it difficult for Jason to feel safe, effective, and able to think clearly and to understand his feelings or other people's feelings. Sorting out medications to help with these problems is one of the goals. Jason's psychological and learning capacities are assessed to better understand how he learns, and how best to use his wonderful intelligence and accommodate the kind of processing that is a relative weakness for him.

The final goal of the hospitalization is to have an opportunity for Jason and the family to prac-tice how to keep one's mind effectively engaged (how to mentalize) in the challenging situa-tions in which it becomes difficult to keep one's mind engaged. Individual, group, and family sessions give an opportunity for this practice in various situations that present different kinds of challenge. Jason and his parents anticipate that the hospitalization will set them on a path to continue after discharge from the hospital on a program of weekly individual and group sessions and once-monthly family sessions for about 1 year. Once a month, the team will also meet with Jason and his parents to review the progress.

Box 2
Successful mentalizing 1: self-representation

- A rich, agentive, internal life
  - This quality is characterized by the person rarely experiencing their mind as being empty or contentless, but feeling real, alive, and aware of the link between one's actions and one's intentional mental states (ownership and responsibility for one's actions vs "my behavior happens to me").
- Autobiographical continuity
  - This quality is the capacity to remember oneself in the past and to experience the continuity of internal states, despite one's changes.
- Advanced explanatory and listening skills
  - These skills denote the person's ability to explain things to others, and the person with these skills is experienced by others as patient and able to listen and to comprehend (talk in ways that others can listen and listen in ways that others can talk).

Box 3
Successful mentalizing 2: 7 strengths of perception of one's own mental functioning

1. Taking a developmental perspective
   a. This strength refers to the ability to appreciate that one's perspective of self and others, as well as other people's perspective of themselves and others, changes as they develop and as maturation and experience provide tools to perceive, think, and feel in more complex ways (eg, Mark Twain's statement that "When I was a boy of fourteen, my father was so ignorant I could hardly stand to have the old man around. But when I got to be twenty-one, I was astonished at how much he had learned in seven years").

2. Awareness of internal conflict
   a. This strength refers to the capacity to recognize that our thoughts and feelings are complicated and may contain multiple, contradictory, and at times incompatible wishes and intentions.

3. Self-inquisitive stance
   a. This strength refers to a stance of curiosity about one's own thoughts, feelings, and perspective, as well as about other people's perspective and the ways their minds work (eg, considering differences of perspective related, for example, to age, gender, culture). This curiosity and interest in differences relates to the openness to question one's assumptions.

4. Realistic skepticism and the playful stance

   a. This strength refers to the recognition of the potential errors, foibles, and even absurdity of one's perspective, and a readiness and ability to engage others in playful exchanges that allow for an immersion in mutually acknowledged and enjoyable pretend scenarios (see Mark Twain).

5. Awareness of the impact of affect

   a. This strength involves a capacity to take a step back and recognize the impact of emotional states on our perspective of ourselves and of others.

6. Acknowledgment of unconscious or preconscious mental states

   a. This strength involves an appreciation and a capacity to tolerate not knowing all aspects of what one thinks and feels and not even fully appreciating one's own intentions.

7. Belief in changeability

   a. This strength involves an appreciation that one's thoughts and feeling are not fixed like physical objects but can be transformed in multiple ways as a result of changes in perspective and exchanges with other people's minds.

Box 4
Successful mentalizing 3: 7 strengths of relational capacity

1. Curiosity/openness of genuine interest

   a. This strength refers to an attitude of interest in other people's thoughts and feelings and respect for the perspectives of others. It is also characterized by an expectant attitude that one's understanding is elaborated or expanded by what is in another person's mind. It also implies openness to discovery and a reluctance to make assumptions, or hold prejudices, about what others think or feel.

2. The stance of safe uncertainty[128] (also referred to as opaqueness)

   a. This strength refers to the open acknowledgment that one frequently does not know what other people are thinking, without being completely puzzled or overwhelmed by what happens in the mind of others. This stance is based on a general sense that the reactions of others are to some extent understandable, given the knowledge that one may have of what others think and feel.

3. Contemplation and reflection

   a. This strength refers to the desire to reflect on how others think in a relaxed rather than a compulsive manner.

4. Perspective taking

   a. This strength is a stance and attitude which are characterized by the acceptance that the same event or experience can look different from different perspectives, which tend to reflect individuals' different experiences and histories.

5. Forgiveness

   a. This strength refers to the understanding of people's actions based on understanding their mental states. An example of this understanding is the dissipation of one's own anger once one has understood why the other person acted as they did.

6. Impact awareness

   a. This strength refers to the awareness of how one's own thoughts, feelings, and actions affect others.

7. A nonparanoid attitude

   a. This strength describes the stance whereby the individual does not assume or expect that the thoughts of others are malevolent or threatening and is aware of the possibility that minds can be changed.

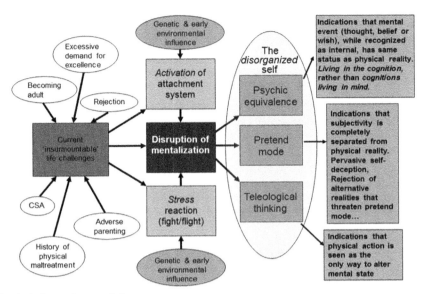

Fig. 8. Failure of mentalizing.

Box 5
Formulation
• Background
• Coping skills
• Personality style
• Engagement in therapy
• Self-destructive behavior
• Effective mentalizing
• Mentalizing problems
• Family mentalizing
• Treatment plan

the emergence of nonmentalizing modes (**Fig. 8**), such as psychic equivalence, the pretend mode, or the teleologic mode, as well as by the markers of misuse or abuse of mentalizing.

The family and the adolescent are thus recruited to construct a formulation that can follow the outline presented in **Box 5**.

THE CORE FEATURES OF MBT-A
The Therapist's Stance: How to Be when Conducting MBT

The foundation of MBT in all of its different applications is the stance that therapists take when engaging with patients and families in treatment (**Box 6**). The stance refers to the skills and attitudes therapists present to facilitate the patients' involvement in a mentalizing process and staying connected with the patient in a developing attachment relationship.

Box 6
Core features

1. Basic good practice
2. The therapist's stance: 4 legs (how to be)
3. Explicit mentalizing: psychoeducation
4. The mentalizing loop: 3 + 3 stations (where to be)
5. Formulating and planning
6. The spectrum of interventions

The therapist's stance involves 4 areas of competence:

1. Maintaining an inquisitive, not-knowing stance
2. Holding the balance
3. Interrupting nonmentalizing
4. Highlighting and marking good mentalizing

The inquisitive/not-knowing stance

The inquisitive/not-knowing stance is one of affirming the value of the mentalizing-promoting attitudes of authenticity, genuineness, respect, interest, curiosity, openness, and tentativeness. The therapist actively enquires about the patient's subjective experience. This inquiry is not an exercise in fact-finding but, instead, is an attempt to open a conversation about the details of the patients' thoughts and feelings and the meanings and relationships in which these thoughts and feelings are generated. Therapists thus seek to invite curiosity about "what is going on in your mind," often asking "What was X like for you?" The competencies involved in adopting an inquisitive/not-knowing stance include:

- An ability to communicate with the patients and families in a direct, clear manner, using simple and unambiguous, nonmetaphorical statements that minimize misunderstandings
- An ability to adopt a stance of not knowing that communicates to patients and families a genuine interest and an attempt to find out about their mental life and experience
- An ability to sustain an active, nonjudgmental mentalizing stance that emphasizes the joint exploration of the patient's mental states

A favorite image teaching the inquisitive/not-knowing stance is to suggest that therapists in training imagine themselves sitting alongside the patient, actively focusing with the patient on a mental map made up of the patient's intentional mental states.

In showing how mentalizing works, therapists do not tell patients what the patients' think or feel, much less what they really think and feel, without being aware of it. Thus, the MBT therapist would not interpret for the patient the underlying unconscious reasons explaining their experience and motivation. Instead, in a mentalizing stance, therapists hold to a position of tentativeness and not knowing. That is, therapists encourage the patients to tolerate not knowing, that is, to avoid certainty and being an expert about what is in the other person's mind. They do so by showing that we can find out about the other's perspective only by enquiring and being open to be surprised (and change our mind) by the information we then gain.

On learning of the patient's perspective, the therapists acknowledge that we all experience interactions subjectively and impressionistically. Thus, in identifying differences between perspectives (between the therapist and the patient or among family or group members), therapists accept and validate individual perspectives before challenging or inviting consideration of multiple perspectives. For example, a therapist could state "I can see how you get to that impression, but when I think about it, it occurs to me that he may have been preoccupied with something rather than ignoring you."

In showing honesty and openness to more than 1 perspective (and the courage required to remain open and nondefensive), MBT therapists monitor and acknowledge their own mistakes and mentalizing failures (ie, "I failed to notice" or "I got confused"), recognizing that in all mentalizing breakdowns, everyone (including the therapist) likely plays a part. This judicious self-disclosure models honesty, courage, and openness and suggests that:

a. Mentalizing breakdowns are inevitable; they are the focus of treatment and follow understandable defensiveness and inevitable mistakes.
b. Mentalizing breakdowns offer the greatest therapeutic opportunity to learn about how to mentalize when it becomes challenging.

Holding the balance

As discussed earlier, the essence of functional mentalizing is the balance between various aspects of mentalizing: automatic and controlled, affect and cognition; external and internal, self and others. Balance is also central in the calibration of the optimal arousal (not too much nor too little) at which mentalizing operates and the degree of attachment activation (the interpersonal distance) that allows for empathic connection and an awareness of one's separateness.

The competences involved in holding the balance include monitoring when there is an imbalance between the various mentalizing aspects and responding to such imbalance with contrary moves, that is: when the patient is mostly focused on introspection, invite consideration of other persons' minds (ie, "What do you think this is like for your mom?"); when overfocused on others, invite consideration of the patient's own perspective; when affect dominates, recruit a controlled, reflective stance, and vice versa.

Holding the balance is also achieved by matching the interventions to the patient's level of mentalizing and arousal, as it is reviewed under the core component of the spectrum of interventions. Holding the balance also entails striking a careful point between promoting, in family and group sessions, natural interactions around problematic issues, and intervening at critical moments to show how problems are perpetuated by misunderstandings and mentalizing breakdowns.

Intervening to interrupt nonmentalizing interactions

A basic premise of the MBT model is that nonmentalizing interactions are at the heart of the impasses generating coercive, defensive and symptomatic behavior and thus, are the primary indication for therapeutic intervention.

The competences involved in interrupting nonmentalizing include

a. Identifying when mentalizing fails (see section on assessing mentalizing)
b. Interrupting nonmentalizing, which includes the therapist's ability to slow down and invite the patient, family, or group to stop and rewind; that is, to look at what just happened, emotionally and interpersonally, at the moment when mentalizing began to fail
c. Helping patients and other family members to identify when their own mentalizing begins to fail and request a pause, before increased stress renders them unable to

hear, understand, or explain their point of view; this request is a signal, to themselves and others, of their need to take a step back to reflect and recruit controlled mentalizing

Highlighting and marking good mentalizing

To deepen people's ability to connect and understand thoughts, feelings, and intentions, therapists practice the following competencies:

a. Actively searching for examples or instances of good mentalizing
b. Marking and positively connoting these instances of spontaneous good mentalizing, for example by saying, "Johnny, when you told your parents how you felt when you were struggling with thinking that you really had screwed up, I was impressed by how clear you were and how you noticed that your parents were actually trying to understand how you were feeling"
c. Enlarge these instances by inviting others to pay attention and review interactions that generate good mentalizing, which in turn allows for effective communication and problem solving

The Mentalizing Loop

The steps involved in the mentalizing loop are depicted in **Fig. 9**. These steps provide a framework to orient the therapist in facilitating a mentalizing process with the adolescents and their families or with the adolescent groups, rather than a rigid sequence that has to be followed.

The first step is for the therapist to notice when there is a break in mentalizing in the family or the group and, applying the skill described in interrupting nonmentalizing, to suggest a pause (adolescents often understand how to pause when offered a pretend pause button to press or a sign they can display when wanting to slow down the action). Therapists then check if their observation matches 1 or more family or group member's experience of a problematic interaction or of a moment in which understanding and communication became difficult. For example, a therapist may say "I noticed that when Johnny said X, mom seemed to get worried and dad began to interrupt him." If 1 or more family or group members agree that a problem was noticed, therapists then invite family or group members to brainstorm about the problematic interaction and figure out how to describe it, for example, "We all walk on egg shells when Johnny...."

In the next step in the loop the therapists check for consensus of every family or group member about the description of the problematic interaction. Checking is the

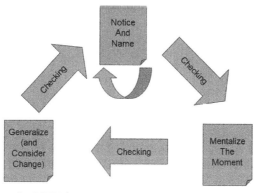

Fig. 9. Core features: the MBT-F loop.

grease that oils that transition from 1 step to another in the loop and the clearest evidence of mentalizing in action.

The following step in the loop is the invitation to all family or group members to mentalize the moment.

The therapist uses the competence of sharing and inviting curiosity among family or group members about the thoughts and feelings associated with mentalizing breaks. Family or group members are invited to disentangle feeling states and concerns associated with relationship impasses, to think about other's perspective (ie, "Dad, what do you think it is like for Sally when...?") and to enquire to find out what she is upset about. The therapists seek to redirect the family's discussion from how to fix behaviors to identifying the hidden feelings and missing perspectives that lead to getting stuck. Individual sessions with the adolescent can serve as practice for family or group sessions, allowing for some slowing down to make room for mentalizing.

More checking after mentalizing the moment serves to show that the aim of the process is not to get it right (we can all anticipate not getting it right more often than not) but to pay attention and try to understand.

The next step in the loop consists of the therapists inviting the family or the group members to move away from discussing a specific interaction and to widen the lens toward generalizing; that is, capturing how particular patterns of problematic interaction repeat themselves. Families are stimulated to generate applications of these understandings by inviting a vision of possible alternatives and of what changes may look like and planning implementation of an application of these changed perspectives.

Before restarting on the loop, the therapists check back with each family or group member what happened in the process for them, giving all the family or group members an opportunity to reflect and talk together about "what this was like for each and all of you" and what conclusions and consequences could be derived from it.

The Spectrum of Interventions

This core feature refers to the therapist's sensitivity and ability (1) to assess the patient's (and the group or family's) mentalizing competence in general, and the changes in mentalizing competence in response to particular affective and interpersonal contexts and levels of arousal and (2) to adjust the mentalizing demands made on the patient by the therapist's interventions and the emotional closeness between patient and therapist to the patient's level of mentalizing competence at any given moment (**Fig. 10**).

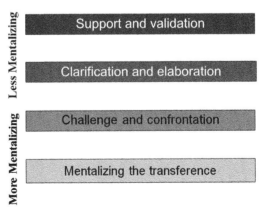

Fig. 10. Interventions: spectrum.

Support and validation
When a therapist identifies a mentalizing break, they intervene with support and validation. Paradoxically, mentalizing-based support involves therapists' increasing the emotional distance with the patients to reduce the arousal triggered in adolescents (particularly adolescents with emerging BPD) by emotional closeness and activation of attachment. As discussed earlier, it is this increase in arousal that brings about a breakdown or defensive inhibition of mentalizing.

Increasing emotional distance by becoming less expressive and shifting the focus away from the patient-therapist relationship seems counterintuitive when patients are more distressed. Yet the aim of MBT is to help the patients regain mentalizing. When therapists respond to the increased distress of adolescents and patients with BPD by becoming more emotionally engaged and sympathetic (becoming gentler, speaking more softly, showing even more interest in understanding the patient's plight, extending sessions, or offering additional meetings), they increase arousal, because dependency and attachment are hyperactivated. The resulting vicious cycle is one in which the patient's crisis leads to greater involvement by the therapist, which generates more crisis and can lead to a catastrophic escalation of the crisis or a loss of therapeutic boundaries.

Supportive interventions respect and validate the patient's narrative and convey a desire to understand the emotional impact of the current situation associated with increased distress and decreased mentalizing. Interventions are presented as simple, clear, and unambiguous statements and questions. Complex interventions, such as those involving symbolic meanings or hypotheses about the origin in the past of current relationship patterns, require the reflective, controlled mentalizing that the patient lacks, at least at a moment of distress or, more persistently, as is the case with adolescents or patients with BPD. Using the competencies described in the core feature of the therapist's stance, therapists mark and praise judiciously patients' good mentalizing and explore the positive effects of mentalizing in increased sense of real control and enhanced ability to receive help and support. The therapists explore these effects from the perspective of both self (eg, "It's impressive how you sorted out what went on between you and…. What was it like for you when you worked it out?") and the other (eg, "How do you think your mother felt when you explained to her how things felt to you?").

Clarification and elaboration
When patients give evidence of less arousal and more mentalizing, therapists can move in the spectrum of interventions to clarification and elaboration.

Clarification involves an active effort to tidy up or reconstruct the emotional and interpersonal context leading to the break in mentalizing. The therapists engage with the patients in an active effort to gather a detailed picture of the behavioral and interpersonal sequence leading to the mentalizing break or the interpersonal impasse and the feelings associated with each step. Actions should be traced to feelings by rewinding the events and establishing, on a moment-to-moment basis, the mental states leading to impulsive, maladaptive, or hurtful actions. The task of the therapist is to help the patient make connections between actions and interactions and thoughts and feelings, and to be able to elaborate the therapist's and the patient's understanding of thoughts, feelings, and other mental states in a way that opens more discourse and curiosity.

For example, Jason could clarify how quickly feeling angry and out of control leads to feelings of self-loathing and shame, whereas Maria could articulate how she looked intently for evidence that she was about to be rejected and could clarify and elaborate how she felt misunderstood and put down when her mother compared her with her brother.

In clarifying and elaborating the connections between feelings, thoughts, actions, and relationships, adolescents are helped to understand that hidden feelings and missing perspectives drive misunderstandings and breakdowns in mentalizing. In elaborating, therapists are alert to the patient's failures to understand their own mind or the mind of others and when such mentalizing failure is apparent, the therapist questions and seeks an alternative understanding.

When a therapist summarizes their understanding after clarifying and elaborating, they are careful, as when presenting the mentalizing formulation discussed earlier, not to suggest that they are sharing the real truth about the patient's mental life, but merely the therapist's own perspective.

Challenge and confrontation
Reaching an increased level of mentalizing competence makes it possible for a therapist to challenge and confront.

In challenging and confronting, the therapist seeks to help the patient grow curious about their own motivations and appreciate the possibility of either concealing, ignoring, or dismissing mental states, or trying to understand mental states and motivations.

Therapists help identify how nonmentalizing and automatic, impulsive, addictive patterns provide relief and a sense (however pretend or illusory) of control, safety, and connection. This feeling was something that Maria could articulate when she recognized how "wonderful" it was to "get rid" of negative feelings by purging and Jason acknowledged that "numbing" himself with drugs helped him when he felt out of control and humiliated. Such discussion allows for an articulation of the understandable reluctance everyone feels to interrupt impulsive and nonmentalizing behavior. It also paves the way for an exploration of the pain and adaptive price associated with impulsivity and nonmentalizing patterns and the courage required to change and seek real mastery.

The aim of the challenge is to stimulate in the patient an interest in taking the risk of learning self-control and effectiveness in relationships through exercising the capacity to understand and represent their own and other peoples' mental states in increasingly more complex and accurate ways.

Mentalizing the transference
The final step in the spectrum of interventions, mentalizing the transference, becomes possible when patients show a capacity to engage in more complex and accurate mentalizing despite increased arousal and greater emotional closeness.

The relationship between patients and therapists inevitably stimulates attachment and thus, distress and mentalizing failure. The therapeutic relationship, therefore, offers a unique opportunity to experience and practice mentalizing in the context of intense affect and emotional closeness.

In MBT, mentalizing the transference does not refer to an interpretation of the past (the there-and-then) based on the current patient-therapist relationship (the here-and-now). Instead, mentalizing the transference involves a well-defined sequence of interventions, along the path reviewed in the spectrum of interventions (**Box 7**) that validate the patient's experience; clarify and elaborate that affect and relationship context; and challenge by offering an alternative perspective. However, in mentalizing the transference, the exploration of the patient's experience is conducted in the current relationship with the therapist.

Clarifying the patient's feelings and the thoughts and interactions associated with these feelings makes apparent the contributions of the therapist to the current

---

Box 7
Components of mentalizing the transference

- Validation of experience
- Exploration in the current relationship
- Accepting and exploring enactment (therapist's contribution)
- Collaborating in arriving at understanding
- Presenting alternative perspective
- Monitoring patient's reaction
- Exploring patient's reaction to new perspective

---

situation. Therapists accept their contribution to the enactment rather than hide behind the premise that patients are distorting. Taking responsibility for one's mistakes and misattunements is particularly significant to show to patients that courage, openness, and authenticity can generate effective agency, control, and relationships. The capacity of therapists to monitor their own mentalizing failures and the resulting contribution to nonmentalizing enactments is a key competence of MBT-A therapists and a central focus of regular supervision and feedback within the MBT-A team.

In the next step in mentalizing, the transference therapists and patients collaborate in arriving at an alternative perspective (eg, "I was thinking that when I missed how upset you felt, you could only imagine that you had to put a lot of distance from feeling hurt and misunderstood. How does that feel to you"?).

This alternative perspective is followed by checking the reaction of the patient to the new perspective and the impact of the changed view on the therapeutic relations, bringing to life the statement of the young woman offered at the start of this article, that you cannot approach minds alone but that it is possible to use a safe therapeutic attachment to break the grip that anxiety, anger, and defensiveness fasten on young people's (and their family's) despair and loneliness.

REFERENCES

1. Allen JG, Fonagy P, Bateman AW. Mentalizing in clinical practice. Washington, DC: American Psychiatric Publishing; 2008.
2. Bateman A, Fonagy P, Luyten P. Introduction and overview. In: Bateman A, Fonagy P, editors. Handbook of mentalizing in mental health practice. Washington, DC: American Psychiatric Publishing; 2012. p. 3–43.
3. Frith CD, Frith U. The neural basis of mentalizing. Neuron 2006;50:531–4.
4. Luyten P, Fonagy P, Lemma A, et al. Depression. In: Bateman A, Fonagy P, editors. Handbook of mentalizing in mental health practice. Washington, DC: American Psychiatric Publishing; 2012. p. 385–417.
5. Luyten P, Fonagy P, Lowyck B, et al. Assessment of mentalization. In: Bateman A, Fonagy P, editors. Handbook of mentalizing in mental health practice. Washington, DC: American Psychiatric Publishing; 2012. p. 43–65.
6. Fonagy P, Gergely G, Jurist E, et al. Affect regulation, mentalization and the development of the self. New York: Other Press; 2002.
7. Satpute AB, Lieberman MD. Integrating automatic and controlled processes into neurocognitive models of social cognition. Brain Res 2006;1079(1):86–97.

8. Lieberman MD. Social cognitive neuroscience: a review of core processes. Annu Rev Psychol 2007;58:259–89.

9. Dimaggio G, Lysaker PH, Carcione A, et al. Know yourself and you shall know the other... to a certain extent: multiple paths of influence of self-reflection on mindreading. Conscious Cogn 2008;17(3):778–89.

10. Lombardo MV, Chakrabarti B, Bullmore ET, et al. Shared neural circuits for mentalizing about the self and others. J Cogn Neurosci 2010;22(7):1623–35.

11. Baron–Cohen S, Golan O, Chakrabarti B, et al. Social Cognition and Autism Spectrum Conditions. In: Sharp C, Fonagy P, Goodyear I, editors. Social Cognition and Developmental Psychopathology. Oxford, UK: Oxford University Press; 2008. p. 29–59.

12. Bowlby J. Attachment and loss, Vol. I. In: Attachment. London: Hogarth Press; 1969.

13. Bowlby J. The making and breaking of affectional bonds II: some principles of psychotherapy. Br J Psychiatry 1977;130:421–31.

14. Bowlby J. Attachment and loss, Vol. I. In: Attachment, 2nd Edition. New York: Basic Books; 1982.

15. Bowlby J. A secure base: clinical applications of attachment theory. London: Routledge; 1988.

16. Arnsten AF. Stress impairs prefrontal cortical function in rats and monkeys: role of dopamine D1 and norepinephrine alpha-1 receptor mechanisms. Prog Brain Res 2000;126:183–92.

17. Arnsten AF. The biology of being frazzled. Science 1998;280:1711–2.

18. Arnsten AF, Mathew R, Ubriani R, et al. Alpha-1 noradrenergic receptor stimulation impairs prefrontal cortical cognitive function. Biol Psychiatry 1999;45:26–31.

19. Mayes LC. Arousal regulation, emotional flexibility, medial amygdala function, and the impact of early experience: comments on the paper of Lewis et al. Ann N Y Acad Sci 2006;1094:178–92.

20. McManus M, Lerner H, Robbins D, et al. Assessment of borderline symptomatology in hospitalized adolescents. J Am Acad Child Psychiatry 1984;23:685–94.

21. Keysers C, Gazzola V. Towards a unifying neural theory of social cognition. Prog Brain Res 2006;156:379–401.

22. Uddin LQ, Iacoboni M, Lange C, et al. The self and social cognition: the role of cortical midline structures and mirror neurons. Trends Cogn Sci 2007;11(4):153–7.

23. Westen D, Dutra L, Shedler J. Assessing adolescent personality pathology. Br J Psychiatry 2005;186:227–38.

24. Lieberman MD. Social cognitive neuroscience: A review of core processes. Annu Rev Psychol 2007;58:259–89.

25. Emde R. A Developmental Orientation for Contemporary Psychoanalysis. In: Person E, Cooper A, Gabbard G, editors. Textbook of Psychoanalysis. Washington, DC: American Psychiatric Publishing; 2005. p. 117–30.

26. Stern D. The Interpersonal World of the Infant: A View from Psychoanalysis and Development Psychology. New York: Basic Books; 1985.

27. Sroufe LA, Waters E. Attachment as an organizational construct. Child Dev 1977;48:1184–99.

28. Sroufe LA. Emotional development: the organization of emotional life in the early years. New York: Cambridge University Press; 1996.

29. Stern D. The present moment in psychotherapy and everyday life. New York: Norton; 2004.

30. Stern DN. The motherhood constellation: a unified view of parent-infant psychotherapy. New York: Basic Books; 1995.

31. Gergely G. The role of contingency detection in early affect-regulative interactions and in the development of different types of infant attachment. Soc Behav 2004;13:468–78.

32. Gallese V, Keysers C, Rizzolatti G. A unifying view of the basis of social cognition. Trends Cogn Sci 2004;8(9):396–403.

33. Garnet KE, Levy KN, Mattanah JJ, et al. Borderline personality disorder in adolescents: ubiquitous or specific? Am J Psychiatry 1994;151(9):1380–2.

34. Sroufe LA. Attachment and development: a prospective, longitudinal study from birth to adulthood. Attach Hum Dev 2005;7(4):349–67.

35. Tronick E. The neurobehavioral and social-emotional development of infants and children. New York: WW Norton; 2007.

36. Gergely G. The role of contingency detection in early affect – Regulation interactions and in the development of different types of infant attachment. Soc Behav 2004;13:468.

37. Csibra G, Gergely G. Social learning and social cognition: the case for pedagogy. In: Johnson MH, Munakata YM, editors. Processes of change in brain and cognitive development. Attention and performance, vol. XXI. Oxford (United Kingdom): Oxford University Press; 2006. p. 249–74.

38. Fearon RM, Belsky J. Attachment and attention: protection in relation to gender and cumulative social-contextual adversity. Child Dev 2004;75(6):1677–93.

39. Winnicott D. Mirror Role of Mother and Family in Child Development. In: Winnicott D, editor. Playing and Reality. London: Tavistock; 1956. p. 111–8.

40. Pronin E, Gilovich T, Ross L. Objectivity in the eye of the beholder: divergent perceptions of bias in self versus others. Psychol Rev 2004;111(3):781–99.

41. Frith CD. The social brain? Philos Trans R Soc Lond B Biol Sci 2007;362(1480):671–8.

42. Bleiberg E. Treating personality disorders in children and adolescents: a relational approach. New York: Guilford; 2001.

43. Chanen AM, Jackson HJ, McGorry PD, et al. Two-year stability of personality disorder in older adolescent outpatients. J Personal Disord 2004;18(6):526–41.

44. Ludolph PS, Westen D, Misle B, et al. The borderline diagnosis in adolescents: symptoms and developmental history. Am J Psychiatry 1990;147(4):470–6.

45. Winograd G, Cohen P, Chen H. Adolescent borderline symptoms in the community: prognosis for functioning over 20 years. J Child Psychol Psychiatry 2008;49:933–41.

46. Offer D, Offer J. From teenage to young manhood: a psychological study. New York: Basic Books; 1975.

47. Angold A, Costello AJ. The epidemiology of depression in children and adolescents. Cambridge child and adolescent psychiatry series. In: Goodyear IM, editor. The depressed child and adolescent. 2nd edition. Cambridge (United Kingdom): Cambridge University Press; 2001. p. 143–78.

48. Moffitt TE, Caspi A, Harrington H, et al. Males on the life-course-persistent and adolescence-limited antisocial pathways: follow-up at age 26 years. Dev Psychopathol 2002;14(1):179–207.

49. Offord D, Boyle M, Szatmari, et al. Ontario child health study, II: Six month prevalence of disorder and rates of service utilization. Arch Gen Psychiatry 1987;44:832–6.

50. Fonagy P, Luyten P. A developmental, mentalization-based approach to the understanding and treatment of borderline personality disorder. Dev Psychopathol 2009;21(4):1355–81.
51. Jogems-Kosterman BJ, de Knijff DW, Kusters R, et al. Basal cortisol and DHEA levels in women with borderline personality disorder. J Psychiatr Res 2007; 41(12):1019–26.
52. Johnson J, Cohen P, Smailes E, et al. Adolescent personality disorders associated with violence and criminal behavior during adolescence and early adulthood. Am J Psychiatry 2000;157:1406–12.
53. Keysers C, Gazzola V. Towards a unifying neural theory of social cognition. Prog Brain Res 2006;156:379–401.
54. Siever LJ, Weinstein LN. The neurobiology of personality disorders: implications for psychoanalysis. J Am Psychoanal Assoc 2009;57(2):361–98.
55. Giedd JN, Blumenthal J, Jeffries NO, et al. Brain development during childhood and adolescence: a longitudinal MRI study. Nat Neurosci 1999;2:861–3.
56. Gogtay N, Giedd JN, Lusk L, et al. Dynamic mapping of human cortical development during childhood through early adulthood. Proc Natl Acad Sci U S A 2004;101(21):8174–9.
57. Goodman M, Hazlett EA, New AS, et al. Quieting the affective storm of borderline personality disorder. Am J Psychiatry 2009;166:522–58.
58. Sowell ER, Peterson BS, Kan E, et al. Sex differences in cortical thickness mapped in 176 healthy individuals between 7 and 87 years of age. Cereb Cortex 2007;17(7):1550–60.
59. Sowell ER, Peterson BS, Thompson PM, et al. Mapping cortical change across the human life span. Nat Neurosci 2003;6(3):309–15.
60. Spear L. The developing brain and adolescent-typical behavior patterns: an evolutionary approach. In: Romer D, Walker EF, editors. Adolescent psychopathology and the adolescent brain. New York: Oxford University Press; 2007. p. 9–30.
61. Toga AW, Mazziotta JC. Brain Mapping: The Systems. San Diego: Academic Press; 2000.
62. Nelson EE, Leibenluft E, McClure EB, et al. The social re-orientation of adolescence: a neuroscience perspective on the process and its relation to psychopathology. Psychol Med 2005;35:163–74.
63. Neumann ID. Brain oxytocin: a key regulator of emotional and social behaviors in both females and males. J Neuroendocrinol 2008;20(6):858–65.
64. New AS, Hazlett ER, Buchsbaum MS, et al. Amygdala-prefrontal disconnection in borderline personality disorder. Neuropsychopharmacology 2007;32:1629–40.
65. Casey BJ, Giedd FN, Thomas KM. Structural and functional brain development and its relation to cognitive development. Biol Psychol 2000;54(1–3):241–57.
66. Chabrol H, Mantovany A, Chouicha K, et al. Frequency of borderline personality disorder in a sample of French high school students. Can J Psychiatry 2001;46: 847–9.
67. Dahl RE. Affect regulation, brain development, and behavioral/emotional health in adolescence. CNS Spectr 2001;6(1):60–72.
68. Pine DS, Grun J, Maguire EA, et al. Neurodevelopmental aspects of spatial navigation: a virtual reality FMRI study. Neuroimage 2002;15(2):396–406.
69. Choudhury S, Blakemore SJ, Charman T. Social cognitive development during adolescence. Soc Cogn Affect Neurosci 2006;1:165–74.
70. Cohen P, Crawford TN, Johnson JG, et al. The children in the community study of developmental course of personality disorder. J Personal Disord 2005;19(5): 466–86.

71. Killgore WD, Oki M, Yurgelun-Todd DA. Sex-specific developmental changes in amygdala responses to affective faces. Neuroreport 2001;12(2):427–33.

72. Kobak R, Cassidy J, Lyons-Ruth K, et al. Attachment, Stress and Psychopathology: A Developmental Pathway Model. In: Cicchetti D, Cohen D, editors. Development and Psychopathology, Vol 1, 2nd edition.

73. Damasio A. The feeling of what happens: body and emotion in the making of consciousness. New York: Harcourt Brace; 1999.

74. Sharp C, Pane H, Sturrek S, et al. Theory of mind and emotion regulation difficulties in adolescents with borderline traits. J Am Acad Child Adolesc Psychiatry 2011;50(6):563–73.

75. Yurgelun-Todd DA, Killgore WD. Fear-related activity in the prefrontal cortex increases with age during adolescence: a preliminary fMRI study. Neurosci Lett 2006;406(3):194–9.

76. Wand AT, Lee SS, Sigman M, et al. Developmental changes in the neural basis of interpreting communicative intent. Soc Cogn Affect Neurosci 2006; 1:107–21.

77. Baird AA, Veague HB, Rabbitt CE. Developmental precipitants of borderline personality disorder. Dev Psychopathol 2005;17(4):1031–49.

78. Koenigsberg HW, Harvey PD, Mitropoulou V, et al. Characterizing affective instability in borderline personality disorder. Am J Psychiatry 2002;159(5):784–8.

79. Ni X, Chand D, Chan K, et al. Serotonin genes and gene-gene interactions in borderline personality disorder in a matched case-control study. Prog Neuropsychopharmacol Biol Psychiatry 2009;33:128–33.

80. Ni X, Sicard T, Bulgin N, et al. Monoamine oxidase a gene is associated with borderline personality disorder. Psychiatr Genet 2007;17(3):153–7.

81. Siever LJ, Torgersen S, Gunderson JG, et al. The borderline diagnosis III: identifying endophenotypes for genetic studies. Biol Psychiatry 2002;51: 964–8.

82. Skodol AE, Siever LJ, Livesley WJ, et al. The borderline diagnosis II: biology, genetics, and clinical course. Biol Psychiatry 2002;51(12):951–63.

83. New AS, Hazlett ER, Buchsbaum MS, et al. Amydgala prefrontal disconnection in borderline personality disorder. Neuropsychopharmacology 2007;32: 1629–40.

84. Battle CL, Shea MT, Johnson DM, et al. Childhood maltreatment associated with adult personality disorders: findings from the Collaborative Longitudinal Personality Disorders Study. J Personal Disord 2004;18(2):193–211.

85. Becker DF, Grilo CM, Edell WS, et al. Diagnostic efficiency of borderline personality disorder criteria in hospitalized adolescents. comparison with hospitalized adults. Am J Psychiatry 2002;159(12):2042–7.

86. Lyons-Ruth K, Yellin C, Melnick S, et al. Expanding the concept of unresolved mental states of mind are associated with atypical maternal behavior and infant disorganization. Dev Psychopathol 2005;17:1–23.

87. Mayes LC. A developmental perspective on the regulation of arousal states. Semin Perinatol 2000;24:267–79.

88. Zanarini MC, Barison LK, Frankenburg FR, et al. Family history study of the familial coaggregation of borderline personality disorder with axis I and non-borderline dramatic cluster axis II disorders. J Pers Disord 2009;23(4): 357–69.

89. Crawford TN, Cohen P, Book JS. Dramatic erratic personality disorder symptoms II: Developmental pathways from early adolescence to adulthood. J Pers Disord 2001;15:336–50.

90. Johnson J, Cohen P, Smalles E, et al. Adolescent personality disorders associated with violence and criminal behavior during adolescence and early adulthood. Am J Psychiatry 2000;157:1406–12.

91. White CN, Gunderson JG, Zanarini MC, et al. Family studies of borderline personality disorder: a review. Harv Rev Psychiatry 2003;11(1):8–19.

92. Bornovaloba MA, Hicks BM, Iacono WG, et al. Stability, change and heritability of borderline personality disorder traits from adolescence to adulthood: a longitudinal twin study. Dev Psychopathol 2009;21(4):1335–53.

93. Distel MA, Trull TJ, Derom CA. Heritability of borderline personality disorder features is similar across three countries. Psychol Med 2008;38(9):1219–29.

94. Torgersen S, Czajkowski N, Jacobson K, et al. Dimensional representations of DSM-IV cluster B personality disorders in a population-based sample of Norwegian twins: a multivariate study. Psychol Med 2008;38(11):1617–25.

95. Belsky J, Caspi A, Arseneault L, et al. A test of diathesis-stress theories of the etiology of borderline personality disorders in a birth cohort of 12-year-old children. Dev Psychopathol, in press.

96. Carlson E, Egeland B, Sroufe L. A prospective investigation of the development of borderline personality symptoms. Dev Psychopathol 2009;21(14): 1311–34.

97. Stiglmayr CE, Ebner-Priemer UW, Bretz J, et al. Dissociative symptoms are positively related to stress in borderline personality disorder. Acta Psychiatr Scand 2008;117(2):139–47.

98. Suchman N, Decoste C, Castiglioni N, et al. The Mothers and Toddlers Program: an attachment-based parenting intervention for substance using women: post-treatment results from a randomized clinical pilot. Attach Hum Dev 2010;12: 483–504.

99. Coid JW. An affective syndrome in psychopaths with borderline personality disorder? Br J Psychiatry 1993;162:641–50.

100. Crawford TN, Cohen P, Brook JS. Dramatic-erratic personality disorder symptoms: II. Developmental pathways from early adolescence to adulthood. J Personal Disord 2001;15(4):336–50.

101. Crick NR, Murray-Close D, Woods K. Borderline personality features in childhood: a short-term longitudinal study. Dev Psychopathol 2005;17(4):1051–70.

102. De Clercq B, De Fruyt D. Personality disorder symptoms in adolescence: a five-factor model perspective. J Pers Disord 2003;17(4):269–92.

103. Fergusson DM, Horwood LJ. Prospective childhood predictors of deviant peer affiliations in adolescence. J Child Psychol Psychiatry 1999;40:581–92.

104. Bradley R, Conklin CZ, Westen D. The borderline personality diagnosis in adolescents: gender differences and subtypes. J Child Psychol Psychiatry 2005;46(9):1006–19.

105. Diamond GS, Liddle HA. Transforming negative parent-child interactions: from impasse to dialogue. Fam Process 1999;38:5–26.

106. Solomon J, George C. Defining the caregiving system: toward a theory of caregiving. Infant Ment Health J 1996;17:183–97.

107. Solomon J, George C, Dejong A. Children classified as controlling at age six: evidence of disorganized representational strategies and aggression at home and at school. Dev Psychopathol 1995;7:447–63.

108. Bateman AW, Fonagy P. Psychotherapy for borderline personality disorder: mentalization based treatment. Oxford (United Kingdom): Oxford University Press; 2004.

109. Bateman AW, Fonagy P. Mentalization based treatment for borderline personality disorder: a practical guide. Oxford (United Kingdom): Oxford University Press; 2006.

110. Bateman AW, Fonagy P. 8-year follow-up of patients treated for borderline personality disorder–mentalization based treatment versus treatment as usual. Am J Psychiatry 2008;165:631–8.

111. Bateman AW, Fonagy P. Randomized controlled trial of outpatient mentalization-based treatment versus structured clinical management for borderline personality disorder. Am J Psychiatry 2009;166(12):1355–64.

112. Asen A, Fonagy P. Mentalization-based family therapy. In: Bateman A, Fonagy P, editors. Handbook of mentalizing in mental health practice. Washington, DC: American Psychiatric Publishing; 2012. p. 107–28.

113. Bateman A, Fonagy P. Antisocial personality disorder. In: Bateman A, Fonagy P, editors. Handbook of mentalizing in mental health practice. Washington, DC: American Psychiatric Publishing; 2012. p. 289–308.

114. Suchman N, Pajulo M, Kalland M, et al. At risk mothers of infants and toddlers. In: Bateman A, Fonagy P, editors. Handbook of mentalizing in mental health practice. Washington, DC: American Psychiatric Publishing; 2012. p. 309–46.

115. Sharp C, Romero C. Borderline personality disorder: a comparison between children and adults. Bull Menninger Clin 2007;71(2):85–114.

116. Slade A, Sadler L. Minding the baby. In: Mayes LC, Fonagy P, Target M, editors. Developmental science and psychoanalysis. London: Karnac; 2007.

117. Skarderud F, Fonagy P. Eating disorders. In: Bateman A, Fonagy P, editors. Handbook of mentalizing in mental health practice. Washington, DC: American Psychiatric Publishing; 2012. p. 347–83.

118. Allen J, Lemma A, Fonagy P. Drug addiction. In: Bateman A, Fonagy P, editors. Handbook of mentalizing in mental health practice. Washington, DC: American Psychiatric Publishing; 2012. p. 445–61.

119. Philips B, Kahn U, Bateman A. Drug Addiction. In: Bateman A, Fonagy P, editors. Handbook of Mentalizing in Mental Health Practice. Washington, DC: American Psychiatric Publishing; 2012. p. 445–62.

120. Bleiberg E, Rossouw T, Fonagy P. Adolescent breakdown and emerging borderline personality disorder. In: Bateman A, Fonagy P, editors. Handbook of mentalizing in mental health practice. Washington, DC: American Psychiatric Publishing; 2012. p. 463–509.

121. Bondurant H, Greenfield B, Tse SM. Construct validity of adolescent BPD. Can Child Adolesc Psychiatr Rev 2004;13(3).53–7.

122. Bornovaloba MA, Gratz KL, Daughters SB, et al. A multimodal assessment of the relationship between emotion dysregulation and borderline personality disorder among inner-city substance users in residential treatment. J Psychiatr Res 2008;42:717–26.

123. Rossouw T, Fonagy P. Mentalization-based treatment for self-harm in adolescents: a randomized control trial. J Am Acad Child Adolesc Psychiatry 2012; 51:1304–1313.e3.

124. Bateman AW, Fonagy P. The effectiveness of partial hospitalization in the treatment of borderline personality disorder–a randomised controlled trial. Am J Psychiatry 1999;156:1563–9.

125. Bateman AW, Fonagy P. Effectiveness of psychotherapeutic treatment of personality disorder. Br J Psychiatry 2000;177:138–43.

126. Bateman AW, Fonagy P. Treatment of borderline personality disorder with psychoanalytically oriented partial hospitalization: an 18-month follow-up. Am J Psychiatry 2001;158(1):36–42.
127. Sharp C, William L, Ha C, et al. The development of a mentalization-based outcomes and research protocol for an adolescent inpatient unit. Bull Menninger Clin 2009;73:311–38.
128. Mason B. Towards positions of safe uncertainty. Hum Syst 1993;4:189–200.
129. Mayes L. A developmental perspective on the regulation of arousal states. Semin Perinatol 2000;24:267–79.

A New Model of Techniques for Concurrent Psychodynamic Work with Parents of Child and Adolescent Psychotherapy Patients

Kerry Kelly Novick[a,*], Jack Novick, PhD[a,b]

KEYWORDS

- Parent work • Psychodynamic psychotherapy • Children and adolescents
- Phase of parenthood • Emotional muscle • Self-regulation

KEY POINTS

- Working with parents increases the effectiveness of child and adolescent psychodynamic therapy.
- All child and adolescent treatments have dual goals: restoring the patient to the path of progressive development and strengthening the parent-child relationship.
- Dynamic concurrent parent work makes use of the full range of techniques and interventions.
- Parent work is most effective when continued regularly throughout the whole treatment.
- Parent work and the child or adolescent's individual psychotherapy are mutually enhancing.

WHY WORK WITH PARENTS?

Children and adolescents do not live independently; they do not bring themselves to treatment. Parents are a big part of the child's world. They are also part of the child's troubles, either primarily, as contributing to the cause, or secondarily, as affected by the impact of disturbance. Parents or other caretaking adults are integral to assessment and treatment of young people. Children continue to live in and will

Adaptive growth in parents promotes child change.

No disclosures.
[a] International Psychoanalytic Association; [b] Department of Psychiatry, University of Michigan Medical School, MI, USA
* Corresponding author. 617 Stratford Drive, Ann Arbor, MI 48104.
E-mail address: kerrynovick@gmail.com

Child Adolesc Psychiatric Clin N Am 22 (2013) 331–349
http://dx.doi.org/10.1016/j.chc.2012.12.005
1056-4993/13/$ – see front matter © 2013 Elsevier Inc. All rights reserved.

return to their family and environment. Adaptive growth in parents supports child change; parental pathologic condition can destroy child treatment gains. However, there has been no articulated model of parent work in psychodynamic psychotherapy.

Most treatments, whether medical or psychological, finish prematurely.[1,2] Most of us have struggled with some treatments that never got started, were interrupted, or terminated suddenly or too soon. We all want child and adolescent therapy to be effective.

WORKING WITH PARENTS MAKES THERAPY WORK

We have been writing since 1990 about an evolving model of parent work and summarized our views in a book[3] and in papers published and presented subsequently.[4–7] The model asserts that parent work is substantive and legitimate and makes use of the full repertoire of psychodynamic interventions. Progression through the phases of the child's treatment affects and is dynamically affected by interaction with the parent work. Parental consolidation in the phase of parenthood may also be profoundly affected by the child's forward developmental movement.

OUR CONCEPTUAL FRAMEWORK

All clinicians bring their own conceptual frames to the work, whether they articulate them explicitly or not. Here are the underlying assumptions from which we derive a therapeutic stance, which then leads to specific techniques.

A Developmental Approach is Essential

Our work with parents issues from a developmental approach to primary prevention and treatment of patients of all ages.

- A developmental approach is a crucial dimension of understanding the complex, multifaceted determinants of personality.
- A developmental approach assumes that all behavior has meaning and a history.
- Development can take place only in the context of relationships.
- A child's history encompasses generations, at the very least the parents and the beliefs and fantasies they bring to rearing the particular child. Cultural influences are transmitted through parents and other relationships and experiences in the child's life.

The Parent-child Relationship is Fundamental

Recent research supports the past years of clinical work and research, which have established that the parent-child relationship is the single most important factor in the growth of the child. As reported by the National Scientific Council on the Developing Child, "Stated simply, relationships are the 'active ingredients' of the environment's influence on healthy human development. They incorporate the qualities that best promote competence and well-being – individualized responsiveness, mutual action-and-interaction, and an emotional connection to another human being...."[8]

- The first determinant of any current behavior is likely to be found in the parent-child relationship, especially in the realms of security/attachment and the pleasure/pain economy.[9,10]
- Behavior evolves through phases in which current levels of psychological and biologic functioning influence and are influenced by previous phases.[11]
- Transformation is the main characteristic of this epigenetic evolution.

- No one phase has more importance than any other and developmental transformations continue throughout the life span.[11]
- Each phase brings something unique to the mix, which may compensate for earlier difficulties or raise prior dormant issues to problematic or even traumatic intensity.[12]

These ideas inform our model of parent work in general, as parents constitute a major, primary environmental influence in ongoing ways throughout the child's development.

Self-regulation is Basic

All developmental research during the past 30 years has converged on the conclusion that the "growth of self-regulation is a cornerstone of early childhood development that cuts across all domains of behavior."[13] Everyone, including parents and children, needs to protect himself/herself against helplessness and potential traumatization from inside or outside.[14] The aim of self-regulation is protection against helplessness. Parents need help in strengthening their own capacities for self-regulation. Then they become better able to foster the growth of competent self-regulation in their children.

Two Systems of Self-regulation

From our clinical work on pathologic power relationships and the defensive omnipotent beliefs and fantasies that organize them, we postulate 2 systems of self-regulation and conflict resolution.[14] One system, the open system, is attuned to reality and characterized by joy, competence, and creativity. The other, the closed system, avoids reality and is characterized by power dynamics, magical thinking, and stasis.

The closed and open systems do not differentiate people, that is, they are not diagnostic categories. Rather, the constructs describe potential choices of adaptation available within each individual at any challenging point throughout development and allow for a multidimensional description of the components of the individual's relation to himself and others. Parents respond throughout their children's development in either open- or closed-system ways.

Rather than characterizing treatment as a progression along a path from pathologic condition to health, we see simultaneous potential for both closed and open systems operating throughout in patients, therapists, and parents.[15] Both aspects have to be addressed in parents and children in each phase of treatment. With a 2-system model, "Restoration of the capacity to choose between closed, self-destructive and open, competent, and creative systems of self-regulation is the overarching goal of all therapies" (**Table 1** and **Box 1**).[1]

Table 1
Two systems of self-regulation in parents and children

The Closed System	The Open System
Avoids and denies reality	Is attuned to inner and outer reality
Repeats old solutions	Constantly expands and changes
Uses static hostile power dynamics in relationship patterns	Is characterized by joy, competence, hope, and creativity
Considers that parents are authoritarian and/or laissez-faire	Creates a positive self-reinforcing cycle of pleasure in mastery
	Considers that parents are authoritative and attuned

Box 1
Closed- and open-system responses in children at different developmental levels[a]

Closed-system responses manifest in symptoms of disturbance or pathology

- Gaze aversion in infants
- Rages and sleep disturbances in toddlers
- Controlling behavior and frequent tantrums in preschoolers
- Obsessional rituals or bullying in school-aged children
- Self-destructive behavior in adolescents

Open-system responses manifest in signs of health or normality

- Predominance of positive affect
- Resilience
- Curiosity and reality orientation
- Capacity for pleasure in work and mastery of impulses
- Increasing capacity to parent self

[a] For more details of age-related manifestations of closed- and open-system functioning see Ref.[1] pp.174–5.

The Therapeutic Alliance Determines Outcome

The quality of the working alliance predicts outcome.

Research in psychiatry, counseling, and psychotherapy finds that the quality of the therapeutic or working alliance is a critical factor in predicting outcome.[16–19] Karon[20] states that this phenomenon is so robust that it seems to work no matter which measure is used.

The therapeutic or working alliance has come in and out of fashion in the history of psychoanalytic thinking. Our revised definition and description of the therapeutic alliance is conceptualized in terms of tasks at each phase of treatment of all parties to the treatment. We have demonstrated its importance in successful therapy for even severe pathologies, which represents an application of a developmental approach to the trajectory of treatment.[21,22] Accomplishment of each therapeutic alliance task contributes to consolidation of open-system functioning.

Using the lens of this formulation of the therapeutic alliance has proved illuminating in examining theoretical and developmental concepts such as the superego or conscience and increases therapeutic effectiveness in work with patients of all ages and types and concurrent work with parents (**Box 2**).[1,3,7,15,23,24]

Box 2
Conceptual framework

- A developmental approach is essential.
- The parent-child relationship is fundamental.
- Self-regulation is basic.
- The therapeutic alliance determines outcome.

OUR THERAPEUTIC STANCE

Our therapeutic stance derives from the conceptual framework described earlier. It expresses in form and content the basic ideas that guide our clinical choices.

Parents and Child are the Unit of Assessment and Treatment

A 2011 volume of the *Journal of the American Academy of Child and Adolescent Psychiatry* contained an editorial by David Reiss, who cited important studies demonstrating the interrelationship of child and parental pathologies. Based on the research he summarized, he called for "better integration of child and adult mental health services. Under ideal auspices, we may consider two levels of integration. First is to make the parent-child dyad the *unit of assessment*.... A second and more complex integration of care is where the parent and child become the *unit of treatment*."[25]

One hundred years earlier, in 1911, Freud said that development in a child can only take place "provided one includes the care it receives from its mother."[26] Many years later, Winnicott said that there is no such thing as a baby, there is only a mother and a baby.[27] Between those 2 psychoanalytic comments and in subsequent years there has been a neglect of the role of parent work in the dynamic treatment of children and adolescents.

With this evolving model of concurrent dynamic work with parents we hope to fill that gap.

Seeing Patients and Parents as Whole People Promotes an Effective Relationship

Psychoanalysis is both general psychology and an overarching guide to therapeutic interventions. Working from our 2-systems model we do not make a sharp dichotomy between health and illness, but rather try to encompass complex choices and solutions throughout development. Assessing both strengths and vulnerabilities in the patient and the family allows for a more comprehensive understanding. When you see parents and children as whole people striving to master the challenges of their lives, it becomes possible to respect their efforts, no matter how pathologic the symptom picture.

> *Psychodynamic assessment should come first.*

Rather than seeing psychodynamic therapy as an add-on or a last stop when other remedies have been exhausted, we suggest that a psychodynamic assessment of patient and parents should be the first step in treatment planning.

Psychoanalytic Thinking Leads to Multimodal Technique

Many approaches are limited by external constraints, largely those imposed by third parties such as insurance carriers or agencies. Some theoretical models mandate limited therapeutic contact or manualize treatment to a one-size-fits-all application. Shortcuts to substantive change, for instance, the vain hope of magic medication, have largely provided disappointing long-term results.

> *Psychodynamic therapy is a strength-building learning experience.*

Psychodynamic therapy not only is directed at dealing with pathology but also is equally a strength-building learning experience. It leads to the development of mastery, competence, joy, and emotional muscle.[24,28] Psychodynamic theory and knowledge attempt to encompass the full complexity of individuals and their families. It follows then that any techniques based in analytic thought must be multimodal, flexible, creative, and individualized.[29]

Therapists' Conviction Matters

Parents who come for assessment and potential treatment of their child have many strong feelings, wishes, and worries about the process. They are going to entrust their child to the therapist's care. They are seeking expert knowledge and help and have a right to expect authoritative feedback. Parents also carry less conscious motivations, transferences from their own parents to the therapist. However, this does not obviate the therapist's responsibility to present a recommendation that is based on conviction of the relevance and effectiveness of the approach, rooted in clinical experience and the growing body of supporting empirical research (see the article by Fonagy and colleagues elsewhere in this issue). This area is where good clinical work with parents throughout a child or adolescent's treatment intersects with empirical evidence.

Numerous studies have shown that the therapeutic alliance with parents has significant correlation with treatment outcome.[30–33] Our general stance is pragmatic, with the question of "what works" foremost. The most reliable measure is whether the parents of a prospective child or adolescent patient accept or reject the recommendation for treatment. If they and the child accept, we ask whether the child or adolescent can remain in treatment; engage in the necessary work; undergo sufficient positive change; end in a manner satisfactory to patient, parents, and therapist; and retain the positive gains some time after treatment.

> Concurrent work with parents significantly improves treatment outcomes.

Using ourselves, our colleagues, and our students as our own controls, we have found significantly greater success on each of these measures after changing our technique to include substantial concurrent work with parents. This lends itself to empirical testing (**Boxes 3** and **4**).

Box 3
An 18-year-old boy treated without parent work

In Jeremy's case, treatment started because of school failure. His parents were seen only briefly during the evaluation. Jeremy made considerable improvement in the first months of work—he was less depressed, his grades improved, and he was feeling better about himself. He had been smoking marijuana since middle school, and at times he seriously abused the drug, staying stoned for days on end. One day he was caught at school with marijuana in his car and he was suspended. His father was in a rage. Both parents felt that treatment had been a failure and peremptorily ended his therapy.

Box 4
A 19-year-old with consistent parent work throughout

Janet presented with serious school problems, depression, and self-destructive behavior. She made significant progress, but when she started college, she began to abuse alcohol, sometimes becoming "wasted" to the point that she could not remember the events the following day. This issue was being addressed in the treatment when Janet had a serious car accident while driving drunk. Her car was totally wrecked, and she was fortunate that no one was seriously hurt. Her mother was furious and wanted to punish Janet to "teach her responsibility."

The therapist had met regularly with Janet's mother and stepfather during the high school years and maintained contact when Janet started college. The mother called the therapist and expressed her rage and frustration, saying how much she wanted to punish Janet but added, "I wanted to talk to you first." A series of meetings with Janet and her parents led to working out a reparative program that everyone could feel comfortable with. It maintained the loving, supportive tie between parents and child. Treatment continued and important inroads were made on Janet's self-destructive rage when she had been left by a boyfriend and the roots of these reactions in her early abandonment by her father.

Establishing a Therapeutic Alliance is the Responsibility of the Therapist

Many practitioners see the therapeutic alliance as residing in the patient. Failures in treatment are often ascribed to the patient's deficiency in motivation or cooperation. Our stance is that therapists are responsible for actively fostering and maintaining the alliance throughout treatment. Disruptions of the alliance are to be expected throughout; these provide opportunities to examine obstacles to change and growth (**Box 5**).[21,34]

Box 5
Therapeutic stance

- Parents and child are the unit of assessment and treatment.
- Seeing patients and parents as whole people promotes an effective relationship.
- Psychoanalytic thinking leads to multimodal technique.
- Therapists' conviction matters.
- Establishing a therapeutic alliance is the responsibility of the therapist.

ESSENTIAL COMPONENTS OF OUR MODEL OF CONCURRENT PARENT WORK
Dual Goals for Every Treatment

Anna Freud defined the goal of child therapy and analysis as restoration of the child to the path of progressive development.[35] We have extended this idea to include a second goal: helping parents achieve the developmental phase of parenthood, that is, restoring parents to the path of progressive adult development, in which parenthood is one phase.

Treatment of children has dual goals:

- Restoration of the child to the path of progressive development
- Restoration of the parent-child relationship to a lifelong positive resource for both

Establishing Multiple Alliances

Parents almost always have strong wishes to do well by their children, no matter what the degree of interference or pathology. This wish provides a powerful motive for entering into a partnership with the therapist on the child's behalf. Although the alliance is not the whole of any therapeutic relationship, it functions as a clarifying lens that helps us see how to enlist parents in the work of treatment and promote growth and change in parents. The model of alliance tasks also gives us a way to approach intense parental resistances.

Maintain an equidistant position within the network of alliances.

In child and adolescent work, therapists are challenged to create and maintain multiple alliances—between therapist and parents, between parents, between parents and child, and with the child patient. One essential task for therapists is to maintain an equidistant position within this network of alliances.

Differentiating Privacy and Secrecy

When we differentiate privacy and secrecy it helps us define confidentiality more precisely. We talk with parents and youngsters about the intrinsic privacy of thoughts

> Thoughts and feelings are private.
>
> Actions are public.

and feelings but state that actions are public. Safety is the paramount clinical requirement, and it will be destructive of the treatment, and perhaps dangerous to the child or adolescent, if unsafe actions are concealed. Confidentiality should be maintained in support of privacy but not as a reflexive collusion with secrecy. Our clinical goal is to make secrecy an object of therapeutic exploration and insight, so that patients and their parents can begin to take pleasure in fruitful sharing and communication.[3,4]

Development as Transformation, Not Separation

We see the major lifelong developmental tasks for both parents and children as involving transformation of the self and the relationship, in the context of separateness rather than separation. Autonomy, independence, responsibility, and emotional muscle all develop in the context of attachment and interdependence in primary relationships. Ruptures in relationships that derive from pathologic conditions, misfortune, or cultural pressures for physical separation can be repaired through concurrent child and parent treatment.

Parent Work Throughout the Treatment

Parents have therapeutic alliance tasks throughout treatment, so it is important to maintain a relationship to address new anxieties and concerns as they arise. Regularly scheduled meetings throughout the treatment and perhaps even beyond the child's ending create a strong and safe relationship that is better able to withstand inevitable crises and pressures.

The frequency of parent meetings is always an individual determination, involving both practical and psychological factors. What matters is a frequency that allows for creating and maintaining a relationship that encompasses good times and bad. There can be internal resistances in parents and therapists to ongoing concurrent parent work, and there is a danger when finances, schedules, or improved functioning are used to rationalize cutting back or discontinuing parent work. A sturdy alliance between parents and therapist, built on the foundation of an ongoing relationship, will protect the treatment from interruption or premature termination.

Using the Full Range of Interventions

In addition to the traditional use of education, support, validation, modeling, facilitating, and so forth that have been staples of parent guidance, we incorporate in parent work interventions traditionally labeled as dynamic therapy. These include analysis of defenses, verbalization, insight, reconstruction, interpretation, and the use of transference and countertransference for understanding and technique (**Box 6**).

Box 6
Essential components of our model of parent work

- Dual goals for every treatment
- Establishing multiple alliances
- Differentiating privacy and secrecy
- Development as transformation, not separation
- Parent work throughout the treatment
- Using the full range of interventions

THE THERAPEUTIC ALLIANCE AS ORGANIZER OF TECHNIQUES OF DYNAMIC CONCURRENT PARENT WORK

This section lists the alliance tasks and challenges for parents, their feelings and anxieties around those tasks, the defenses and resistances they may mobilize in response, and the therapist's interventions to address those. The parental therapeutic alliance tasks provide a shared arena for working on interferences with aspects of psychological parenting. Each phase of treatment presents parents with new alliance tasks the accomplishment of which consolidates progressive development in the parents. Parallel with the child's internalization of the therapeutic alliance is the parents' internalization of ways of functioning that foster and maintain mutual respect, support, love, attunement, and continued growth. This constitutes the goal of open-system, competent, authoritative parenting.

As we proceed through describing the phases of treatment, we highlight a few of the features summarized in each table (**Table 2**).

Table 2 Evaluation and beginning phases of dynamic concurrent parent work		
	Evaluation	**Beginning**
Alliance tasks for parents	Engage in transformations	Allow child to be with another
Parental affects/anxieties	Guilt, helplessness, failure, shame, irrelevance Hatred of child Fear of hostility Fear of exclusion	Loss of child Loss of love Guilt over lack of authentic love
Parental reactions— resistances/defenses	Blaming the child or external factors Push for immediate relief Abdication of parental role	Uninvolved/too involved Externalizations
Therapist's techniques, interventions, goals	Emphasize continuing importance of parents Present dual goals Access primary parental love Clarify contract Differentiate privacy and secrecy Resist urgency Articulate learning/ strengths-building model (emotional muscle)	Help parents see child as unique Psychoeducation redevelopment Link parental past to present Interpret sadomasochistic power relationships Generate alternatives
Parental emotional muscles	Bravery Putting child first	Flexibility Sharing child's love with another Competence, not dominance
Parenthood phase components	Integration and ownership of parental role	Secure in primacy as parent despite physical separation

Evaluation and Beginning

We often extend the evaluation longer than is standard for many. We do this because it

- Helps establish the basis for an alliance with the parents
- Allows for the emergence and acceptance of a jointly created, individualized treatment plan

---

Box 7
Four-year-old George

George's parents called and asked the therapist to see him right away because he wanted to dress up in girl's clothes. The therapist suggested first meeting with them to explore George's history and see if together they could begin to make sense of the mystery. "Perhaps," he said, "you will be able to help George through this confusion yourselves if we understand what it means to you all." George told them that it would be safer to be a girl.

Exploring George's development to find out what might feel so dangerous revealed a serious medical history. George had undergone major surgeries from infancy. The operations themselves had been frightening, and after each one, they had to restrain George and prevent any gross motor activity. Both parents worried about George's future, as he would never be able to play contact sports, the way his daddy had. This work helped them realize that they were conveying to George that being a boy exposed him to serious danger, since boys are drawn to rough sports.

Parent sessions clarified the history and the prognosis. The parents practiced how to talk with George about the scary things that had happened when he was a baby and give him appropriate explanations of his condition. George said he could remember being held down and restrained. He recalled his frustration, terror, and rage and revealed his idea of being punished for being a bad boy. The parents also remembered that his 6-year-old sister, out of her own terror, had told George that girls never needed that kind of operation.

The final piece of work related to George's pleasures in masturbation and his oedipally-tinged conclusion that having boy feelings in his penis for his mother and sister would bring further medical trauma upon him. The parents themselves had been traumatized, first by having a damaged child, then by unsupported medical experiences. After the initial period of sharing, sorrow, and reliving of their panic and distress, they worked together with each other and the therapist effectively on George's behalf. George responded quickly. After some months of working via the parents, George was functioning in an age-appropriate masculine way at home and at school. He played with boys, loved fire trucks, never talked about wanting to be a girl, and still loved ballet.

The case of 4-year-old George (**Box 7**) illustrates the centrality of working with parents to initiate transformations in their feelings and interactions with their child. Their efforts at self-help needed to be transformed into a joint effort with a professional. Their guilt and frustration had to be changed into usable concern, so that they could regain a feeling of effectiveness as parents. The parent work helped them embrace their continuing importance as they realized the powerful impact of their image of George. They developed the emotional muscles to see George realistically and hold on to their primary parental love for him.

Often, this most economical intervention, treatment via the parent, to help the child move forward and restore a positive attachment between parents and child, is effective in itself. However, even if a child eventually needs therapy in his own right, the first period of parent work creates a strong collaborative working relationship between the parents and the therapist. The shared experience of working effectively is an essential foundation for a therapeutic alliance that sustains a treatment to a good goodbye.

In contrast to George, the 4-year-old where all the work was accomplished only with his parents, Melinda was a late adolescent whose parents were never actually seen in person (**Box 8**). However, they were very much part of the treatment. We work in a college town, where many older adolescent patients are students from far away. The dual goals apply just as much with these late adolescents as they do with preschoolers and schoolchildren.

The work with Melinda and her family illustrates the dynamic interaction of individual and parent work, even at the beginning of treatment. Melinda's mother feared losing her child. The dual goals and the alliance with the therapist reassured the mother that she would not be extruded. Without the concurrent parent work on the open-system

---

Box 8
Eighteen-year-old Melinda

Melinda's mother called from a distant city because her daughter was having panic attacks. She asked about Cognitive Behavior Therapy (CBT). The therapist said that she uses a multimodal technique; specifics would depend on getting to know Melinda and what she needed. The therapist also noted that any treatment would also include her parents, in a partnership among them all. The mother was relieved, as she felt helpless being so far away.

The therapist explained the dual goals and how this would help Melinda make the developmental transition to young adulthood, currently blocked by her intense anxiety. They arranged to talk on the phone again to learn more about the family history and Melinda's development. The mother said that she herself had had tried many therapeutic modalities for her lifelong anxiety. Everyone in the family, except Melinda, was currently on medication, and the mother wondered if that would be helpful. The therapist said that the first approach with Melinda and her family would be to get to know what strengths everyone might be able to draw on to handle challenges.

During Melinda's evaluation sessions, Melinda understood that anxiety was her way of dealing with troubles over other feelings and thoughts. At the same time, in phone conversations with her mother, the therapist learned that Melinda and her mom spoke daily on the phone, trading tips for dealing with panic. Reminding mother of the dual goals, the therapist suggested that it would help Melinda's growth if the mother found more mature topics to share, referring Melinda's anxious queries to the therapy. The mother realized how anxious she felt about giving up this bond with her daughter.

In the meantime, Melinda worked to disentangle the stresses of ordinary life choices from neurotic defensive anxiety. She began to enjoy herself more and started sharing that pleasure with her mother. The transformation of the exclusive anxious tie between Melinda and her mother to a richer relationship between 2 separate people created new space for both of them to truly include others, especially Melinda's father. He had supported Melinda's treatment but never participated in the parent sessions. Melinda said she had always felt he really did not understand her. The therapist's impression was that he had been squeezed out. Soon after this, he spontaneously called and joined the parent phone sessions. Melinda's treatment and growth were something he could now feel part of.

---

strengths of their relationship, as well as the closed-system belief that shared anxiety was what kept them attached, she would not have been able to let her daughter make a significant independent relationship with anyone else (**Table 3**).

Table 3
Two-systems techniques with parents—evaluation and beginning phases

Addressing the Closed System	Engaging the Open System
Respect the need to find solution to conflicts	"Feel with"[21] to foster therapeutic alliance
Take up symptoms as solutions	Listen for pleasure, admiration, and creativity with the child
Determine what needs are being met by dynamic power struggles with child	Begin transformation from closed- to open-system solutions
	Introduce relevant emotional muscles and idea of steps and practice
	Generate alternatives

Middle Phase

The middle phase is often when therapists turn more to the child's inner life and let parent work lapse, but it is actually crucial to a series of important tasks in the alliance with parents. When these are engaged with, they consolidate parenthood, address

Table 4
Middle phase of dynamic concurrent parent work

Alliance task for parents	Allow psychological separateness, individuation, autonomy
Parental affects/anxieties	Abandonment, loneliness, loss of love Fear of child's assault on parent's personality
Parental reactions—resistances/defenses	Reactive hostility Withdrawal from child Denial of child's growth Competition with therapist Protection of character defenses and superego Protection of dysfunctional marriage Resistance to revival and revision of past
Therapist's techniques, interventions, goals	Consolidate parental strengths Interpret pathologic beliefs Reinforce that growth is not loss Support reality testing Engage with resistance to change
Parental emotional muscles	Differentiate assertion and aggression Limit aggression to signal Support enjoyment of assertion Differentiate authoritative from authoritarian stance
Parenthood phase components	Continuity of parent-child relationship in context of psychological separateness

resistances that can stalemate or end the child's therapy prematurely, and help ensure that the treatment will proceed to a useful termination (**Table 4**).

The case of John (**Box 9**) illustrates how the child's progress can evoke a parent's fear that he is being abandoned. Parents may react by withdrawing. The therapist

Box 9
Eight-year-old John

When John was brought to his session by his father, there was a lot of giggling, wrestling, and physical contact whenever they were together in the waiting room. During the initial phases of treatment, the therapist had worked with John around new ways of making friends and doing better at school. The therapist noticed that, every time father brought John, he entered the session regressed, provocative, and unable to work. When his mother brought him he functioned at his most advanced level.

In John's session, the therapist remarked on this contrast and wondered aloud if all the physical activity with his dad was upsetting to John. John denied this in the session but asked his father to stop wrestling. In the next regular parent session, John's father told the therapist that he thought his son did not love him anymore but that he did not mind so much because he had his younger son and could now love him.

In this situation, the therapist could clearly track the sequence of the oversexualized, pathologic mode of relating, John's effort to separate himself from his father's use of him, the withdrawal of investment in John by the father, and the subsequent reexternalization of excitement on to his next child. First, the analyst questioned the father's assertion that John did not love him. The father's belief that love is equivalent to sadomasochistic enmeshment (closed-system love) could be made explicit. The father then volunteered the memory that this was the way he related with his own father and older brothers.

The father and the therapist then began to explore other ways of loving, more in tune with John's own interests. For instance, he took John to a car dealer with him when he was shopping for a new car, and they shared their likes and dislikes. The relationship began to change to a warmer, more age-appropriate interaction. Soon after this, the father asked for a referral to begin his own therapy while continuing in parent work.

focused on the father's closed-system belief that love is equivalent to sadomasoch-istic excitement. With this work, the father was able to differentiate his own past history of abuse from his newly formed open-system interactions with his children.

Twelve-year-old Nathan's parents were knowledgeable and supportive of his treat-ment. When parents seem positive and healthy, therapists often take them for granted and minimize contact. This case illustrates that parental anxieties and the defenses against them are always active. Nathan's parents denied his prepubertal increase in sexuality, impulsivity, and secretiveness in the service of maintaining their psycholog-ical tie to a little boy. The tendency of younger adolescents to use secretiveness as a way to assert their autonomy creates pressure for therapists to collude. Rather than reflexively go along with the conventional blanket imposition of "confidentiality" it is important for therapists to find tactful, honest ways to promote communication within families and so enhance authentic open-system growth to independence (**Box 10**).

In the case of 14-year-old Steven we see how concurrent, substantive therapeutic work with the parents' authoritarian, closed-system defenses allowed the adolescent patient to undergo a major transformation of his own defenses and then engage fully in

---

Box 10
Twelve-year-old Nathan

Nathan talked in his sessions about his excitement in setting fires. He and his friends used butane candle lighters to scorch various materials. The sexual excitement represented in this behavior was explored in treatment, and the therapist also raised the question of safety for Nathan and the house, asking if Nathan was being a good parent to himself by keeping every-thing safe enough. Nathan began to think through how to make it safer, but this material also signaled a possible lack of parental vigilance. The parents were still seeing Nathan as a little boy, rather than as an impulsive pubertal adolescent.

Here is a familiar dilemma—does the therapist respect Nathan's confidentiality and say nothing, even though the boy may be endangering himself, not to mention the whole house? Keeping in mind the hierarchy of clinical values that puts safety at the top of the list, he began to listen closely in parent sessions for an opportunity to address the issue of parental disen-gagement from Nathan.

In a parent session, this issue arose first in relation to the parents having no qualms about Nathan babysitting for a neighbor's little girl. Babysitting represented in part a progressive impulse for Nathan, in that he was seeking responsibility and earning capacity for the first time, but neither the boy nor the parents allowed themselves to think of any potential pitfalls. The therapist asked them what they thought of a pubertal boy caring intimately for a 4-year-old girl. This question allowed for a discussion of general difficulties in impulse control at Nathan's age and the continuing need for parental involvement and monitoring of activities to support the development of appropriate controls. The mother then remembered her 13-year-old cousin approaching her inappropriately during a family vacation and her parents intervening. Part of the parental denial may have been protection of their own past histories. The result of this work was a greater recognition on the part of the parents for Nathan as who he presently was—a person with growing strengths *and* continuing needs for his parents.

In this instance, the therapist did not have to raise with the parents the specific behavior of fire setting described in Nathan's sessions but could address more importantly the general issue of impulsivity and Nathan's ongoing need for supportive supervision. If the therapist had shut down his mind to protect a conventional wall of confidentiality, he might not have been open to hearing the opportunity to address the parents' continuing denial of both Nathan's reality and their own responsibility. Feeling comfortable with the idea of addressing Nathan's vulnerabilities in general ended up making it unnecessary to describe the specifics; this was an important shared experience for the parents and for the therapist that was put to good use later in the treatment when Nathan briefly stole and shoplifted.

the work of his own treatment. Concurrent work is important, because parallel and interactive dynamic changes in child and parent replace negative, static relationship patterns with open-system, progressive, positive cycles of interaction (**Box 11, Table 5**).

Box 11
Fourteen-year-old Steven

Steven began treatment because of lying and confabulation, lack of anger management, not wanting to try anything new, and doing poorly in school. Other self-destructive symptoms, such as frequent injuries and bulimia, soon emerged. He made substantial progress in the first year but then began missing sessions and hanging out with drug users at school. There was some parent work at the beginning of the treatment, but it had tapered off. The therapist had never discussed dual goals for the treatment.

The therapist consulted us because he was afraid that both Steven and his parents were on the verge of leaving treatment. After we discussed the relevance and techniques of parent work for this adolescent case, he invited the parents for a meeting.

Learning more about the emotional muscle of distinguishing an authoritative stance from an authoritarian one helped him feel able to tell Steven's parents that Steven was at real risk and that they needed to act before it was too late. They became angry. His mother resented the responsibility and his father was holding back in a struggle with his own rage at Steven. The therapist noted the breakdown in communication between Steven and his parents and then articulated the dual goals. The parents were relieved to feel it was all right to try to have a closer relationship with Steven and not let him drift off just because he was an adolescent. The therapist began meeting weekly with one or both parents.

As he worked with Steven on how he disconnected his thoughts and feelings from his lies and actions so as to not feel anxious, the therapist realized that there was a parallel issue with the parents. For them, it was safer to not know than to reveal the secrets they kept from themselves, each other, and the therapist. In parent sessions, they talked about the mother tricking the father into conceiving Steven to preserve the marriage. When their constant anxiety about poverty was interpreted as a defense against the imagined envy of others, they revealed that they had been deceiving their children and the therapist about the extent of their wealth.

As this substantive parent work progressed, Steven began attending his sessions regularly and bringing fruitful material to work on. He no longer engaged in secretive, dangerous acting out. Gradually, Steven showed progress in being more organized, performing better at school, and being less temperamental and more able to look at and elaborate on his thoughts and feelings.

Table 5
Two-systems technique with parents—middle phase

Addressing the Closed System	Engaging the Open System
Articulate omnipotent beliefs	Verbalize conflict between 2 ways of relating to child
Interpret externalizations (positive and negative) and transferences	Note pleasure in joint work with child
Reconstruct deferred action and impact of parents' histories	Articulate partnership with child and therapist
Address authoritarian or other pathologic parenting styles	Reinforce pleasure in mastery by verbalizing it explicitly
Develop a narrative	Address balancing the influence of culture, family, and friends on parenting choices
	Work on parental emotional muscles

Pretermination and Termination

Whether the end of a treatment is mandated by insurance companies, a clinic's guidelines, or, ideally, by internal factors, there is always a challenge in assessing when and how it should take place. How do we know a patient is ready to end? What about the patient's parents—have they also changed enough for everyone to move forward together in a stronger way?

Pretermination is seldom discussed and not discussed at all in relation to parents. A bad ending can destroy an otherwise good treatment, leading even to catastrophic results, such as major illness or death in some cases. We think it is important to define a pretermination phase of treatment in which patient, parents, and therapist can explore what is left to be accomplished and whether they are ready to enter into and make maximum use of the termination period.[15,21,22] The pretermination phase has its own specific features, tasks, anxieties, and conflicts for all parties. It is a therapist's responsibility to take this phase seriously and give it the time and attention it needs.

Parents may react to a fear of being rejected or no longer needed by a dependent child with a preemptive recapturing of control. Fearing abandonment, parents may turn the tables and suddenly end the treatment. The therapist is then left feeling helpless and useless. Therapists may defend against the hurt and pain of this, as well as their own anger, by rationalizing a sudden or premature ending as a normal aspect of development, particularly when the patient is an adolescent. All parties in the treatment have to develop the open-system emotional muscles to bear the real sadness of parting while holding on internally to the positive relationships formed (**Table 6**).

Table 6
Pretermination and termination phases of dynamic concurrent parent work

	Pretermination	Termination
Alliance tasks for parents	Enjoy and validate progression	Allow child to mourn Internalize relationship with therapist
Parental affects/ anxieties	Fear of abandonment Feeling useless	Fear of sadness, love, and loss Fear of reliving core conflicts

Parental resistances and defenses	Reversion to old, pathologic
	  patterns
	Preemptive premature
	  termination—passive to active
		Avoidance
		Premature leaving or withdrawal

Therapist's techniques, interventions, and goals	Interpret repetition of old
	  patterns
	Do not rationalize a bad goodbye
	  as normal
	Address need to learn about
	  parting
	Support transformation
		Acknowledge deep bond
		  between parents and therapist
		Work until end
		Stay available in the therapeutic
		  role

Parental emotional muscles[a]	Flexibility Stamina Self-reflection Persistence	Bearing sadness Taking pleasure in child's new capacities

Parenthood phase components	Capacity to transform the
	  parent-child relationship
	  throughout life
		Maintain love and connection
		  despite physical and
		  psychological separateness

[a] For more details on parental emotional muscles, see Ref.[33]

Box 12
Eighteen-year-old Luke

Luke, who nearly died following a suicide attempt, had made substantial progress. Both he and his therapist began to think about finishing treatment. They worked together to get ready for the intense work of termination. However, Luke found himself unable to set the end date that would actually initiate the termination phase.

Concurrent work with his parents, especially his father, continued. The therapist talked to the father about this time of getting ready to say goodbye. The father's initial reaction was anxiety that Luke would slip back. The therapist reassured him that nothing would be decided until they had more understanding of the reasons for his concern. In going over what he had learned from the treatment, the father realized that he had stood by passively in the past while his son had been abused. The treatment had helped him become more appropriately protective.

At the same time that Luke was in his stalemate about picking the date, his father expressed the feeling that he would be out of a job as a parent if Luke were all better. This father's work on the emotional muscles of stamina and self-reflection allowed for crucial changes in his personality and in Luke's therapeutic progress. As Luke's father worked through the idea of keeping Luke a helpless child so that he could be a valued father, he began to enjoy spending time with Luke on age-appropriate positive shared interests.

Soon after, Luke cleared the last hurdle of the pretermination phase. He felt ready and confident to start a time of saying goodbye. In the next week he chose a date 3 months ahead for finishing his treatment.

The case of Luke (**Box 12**) illustrates the dynamic interaction between the individual child or adolescent work and the substantive treatment of parental obstacles to forward progress. Both Luke and his father stalled, invoking old closed-system defenses against the anxiety of what progress meant to each of them at this stage of treatment. Luke could not move forward until the therapist worked with the father on his closed-system belief that he could only stay connected to Luke by keeping him helpless. This kind of work is needed at the pretermination phase to ensure consolidation of gains in both parents and patient during termination.

Termination work with parents is crucial to consolidating their autonomous capacity to use the positive parenting skills they have developed. It helps them support their child's adaptive use of the termination work. Then they are able to meet the child's legitimate need for a supportive, validating person when the therapist is no longer available.

Tamara's parents needed more work during the termination period on their open-system emotional muscles of tolerating their child's sadness and acknowledging their own (**Box 13**). Mourning is only possible when there are loving feelings, and

---

Box 13
Twelve-year-old Tamara

Throughout Tamara's treatment, her parents had difficulty in allowing her psychological autonomy. Near the end of her successful treatment, the decision to terminate was made jointly by child, parents, and therapist. Both parents reverted to emotional patterns seen at the beginning—Tamara's mother became angry and depressed, and her father seemed unable to manage his bad temper.

After a period of intense work on these issues, the father noted that it would be strange not to meet any more. The therapist said, "Yes, we will miss each other." This intervention allowed the parents to acknowledge and own their positive feelings about the work and the therapist. The therapist suggested that they share their thoughts and feelings with their daughter. Both parents smiled and said, "That will help us all!"

Table 7
Two-systems technique with parents—pretermination and termination phases

Addressing the Closed System	Engaging the Open System
Be alert to reversion to closed-system responses to the stress of finishing	Address disappointments and limitations
	Describe achievements explicitly
Listen for wishes/fantasies of different relationships after ending	Consolidate other sources of support
	Engage with real sadness at ending the therapeutic relationship

internalization does not take place without mourning. Hence the critical importance of a good termination to the consolidation of therapeutic work and the parents' capacity to continue growing and fostering their child's growth subsequently (**Table 7**).

SUMMARY

- Concurrent work with parents significantly affects treatment outcome with children and adolescents.
- Treatment of children and adolescents has dual goals:
  - Restoration of the child to the path of progressive development
  - Restoration of the parent-child relationship to a lifelong resource for both
- The therapeutic alliance is a conceptual framework for parent work.
  - Treatment has phases.
  - There are highlighted tasks at each treatment phase for all parties.
- Mastery and internalization of the therapeutic alliance tasks moves parents through the subphases of parenthood; this also represents a movement toward greater competent, authoritative, open-system parenting.
- Parental movement from the closed to the open system of self-regulation in their parenting is the overarching criterion of change.
- Parent work is substantive, making use of the full range of psychodynamic techniques and interventions.
- Parent work is crucial through all phases of treatment from evaluation to posttermination.

> Working actively with parents throughout their child or adolescent's therapy increases effectiveness and promotes genuine and lasting changes.

REFERENCES

1. Novick J, Novick KK. Good goodbyes: knowing how to end in psychoanalysis and psychotherapy. Lanham, MD: Jason Aronson/Rowman and Littlefield; 2006.
2. Novick J. Comments on termination in child, adolescent and adult analysis. Psychoanal Study Child 1990;45:419–36.
3. Novick KK, Novick J. Working with parents makes therapy work. Lanham (MD): Jason Aronson/Rowman and Littlefield; 2005.
4. Novick J, Novick KK. Expanding the domain: privacy, secrecy and confidentiality. Annu Psychoanal 2008–2009;36–37:145–60.
5. Novick J, Novick KK. Mastery or trauma: the adolescent choice. Keynote address presented at the quadrennial Conference of the International Society for Adolescent Psychiatry and Psychology. Berlin, September 17, 2011.
6. Novick KK, Novick J. The dynamic interaction of transformations of parental and adolescent defenses: the importance of parent work concurrent with adolescent analysis. Workshop presented at the Annual Meeting of the Association for Child Psychoanalysis. St Louis, May 2, 2008.

7. Novick KK, Novick J. Concurrent work with parents of adolescent patients. Psychoanal Study Child, in press.

8. National Scientific Council on the Developing Child, cited in Luthar and Brown, p. 943; Young children develop in an environment of relationships. Available at: www.developingchild.net/pubs. 2004.

9. Novick KK, Novick J. The essence of masochism. Psychoanal Study Child 1987; 42:353–84.

10. Novick J, Novick KK. Fearful symmetry: the development and treatment of sadomasochism. New York: Aronson; 2007 [1996].

11. Novick KK, Novick J. Post-oedipal transformations: latency, adolescence and pathogenesis. J Am Psychoanal Assoc 1994;42:143–70.

12. Novick J, Novick KK. Trauma and deferred action in the reality of adolescence. Am J Psychoanal 2001;61:43–61.

13. Shonkoff J, Phillips D. Introduction. From neurons to neighborhoods: the science of early development. In: Shonkoff J, Phillips D, editors. National Research Council and Institute of Medicine. Washington, DC: National Academy Press; 2000. p. 3.

14. Novick J, Novick KK. Two systems of self-regulation. Journal of Psychoanalytic Social Work 2002;8:95–122.

15. Novick J, Novick KK. Two systems of self-regulation and the differential application of psychoanalytic technique. Am J Psychoanal 2003;63:1–19.

16. Frieswyk SH, Allen JG, Colson DB, et al. Therapeutic alliance: its place as a process and outcome variable in dynamic psychotherapy research. J Consult Clin Psychol 1986;54:32–8.

17. Gelso CJ, Carter J. The relationship in counseling psychotherapy. Counsel Psychol 1985;13:155–244.

18. Heinssen RK, Levendusky PG, Hunter RH. Client as colleague: therapeutic contracting with the seriously mentally ill. Am Psychol 1995;50:522–32.

19. Horvath AO, Greenberg LS. The working alliance: theory, research and practice. New York: John Wiley and Sons; 1994.

20. Karon BP. The state of the art of psychoanalysis: science, hope, and kindness in psychoanalytic technique. Psychoanal Psychother 1989;7:99–115.

21. Novick KK, Novick J. An application of the concept of the therapeutic alliance to sadomasochistic pathology. J Am Psychoanal Assoc 1998;46:813–46.

22. Novick J, Novick KK. Love in the therapeutic alliance. J Am Psychoanal Assoc 2000;48:189–218.

23. Novick J, Novick KK. The superego and the two-system model. Psychoanal Inq 2004;24:232–56.

24. Novick KK, Novick J. Building emotional muscle in parents and children. Psychoanal Study Child 2011;65:131–51.

25. Reiss D. Parents and children: linked by psychopathology, but not by clinical care. J Am Acad Child Adolesc Psychiatry 2011;50(5):431–4, 432, 433.

26. Freud S. Formulations on the two principles of mental functioning. Standard Edition 1911;12:213–26.

27. Winnicott DW. The theory of the parent-infant relationship. In: The maturational processes and the facilitating environment. New York: International Universities Press; 1965. p. 37–55.

28. Novick KK, Novick J. Emotional muscle: strong parents, strong children. Bloomington, IN: XLibris; 2010.

29. Novick KK, Novick J. Reclaiming the land. Psychoanal Psychol 2002;19(2): 348–77.

30. Kazdin AE, Whitley M, Marciano P. Child-therapist and parent-therapist alliance and therapeutic change in the treatment of children referred for oppositional, aggressive, and anti-social behavior. J Child Psychol Psychiatry 2006;47:436–45.
31. Garcia J, Weisz J. When youth mental health care stops: therapeutic relationship problems and other reasons for ending youth outpatient treatment. J Consult Clin Psychol 2002;70:439–43.
32. McCleod B, Weisz J. The therapy process observational coding system - alliance scale: measure characteristics and prediction of outcome in usual clinical practice. J Consult Clin Psychol 2005;73:323–33.
33. Novick J, Benson R, Rembar J. Patterns of termination in an outpatient clinic for children and adolescents. J Am Acad Child Psychiatry 1981;20:834–44.
34. Novick KK, Novick J. Some suggestions for engaging with the clinical problem of masochism. In: Holtzman D, Kulish N, editors. The clinical problem of masochism. Lanham, MD: Jason Aronson/Rowman and Littlefield; 2012. p. 51–75.
35. Freud A. Problems of termination in child analysis. Writings 1970;7:3–21.

Psychodynamic Perspectives on Psychotropic Medications for Children and Adolescents

Peter Chubinsky, MD[a,b,c,]*, Horacio Hojman, MD[d]

KEYWORDS

- Psychodynamic psychopharmacology • Therapeutic alliance
- Meanings of medication • Medication management • Split treatments
- Psychopharmacotherapy

KEY POINTS

- The use of medication in children and adolescents has expanded beyond evidence-based findings.
- Understanding the meaning of medication may result in better outcomes for children and families.
- Child psychiatrists need to be aware of the complexities created by split treatments.
- Medication consultations may be better understood as consultation to the overall treatment.
- The prescribing of medication to children and adolescents is an individual family and systems intervention.
- Child and adolescent developmental issues need to be considered for successful intervention.

RECENT TRENDS IN CHILD AND ADOLESCENT PSYCHIATRY

Over the past 30 years, psychopharmacological intervention to treat psychiatric disorders in children and adolescents has increased, with a steep incline in the numbers of prescriptions in the late 1990s.[1–3] This increase partly stemmed from a greater effort to diagnose attention-deficit disorders and treat them with medication as well as from developments occurring in adult psychopharmacological treatment whereby research on new medications for disorders of mood, anxiety, and psychosis had given rise to therapeutic optimism. Apparently safer and with fewer side effects, new medications

[a] Department of Psychiatry, Harvard Medical School, 25 Shattuck Street, Boston, MA 02115, USA; [b] Division of Child and Adolescent Psychiatry, Cambridge Health Alliance, 1493 Cambridge Street, Cambridge, MA 02139, USA; [c] Boston Psychoanalytic Society and Institute, 169 Herrick Road, Newton Centre, MA 02459, USA; [d] Department of Psychiatry and Human Behavior, Brown Alpert Medical School, 222 Richmond Street, Providence, RI 02912, USA
* Corresponding author. 1419 Beacon Street, Brookline, MA 02446.
E-mail address: pchubinsky@msn.com

Child Adolesc Psychiatric Clin N Am 22 (2013) 351–366
http://dx.doi.org/10.1016/j.chc.2012.12.004
1056-4993/13/$ – see front matter © 2013 Elsevier Inc. All rights reserved.

(and old medications with new indications) were increasingly prescribed, often in combinations, including 4 or more at a time. With reportedly milder side effects, decreased stigma associated with medication, and a supportive popular literature and culture, it was possible to consider the treatment of wider numbers of conditions.

Following advances in research design, including measurement tools modified for children and adolescents, and the recognition of symptom profiles and diagnoses similar to adults, it seemed possible to expand the use of medication in pediatric populations.[3–5] Trials of these same medications on emotionally volatile children and adolescents initially showed some benefit and few side effects. Excited and hopeful about understanding the biologic aspects of mental disorders and aware of their poor prognosis when untreated, there was a huge increase in psychopharmacological consultations, almost always resulting in prescriptions for medication, with an optimism and enthusiasm not fully justified by the few double-blind placebo-controlled studies.[6,7] In the last few years, concerns from many directions have slowed the process down long enough to reconsider the costs and benefits of the path we were on.[3,6–14]

In discussing the psychodynamic perspective on prescribing medication to children and adolescents, we are inevitably drawn into some of the fundamental clinical, practical, and research-oriented concerns that emerge when psychopharmacological interventions occur without sufficient attention given to the biopsychosocial model in general and to the psychodynamic perspective in particular.

THE PEDIATRIC PSYCHOPHARMACOLOGIST

Unfortunately, the history of psychiatry, even more than other fields in medicine, has shown a tendency to use any treatment method with some positive effect on some patients until it has been shown to do more harm than good. Sometimes our failure derives from our efforts to be a healer, sometimes it is our narcissistic need to succeed and prove ourselves correct, failing to reexamine underlying suppositions. It seems we are at greatest risk when we have succeeded and been admired for it. So, accepting that medications can sometimes be helpful, it is worth stepping back to ask the following question: where does the urge to prescribe come from?

It comes in part from training. Child and adolescent psychiatry fellowship training began to emphasize attending to diagnoses and symptom clusters that might respond to pharmacologic intervention.[1,3] This aspect of training seems to have grown from one of many core competencies to taking center stage as the introduction to one's future professional role and job description as a pediatric psychopharmacologist.

This shift was consistent with a high demand for prescribers, which has led it to become a profitable sub-subspecialty. Child and adolescent mental health services have been willing to pay the higher rates of psychiatrists only for prescribing medication. As the medications became more complicated, pediatricians became more reluctant to share this role with child psychiatrists. The relative shortage of child psychiatrists resulted in clinics and health maintenance organizations using them almost exclusively for diagnostic evaluations and medication monitoring. Most of the psychiatric care, including psychotherapy for children in the United States, is provided by clinicians with varying backgrounds and experience in child and adolescent therapy.[8,9] They are constrained by managed care and other insurance and cost pressures to limit the number of therapy sessions that can be offered to children and families. Targets that are, in effect, set by insurance companies influence their choice of therapeutic goals. These goals are usually based on symptom reduction and behavioral improvements at school and at home.[3,8,9] Thus, therapists and psychiatrists move toward a medical, reimbursable model.[8]

METHODOLOGICAL ISSUES IN RESEARCH AND PRACTICE

A lack of attention to the complexity of the biopsychosocial model[3,10] can be seen in the neglect of the importance of mediating and moderating factors in assessing treatment outcome. Hinshaw's[11] review of the Multimodal Treatment Study of Children with attention-deficit/hyperactivity disorder (ADHD) showed the impact of moderating factors, such as comorbid anxiety disorder, public assistance, severity of ADHD, parental depressive signs and symptoms, and IQ, as well as mediating processes, such as negative and ineffective discipline; these findings dramatically altered the meaning of the results and led to a reassessment of the study.[11] Studies like Hinshaw's raise important questions about what we mean by evidence based for the use of stimulant medication for ADHD: at what point is all the evidence in? Do partial analyses along the way constitute evidence? Do we have to wait until all the mediating and moderating factors have been analyzed before we can make recommendations based on the evidence?[11,15–17]

Other systemic flaws emerged from efforts to expand medication usage in the pediatric population based on analogies with adults. Similar diagnoses, medication algorithms, and principles of therapeutic prescribing have been used for children and adolescents, which often neglect thorough developmental formulations, create difficulties with using the therapeutic alliance with parents, and ignore family dynamics. Jellinek and McDermott[3] thought it important to remind child psychiatrists that we had strayed far from the biopsychosocial approach with structured interviews, symptom checklists, and the willingness to medicate, all of which might entail missing important data that emerges from more open-ended evaluations.

In evaluating all patients, we use our caregiving selves to make a connection. We use our capacity to put ourselves in someone's place and our empathy to understand their experience. With children and adolescents, we may use play and open-ended questions to facilitate communication. We often combine this information with other data, such as symptom profiles documented in the *Diagnostic and Statistical Manual of Mental Disorders* (Fourth Edition)[18] to see the child from multiple perspectives.[3,10] This situation is not necessarily an either/or situation. Structured interviews and symptom checklists offer reliability and consistency. Evidence obtained through the empathic clinician's observation of dollhouse play themes, an adolescent's storytelling, or nonverbal emotional interactions with the clinician is inherently subjective but can be highly revealing and sensitive to the child's life. Furthermore, attention to these matters in an exploratory, open-ended way is more likely to impact the therapeutic relationship in ways that have much to do with the magnitude of the placebo effect.[9,19–30]

The individual variation in the data obtained using more subjective methodologies will likely complicate matters and may decrease the reliability between clinicians. However, what does evidence based mean if it is based on discarding or ignoring methods needed to obtain other types of evidence (including potential moderating and mediating factors) because they take longer or reveal complexity?

DEVELOPMENTAL MODELS

We are also concerned about the divided approaches to evaluation, formulation, diagnosis, and treatment models. Current medication evaluations tend to focus mainly on diagnostic categories, medical history, past medication, and symptom response to medication. Family psychiatric history is important to assess if there is a genetic basis for the current diagnosis and impairing side effects. These evaluations on children and adolescents are based on adult evaluations, minimizing the role of development, family dynamics, and culture. In particular, the dynamic aspect of development is neglected as well as its pervasive impact in childhood and adolescence.[3]

A primary concern is that as the field moves toward psychopharmacology, there will be a diminished understanding of patients in general and children and adolescents in particular. Models of pathology and treatment that are not sensitive to developmental processes are profoundly concerning. A traditional psychoanalytic model, such as Anna Freud's described "lines of development,"[31] was understood to indicate age-appropriate linear paths of developmental mastery involving the achievement of discrete milestones. These developmental lines spanned multiple realms of development, from increased reality testing and improved motor development to learning to modulate aggression. Even a traditional linear view of development requires a sophisticated and close exploration of the course of a child's development and areas of struggle. Discussion with parents, psychotherapists, as well as school and camp reports may reveal how a child has fallen out of step with peers. For example, a once-popular 12-year-old girl, the youngest of her group, is not yet interested in the fashion, dance, and music of, what she calls, her boy-crazy girlfriends. Her depressed mood or irritability, social withdrawal, and decreased energy might be primarily explained by a feeling of being stuck rather than a result of a mood disorder.

Psychopharmacology is not the only area where advances have affected our field. The linear model of development, which is already complicated, may become even more complicated by models like dynamic systems theory that do not assume the system is in equilibrium.[32–37] Prevailing views of development, especially for the periods of intensity and change, have shifted to nonlinear dynamic models, based on chaos and complexity theories that can help make sense of the lack of predictability at the point of change.[32–35] They offer a way of conceptualizing a paradox that we regularly observe in our work. From one perspective, we observe continuity, incremental growth, and steady mastery in a child's development; simultaneously or alternating with this, we observe in the same individual discontinuous, disjunctive growth whereby qualitative change or mastery of a task may seem to come from out of the blue.

Another complication in the models of development, alluded to in the previous paragraph, is that diagnosis and treatment is a complex phenomenon with changing meanings for the children, their families, their schools, and their friends (not to mention their enemies). Although the goal may be to recover a developmental trajectory that is being lost because of impairment, the interventions do not simply put the child back on the same developmental trajectory but can change the developmental trajectory. (As a concrete example, consider how stimulants may help a child get back onto a social and academic trajectory but may affect the child's growth curve.) Children being prescribed medications for a problem of the mind, the brain, or their behavior are likely to be affected (if not immediately, then over time) more than an adult in terms of their developing self-image and self-esteem.[9,38,39] Not intervening psychopharmacologically with a child or adolescent to reduce symptoms may also have negative effects on the child, family, and his or her future development. Indeed, some symptoms are distressing in ways that interfere with the relationship with the psychotherapist and slow the psychotherapeutic work and play. The authors have found that helping reduce symptoms as well as listening for and exploring the meanings of the medication has been very helpful. These meanings are related to feelings, moods, and self-representations that may potentiate the child's problems.[38,39]

A secure setting and a therapeutic alliance is often a prerequisite for accessing these meanings.[9,38–43] It is important to understand that children and adolescents may require the parent's presence or the parent's absence to feel secure enough to communicate to the clinician what role environmental realities or fears are contributing to the symptoms. Conversations with parents about medication by the prescribing psychiatrist can alter the therapeutic alliances, teach us about the meanings of their child's disorder to them, and help them acknowledge fears or guilt that might not have emerged otherwise.[38,39]

FAMILY THERAPY MODELS

The fact that parents need to be involved in most aspects of medication for their child allows the pediatric psychopharmacologist a unique opportunity to integrate family therapy. As Sprengler and Josephson[44] reported, "Many child and adolescent psychiatrists pragmatically treat children and adolescents with both pharmacology and family therapy." It becomes evident that prescribing medication however individualistic it may seem is a family intervention.[38,39] Positive (placebo) effects may be mediated more by the meanings of the medication than by the biologic effect.[20,45] As an example, an adolescent is performing poorly and his or her parents are highly critical, seeing their child as lazy. If the adolescent is diagnosed as clinically depressed, however, and prescribed antidepressant medication by the adolescent psychiatrist, his or her parents may now revise their view of their child. If they choose to see their child as biologically ill rather than lazy, the return of their faith and concern for their child may have a greater impact on the adolescent's mood and future performance than any biologic effect of the medicine. Strategic family therapists Montalvo and Haley,[46] in their classic article "In Defense of Child Therapy," describe child therapy as a way of joining the family. The parents are opened to trusting you and allow you to be an agent of change. One can see medication prescribing as a similar intervention.

REALITIES OF CHILD AND ADOLESCENT PSYCHOPHARMACOLOGY PRACTICE
Split-Treatment Models

Psychoanalysts, too, have been convinced of their theories; after having had success with their method, some psychoanalysts refused to recommend medications at all. Now more than half of patients in psychoanalysis are also on medications.[47] Most psychiatrists who do behavioral or psychodynamic treatment integrate therapy with psychopharmacology.

There are some special issues regarding the benefits of splitting treatments, specifically when adults or children are in psychoanalytic psychotherapies with a high frequency of sessions and intensive work in the transference. There are also some analysts who think that communication and consultation between themselves and other treating clinicians should be avoided because it intrudes into the analytic work.

In recent years, the model of psychiatric care for adults requiring medication has increasingly been the split model whereby medication is prescribed by a psychopharmacologist while psychotherapies of different kinds are provided by a clinician, typically a psychologist or social worker. For this to work, there must be clarity of roles, a compatibility of treatment philosophy, and communication between the caretakers.[48] Lapses in communication are worrisome. As one pilot study[49] showed, less than 15% of the time had there been even quarterly communication between a psychopharmacologist and the psychotherapist. No communication had occurred at all in 22% of cases. It is not clear whether this is because of pragmatic issues of time, billing, or a treatment model whereby patients are responsible for communication. It may be more common in the particular private practice setting studied. However, it contradicts recommended practice. Certainly, with children and adolescents, lack of communication carries additional risk.

Child-Guidance Model

For many years, psychotherapy of children and adolescents was a split model of a different kind whereby a psychiatrist or psychologist met with the child, and another clinician, often a social worker, met with the parents. This child-guidance model is used less often now.[48] However, with the number of children and adolescents being prescribed medication, child psychiatrists and often pediatricians began providing just medication as part of split treatments often modeled on those of adult patients.

Dynamic Common Goals

Therapeutic alliances are based on the assumption of common goals among the therapists, the child or adolescent and the parents, the school, and other systems. However, even if there is consensus at the outset, as treatment unfolds, different priorities may lead to tension. The therapeutic alliance, so crucial for good treatment, is not so straightforward when multiple alliances may need to be negotiated (and renegotiated) for treatment to succeed.

In many therapies, there are times when there is a press for behavioral change emerging from difficulties at home or at school that the therapist may be viewed as supporting. This circumstance may leave the child feeling betrayed. The understanding therapist seems like other adults in the child's life. The behaviors at home and at school worsen and test everyone. A psychopharmacological consultation is requested to take the edge off. What is needed is a consultation to the treatment as a whole, including the diagnosis, type of therapy, progress and setbacks, and a formulation about what forces are at work. Is this even a setback or is it just an inevitable resistance? Is this a negative transference that requires time and tolerance to understand and is at the core of the difficulties such that it will inevitably undermine every intervention?

In general, whatever the setting, certain questions are pertinent to such medication consultations, such as the following: Who is requesting the consultation, the therapist, the parents, the adolescent, or the school?

1. Why now? Is it a new patient? Is the treatment stuck? Are there new symptoms or history?
2. Is this a consultation to the overall treatment plan, to the psychotherapy, about the diagnosis, or symptom relief?
3. Is there trauma, a learning disability, a recent loss, or specific family dynamics? Are they being overlooked?
4. How much communication will there be before and after a decision to treat and during the medication treatment? What if patients stop taking medication or reveal information to the psychiatrist that the therapist does not know?
5. Who will explore and communicate the meaning of the medication?
6. Who will patients and families call if there are side effects, if the symptoms worsen, or if patients become suicidal?

Perhaps there is a place for direct psychopharmacological intervention, insecure prescribing, either because a clinical depression has emerged, or attention-deficit disorder is diagnosed or medications are needed to help with an acute sleep disorder. In these cases, diagnoses would need to be very straightforward and highly medication responsive. There would need to be a presumption of trust in the prescribing child psychiatrist by the family. A treatment team, whereby the prescriber has a minimal role, would need to oversee the overall treatment plan. Despite his or her experience or training, this prescriber would have a tunnel-vision view of a complex phenomenon. Poor response to medication might easily be misinterpreted.

Secure prescribing is difficult to achieve if a therapeutic alliance has not been developed. This alliance, which is so crucial to all doctor/patient relationships, takes time to evolve. This time includes time with patients and parents, time to communicate with the other clinicians, and ultimately the time to arrive at an adequate working diagnosis and formulation.

The follow-up also takes time and must deal with communicating with other clinicians, parents, and schools. It must soften the impact of side effects, medication failures, and the complex roles of language and cultural factors. Finally, over time, the prescriber must remember the changes that normal development brings and the effects of life events and stressors. The meaning of the medication will change over time, something that emerges in the relationship and often in the transference.[39] Some of this can be ascertained through the parents or therapists, but this cannot be relied on.

The Meaning of Medication to the Therapist and Psychiatrist During Split Treatment

Split treatment occurs when the child psychiatrist takes over the medication of patients and a nonmedical clinician takes over the psychotherapy piece of treatment. Liability, clinical, boundary, transference-countertransference, and system issues bring these two aspects of the treatment together. The only way to make sure that split theaters do not split is through effective communication.[1,8,9,21,48,49]

The therapist can trigger the psychiatrist to prescribe medication if he or she acts out of frustration when other treatment modalities, such as individual or family intervention, have not been efficacious and patients continue to show the initial symptoms. In this instance, the child psychiatrist needs to communicate with the therapist to make sure that there is consistency in the psychotherapeutic process, think together with the therapist toward issues around transference and resistance, and question if the family has collaborated enough with the treatment. Shared information should be addressed as 2-way supervision whereby the psychodynamically trained psychiatrist can bring psychodynamic insight to the case. This process is extremely important and can be successful if both colleagues know each other well through the years.

The child psychiatrist might be overidealizing the treatment when the medication is helpful and, thus, might not know some of the residual conflicts the therapist is working on. The therapist might have become a *bad object* as a result of a split by patients who idealize the child psychiatrist as the *good object* because the medicine works. At times, medication can be a double-edged sword because it can be effective; but when the parents and the patients rely on medication success, psychotherapy can be undermined and resistance to analyzing conflicts can occur. Parents may conclude that they will call the therapist again only if there is the need to and the patients stay just with the child psychiatrist. The cycle reappears later when the family realizes that medication cannot cure it all or when side effects arise and the child psychiatrist, as a result, is downgraded; but this time, he or she has no therapist to communicate with.

If the therapist and medical prescriber are synchronized, improvement can be achieved due to the impact of medication on the psychotherapeutic process. Patients reduce their externalization of behavior and that leads to heightened insight as well as greater capacity to tolerate negative feelings. Family functioning also can improve due to less need for parental limit setting and less negative parent-child interactions.

PSYCHODYNAMIC PSYCHOPHARMACOTHERAPY

Beginning in 2005, several adult psychiatrists[20,21,23,25–27,45] rehabilitated the concept of psychodynamic psychopharmacotherapy to highlight the combined use of psychoactive medications and psychotherapy, specifically the psychodynamic aspects of the prescribing of medication.[9,38,39,42] Psychodynamic concepts, such as therapeutic alliance, unconscious fantasy and symbolic meaning, transference and countertransference, impact psychopharmacological treatment. The authors understand these factors to be significant to our understanding of the placebo effect (adult placebo) increasingly found to be responsible for positive treatment response and related more to the strength of the therapeutic alliance than the potency of the medication.[24–26] Less well documented but clinically observed is the *nocebo response*.[30,50] This term refers to a reaction in patients whose response is less than expected because of the psychodynamic factors that elicit resistance to improvement. These factors are usually related to expectations of harm from authority figures. According to Mintz, it is more likely with histories of child abuse and sometimes presents as extremely severe side effects to medication.[45,50]

Child and Adolescent Psychodynamic Psychopharmacotherapy

Beginning as early as 2000, child and adolescent psychiatrists had reported on the profound effects that the meaning of medications had for children, adolescents, and their families.[9,38,39] Many were also increasingly concerned that psychodynamic aspects of prescribing were being neglected.[9,38,39] They also emphasized the importance of establishing a therapeutic alliance and recognizing the meanings, both conscious and symbolic, of medication to everyone in the system. Other key variables include the timing of the intervention, advantages and disadvantages of splitting the treatment, meanings of side effects, fears, and fantasies related to the mechanics of prescribing (pill swallowing, taste, color, blood tests, electrocardiogram [EKG] and electroencephalogram [EEGs]), impact on a child's sense of self, and social stigma.[9,38] The authors briefly review some of these factors.

The Role of the Therapeutic Alliance in Prescribing

The framework within which psychopharmacological management should be discussed is not the 20-minute med check but rather within the therapeutic relationship itself, the fundamental dimension of care.[9] It is hard to imagine the way in which this type of split-treatment approach with such limited time can allow for the kind of alliances that will meet the needs of children and families. Families unfamiliar with these diagnoses and the medication used to treat them need time to have them explained. Families from other cultures or whose native language is different or require translation will require more time. The rush to medicate, even when medication is indicated, without establishing an alliance can lead to a premature termination of care. The child or adolescent can feel pressured into taking a medication in response to the parental anxiety and the psychiatrist's certainty. The parents and therapist who referred the child may want something to be done quickly. However, it takes time to find the right medication, deal with side effects, and adjust the dose. The precipitant for the crisis, such as a family conflict over finances or an impending loss of a beloved grandparent who is requiring more care, may go unattended.[9]

Symptom Relief

Symptoms are often treated before they are understood. To know if symptoms should be relieved first, ideally the clinician should have a clear understanding of the individual and family dynamics of that child.

- Are the symptoms reactive to stressors or conflicts or were they already imbedded in the child's character structure?

- Do these symptoms run in their families as part of a psychiatric diagnosis?
- Are the symptoms a combination of the two?

The answers of these questions will arise after a careful review of biopsychosocial factors revealed in the context of a therapeutic alliance. If these questions are not clarified, a premature medication introduction may undermine the patients' sense that they can cope with the symptoms without the help of chemicals.[9,38,39] On the other hand, procrastinating in medicating troubling symptoms may not only cause unnecessary suffering but also impair the patients' ability to gain more insight through the psychotherapy process.

Parental Attitudes on Medications

Understanding parental attitudes is necessary before the possible medications are discussed and the side effects are reviewed.

- They come with many ideas about this based on theories of causation.
  Parents have no difficulty in understanding that a child with an infection or diabetes is in need of antibiotics or insulin. They are straightforward in understanding concretely that physical diagnosis has a specific treatment for immediate recovery. The *makes-sense* or *input-output* concept is not very clear to them when it is related to their child's behavior. They are understandably much more apprehensive at the prospect of giving medications to alter their child's mood and behavior[38] because they have a more subjective opinion about behavioral outcomes compared with physical outcomes.
- They have worries about blame and guilt.
  Parents can experience a sense of loss and grief if the child has to undergo a medication trial. They fear their child might have a chronic psychiatric illness that could originate from their own history. Parents in this case can feel guilt and shame for causing an inherited disorder.[38]
- They are affected by what they have heard from friends, family, and the media
  Parents are prone to respond more to anecdotal cases of treatment failure with a particular medication that could have been given for a totally different diagnosis than their own child. Parents could also ask the child psychiatrist to use a particular medication that has been successful among their friends or family. Parents are also affected by what they hear from the media rather than requesting scientific and evidence-based information from the child psychiatrist. The child psychiatrist must not only recognize inaccurate or irrelevant information but also what the information means to families.
  Child psychiatrists should always try to be aware and respond to parents' concerns generated by the media.
- They are worried about immediate and long-term side effects, inheritance, and social stigma.
  Understandable worries about side effects and long-term neurobehavioral effects need to be addressed not just by pointing out advantages or disadvantages of the medication to be used but also by analyzing the parents' own fear and guilt of damaging their child if side effects occur.
- In some cultures, for example, mental illness affects one's desirability for marriage.
- The parents will be assessing you and your answers for trustworthiness.
  Trust generally flourishes when a therapeutic alliance not only with the child but also with the parents has been established. Parents also become trusting when the child psychiatrist validates that some uncertainty is inevitable.

They will respond to your understanding of what they as parents have gone through already and what is now required of them in trust, communication, and adherence to the medication protocol. Obtaining informed consent and compliancy with medication as well as clear communication about target symptoms will depend on this early alliance building.[9]

Validation of problem

Some parents are relieved by a recommendation prescribing medication for their child because it validates their concerns about the seriousness of their child's problems. They may no longer think that they are overreacting or exaggerating their child's difficulties but rather are responsible parents who had recognized their child's need for medical help.[38,39] They subsequently may place all their hopes in the medication, even feeling angry at the therapist for not referring their child sooner. Biologic treatment of psychiatric illness does not imply biologic causation but it may seem so to parents. This tendency is encouraged by quasi-scientific discussion of chemical imbalances and other media and cultural forces.

Sense of loss

Parents can also experience a sense of loss if they had the fantasy of an ideal, perfect, and healthy child—a fantasy shattered by the doctors' discussion of diagnosis, mental illness, and potent drugs. Loss will be followed by grief if improvement is slow. Possibilities for guilt and blame abound. Greater family conflict will only exacerbate the child's problem and the child's sense of being responsible for the family strife. The child's psychiatric problems may be seen as a reflection on the parents' competency or proof of their own damaged sense of self. They can feel angry with their child for bringing this on them all.

Cultural factors

Cultural factors can play a role in the way a family sees this kind of situation and whether they can accept what they are being told and comply with recommended treatment. Among the Latino population, for example, some fathers think that giving medicine to their children will impair their sense of self and diminish their capacity for independence. It is as if the father feels like he is damaged if his child needs to take medication.

Case example of cultural factors

I (HH) worked with one of these fathers for almost 2 months around this issue psychodynamically. The father would not give his consent, even though he fully understood the rationale for prescribing a medicine for his son's ADHD. When we worked together on the nature of these feelings, I also accepted his role in his culture as the father who would decide this for his son. I respected his willingness to understand and to put aside some of his beliefs and then to choose to do right by his son. I thought by not trying to pressure him but allowing him time, I showed him respect. He could then acknowledge his own worries and his discomfort with having a son with a problem he did not even understand. It made him feel like a weak father who could not protect his son. The father agreed to a brief trial on the basis that he would judge whether the medicine helped. When his son improved, he regained his self-esteem as a father, at the same time making sure his son never missed a dose.

Understanding parental attitudes is a prerequisite for discussing medication choices, potential side effects, and obtaining informed consent for on- and off-label medications. Ultimately, medication compliance does not depend as much on the child as on their parents' attitudes.

THE MEANING OF MEDICATION TO CHILDREN AND ADOLESCENTS
Meanings of Psychotropic Medications from a Developmental Perspective

A child's or adolescent's fear of taking a pill may have a variety of meanings. From a traditional model of psychosexual stages of development, one can see oral issues, such as the resistance of patients with bulimia to swallowing a pill or sexual meanings in the fear of oral impregnation. In Erikson's model of psychosocial stages[51] of development, one can see that this refusal may represent issues of basic trust versus mistrust, issues of autonomy versus shame and doubt, or issues of identity versus role confusion. Also compelling are theories of the development of the self[52,53] whereby the youngster may see the medication as an impingement on their evolving personhood, failing to validate who they are and who they are becoming. An example of this occurred when Sherry, a 14-year-old girl whose depression and its expression in arguments with her parents, responded well to antidepressant medication. She was getting along at home and at school quite well when she unilaterally stopped the medication. She acknowledged that she felt better and was less angry on the medication but that this was not the real Sherry. She wanted the real Sherry to be accepted for who she was. The specific meaning to a child or adolescent needs to be assessed in the context of discussing the medication recommendation and in the actual prescribing process. It also needs to be considered in the explanation for refusal to take the medication at home or sometimes for the failure of a positive response.

From the research perspective, Floresch and colleagues[54–56] review the subjective experience of adolescents being prescribed psychotropic medications. They conclude that there is an "interpretive gap" between the desired and the actual effects of prescribing psychotropic medication. This gap is related to the concept of adolescent identity and the meaning of medication to youth. In 2009, using semistructured and open-ended interviews with 20 adolescents, they identified different points of view from which adolescents understood their illness and the medications used to treat it. Their findings suggest "that medicating adolescents is symbolically medicating a family because the effects of medication generate meanings that implicate an entire family system."[38,39,54,55]

Clinicians need to be attuned to the kinds of concerns that children of different developmental periods may have about medications before prescribing. The authors now review some psychodynamic themes that may emerge.

Sex and Aggression Anxieties

Children steeped in the pretend fantasies of early childhood (oedipal 3–6 years old) have anxieties about sex and aggression that may result in fears of penetration, castration, or even oral impregnation. The size, shape, color, and time of administration may aggravate or stimulate these fantasies and accompanying anxieties. According to their capacity for reality testing, they might think that they are being poisoned or are being given a magical potion to strengthen or diminish their feelings.[43] For older children, there can be a control struggle like their toilet training. In the worst case, medications can trigger a sadomasochistic struggle whereby a child or adolescent begins to take pleasure in withholding behaviors or taking pleasure in being overly submissive to please a parent.[43]

Intrusion

The sense of being intruded on, seduced, or having one's manhood or femininity taken away are all possible interpretations (phallic) of a vulnerable child who has been made to feel inadequate by his or her clinical symptoms requiring psychopharmacological intervention.[38,43]

Loss of Personality

Adolescents may also fear that medications might take away their sense of self and a loss of their spontaneous personality. They may stop taking medicine because it interferes with their image of themselves as autonomous, perfect, or invulnerable.[38] In many cases, they concretely understand that the medication might help them and their symptoms might lessen in intensity. However, they insist that they want to prove that they can be who they were meant to be without the medicine even if they have to bang their heads against the wall to make it so. A common clinical example is treating an adolescent for mood dysregulation whose irritability decreases and mood becomes more stable, but the adolescent thinks that there is no more excitement in his life.

Loss of Control

Loss of control can be an issue at any age. Clinically, the authors find it to be an important psychodynamic issue in medicating children and adolescents with childhood trauma, obsessive-compulsive disorder, and eating disorders. A particularly complex example is seen with female adolescents who have been sexually abused. They have major concerns about losing control of their body. Medication's unknown effects may generate feelings of danger or panic. Medication prescribing may be perceived as blaming them for their traumatic experience. Efforts to convince them to try medication to alleviate symptoms may be perceived as coercive.[43]

Natural Maturation

Clinicians need to consider the natural force of maturation itself. We need to ask ourselves if the medication is the key to provide the change in behavior and how development and maturation can assist in this process.[43] This consideration is directly related to questions many patients and parents ask: *how long will I be on the medication?*

Medical Issues

Other factors involved in the meaning of medications are the tests, such as EKGs, EEGs, blood draws, that breed their own anxiety, exacerbate the internal fantasy of damage, and can induce fear of serious reactions from medications that need special tests.[3,9,38]

Social Stigma

Children and adolescents with interpersonal problems and self-esteem issues are affected by the timing of the medication in school settings because they feel embarrassed about being seen by peers in the nursing office. Even if they have accepted their need for medication, they may be aware of the social stigma of taking a psychotropic medicine.

Patients with bodily concerns, such as being overweight, sexual performance, and skin appearance, require a sensitive and realistic discussion of these side effects and how they can be managed.[9,38,57]

THE SYMBOLIC VALUE OF MEDICATIONS AND COMPLIANCE

The meaning of prescribing medications has led recent psychoanalytic scholars to look into the transference-countertransference interplay when the therapist also writes a prescription to patients.[42] Medications can represent transitional objects symbolizing a transition from dependency to autonomy in patients with separation anxiety disorder or panic symptoms, as an example. In this case, selective serotonin reuptake inhibitors can represent the psychopharmacologist's nurturance to patients through the prescribing act.[42]

Positive and negative feelings can arise in the clinician whose countertransference against patients' projections can be seen as the action of writing a prescription.[42]

In this case, the therapist/psychiatrist needs to carefully analyze this interplay to make sure that by prescribing a medication he or she is making the right choice for the patients and not for himself or herself.

Psychopharmacologists need to make sure that prescribing to patients is not seen as a prescription to their own anxiety when they cannot hold the patients' feelings enough to understand how to proceed in the treatment process. Calming down the prescriber's anxiety so as to have the unconscious satisfaction that something has been done will not benefit patients.

Compliance can represent placing medication at the center of the therapeutic action, relegating the therapeutic alliance to a secondary role.[50] Patients can become submissive to the authority of the prescriber in an effort to please a parental imago. At times, patients make an effort to minimize side effects either to avoid retaliation or to establish an ongoing idealization of the prescriber. Understanding the symbolic function of psychotropic medications can augment communication during doctor-patient prescription interactions. Finding the right drug for the right patient in terms of diagnosis, internal world, and cultural upbringing is the ultimate goal of the doctor-patient interaction.[42] This approach enables patients to become more active participants in a conversation with the prescriber.[42]

SUMMARY

Recent trends in prescribing in child and adolescent psychiatry have raised questions about the best way to integrate psychopharmacology with other treatment modalities. The increasing specialization and medicalization of pediatric psychopharmacology has led to difficulties at many levels. Choices about the treatment model have been dictated by financial pressures, time pressures, insurance companies, and shortages of child psychiatrists. Research methodology has been flawed in ways that may tend to favor psychopharmacological interventions by downplaying mediating and moderating variables, developmental paradigms, familial factors, and psychodynamic aspects of prescribing. These factors may be particularly important in child and adolescent psychopharmacology. The authors emphasize the importance of the therapeutic alliance, the meanings of medication to everyone involved in the prescribing process, and the dangers inherent in split treatment. Mutual knowledge of the psychodynamic aspects of prescribing is critical to improving collaboration between the therapist and prescriber as well as maximizing the therapeutic benefit to children and adolescents.

REFERENCES

1. American Academy of Child and Adolescent Psychiatry. Practice parameters on the use of psychotropic medication in children and adolescents. J Am Acad Child Adolesc Psychiatry 2009;48:9963–73.

2. Zito J, Slafe R. Psychotropic practice patterns for youth. Arch Pediatr Adolesc Med 2003;157(1):17–25.
3. Jellinek M, McDermott J. Formulation: putting the diagnosis into a therapeutic context and treatment plan. J Am Acad Child Adolesc Psychiatry 2004;43(7): 913–6.
4. Walkup J. Clinical decision making in child and adolescent psychopharmacology. Child Adolesc Psychiatr Clin N Am 1995;4(1):23–40.
5. Wozniak J, Biederman J, Kiely K, et al. Mania–like symptoms of childhood-onset bipolar disorder in clinically referred children. J Am Acad Child Adolesc Psychiatry 1995;34:867–76.
6. Harris J. The increased danger of "juvenile bipolar disorder:" what are we treating? Psychiatr Serv 2005;56(5):1–3.
7. Harris J. A selective review of research on juvenile bipolar disorder: implications for struggling clinicians. Adolesc Psychiatry 2011;1:1–6.
8. Dell M. Child and adolescent depression psychotherapeutic, ethical, and related nonpharmacologic considerations for general psychiatrists and others who prescribe. Psychiatr Clin North Am 2012;35(1):181–201.
9. Pruett D, Martin A. Thinking about prescribing: the psychology of psychopharmacology. In: Martin A, Kratochvil C, editors. Pediatric psychopharmacology, principles and practice, vol. 33. New York: Oxford University Press; 2010. p. 417–25.
10. Gabbard G, Kay J. Whatever happened to the biopsychosocial psychiatrist? Am J Psychother 2001;158(12):156–63.
11. Hinshaw S. Moderators and mediators of treatment outcome for youth with ADHD: understanding for whom and how interventions work. J Pediatr Psychol 2007;32(6):664–75.
12. Kirsch I, Moore T, Scoboria A, et al. The emperor's new drugs, an analysis of antidepressant medication data submitted to the U.S. Food and Drug Administration. Prev Treat 2002;5:1–11. Article 23.
13. Sroufe A. Ritalin gone wrong. New York City, NY: New York Times; January 28, 2012.
14. Perlis R, Perlis C. Industry sponsorship and financial conflict of interest in the reporting of clinical trials in psychiatry. Am J Psychiatry 2005;162:1957–60.
15. Messer S. Empirically supported treatments cautionary notes. Medsc Gen Med 2002;4(4):1–4.
16. Sabo S. Does evidence –based medicine discourage richer assessment of psychopathology and treatment? Psychiatr Times 2012;4(5):1–4.
17. Parens E, Johnston J. Understanding the agreements and controversies surrounding childhood psychopharmacology. Child Adolesc Psychiatry Ment Health 2008;2:51–9.
18. American Psychiatric Association. Diagnostic and statistical manual of mental health. 4th edition. Washington, DC: American Psychiatric Association; 1994.
19. Mintz D. Teaching the prescriber's role: the psychology of psychopharmacology. Acad Psychiatry 2005;29(2):187–94.
20. Mintz D, Ryan D. How (not what) to prescribe: nonpharmacologic aspects of psychopharmacology. Psychiatr Clin 2012;35(1):143–53.
21. Busch F, Gould E. Treatment by a psychotherapist and a psychopharmacologist: transference and counter- transference issues. Hosp Community Psychiatry 1999;44(8):772–4.
22. Kontos N, Querques J. The problem of the psychopharmacologist. Acad Psychiatry 2006;30(3):218–25.
23. Wing Li TC. Psychodynamic aspects of psychopharmacology. J Am Acad Psychoanal Dyn Psychiatry 2010;38(4):655–74.

24. Brookman R. Aspects of psychodynamic neuropsychiatry III: magic spells, the placebo effect, and neurobiology. J Am Acad Psychoanal Dyn Psychiatr 2011; 39:563–72.
25. Kapchuk T. The placebo effect in alternative medicine. Can the performance of a healing ritual have clinical significance? Ann Intern Med 2002;136:817–25.
26. Aldonso C. Dynamic psychopharmacology and treatment adherence. J Am Acad Psychoanal Dyn Psychiatr 2009;37(2):269–86, 32.
27. Gutheil T. The psychology of psychopharmacology. Bull Menninger Clin 1982; 48(4):321–30.
28. Lewis O. Psychological factors affecting pharmacological compliance. Child Adolesc Psychiatr Clin N Am 1995;4(1):1–22.
29. Showalter J. Psychodynamics and medications. J Am Acad Child Adolesc Psychiatry 1989;28:681–4.
30. Kennedy W. The nocebo reaction. Med World 1961;95:203–5.
31. Freud A. The concept of developmental lines. Psychoanal Study Child 1963;18: 245265.
32. Thelen E. Dynamic systems theory and the complexity of change. Psychoanalytic Dialogues 2005;15:255–85.
33. Jaffe CM. Organizing adolescents(ce): a dynamic systems perspective on adolescence and adolescent psychotherapy. Adolesc Psychiatry 2000;25:17–43.
34. Galatzer-Levy R. Chaotic possibilities: toward a new model of development. Int J Psychoanal 2004;85:415–42.
35. Galatzer-Levy R. Emergence. Psychoanal Inq 2002;22:708–27.
36. Sander L. Thinking differently: principles in living systems and the specificity of being known. Psychoanalytic Dialogues 2002;12:11–42.
37. Mayes L. The twin poles of order and chaos. Psychoanal Study Child 2001;56: 137–70.
38. Rappaport N, Chubinsky P. The meaning of psychotropic medications for children, adolescents and their families. J Am Acad Child Adolesc Psychiatry 2000;39(9):1198–200.
39. Chubinsky P, Rappaport N. Medication and the fragile alliance; the complex meanings of psychotropic medication to children, adolescents and families. J Infant Child Adolesc Psychother 2006;5(1):111–23.
40. Silvio J, Condemain R. Psychodynamic psychiatrists and psychopharmacology. J Am Acad Psychoanal Dyn Psychiatr 2011;39(1):27–40.
41. Fine P, Fine S. Psychodynamic psychiatry, psychotherapy, and community psychiatry. J Am Acad Psychoanal Dyn Psychiatr 2011;39(1):93–110.
42. Metzl J, Riba M. Understanding the symbolic value of medications: a brief review. Prim Psychiatr 2000;10(7):45–8.
43. Shapiro T. Developmental considerations in psychopharmacology: the interaction of drugs and development. In: Weiner J, editor. Diagnosis and psychopharmacology of childhood and adolescent disorders. New York: Wiley; 1996. p. (3) 79–95.
44. Sprengler D, Josephson A. Integration of pharmacotherapy and family therapy in the treatment of child and adolescents. J Am Acad Child Adolesc Psychiatry 1998;37:8.
45. Mintz D, Belnap B. What is psychodynamic psychopharmacology? An approach to psychopharmacological resistance. In: Plakun EM, editor. Treatment resistance and patient authority: an Austin Riggs reader. New York: Norton; 2011. p. 42–65.
46. Montalvo M, Haley J. In defense of child therapy. Fam Process 1973;12(9): 227–44.

47. Donovan S, Roose S. Medication use during psychoanalysis: a survey. J Clin Psychiatry 1995;56(5):177–8.
48. Riba M, Balon R. Competency in combining pharmacotherapy and psychotherapy: integrated and split treatment. Washington, DC: American Psychiatric Publishing, Inc.; 2005.
49. Avena J, Kalman T. Do psychotherapists speak to psychopharmacologists? A survey of practicing clinicians. J Am Acad Psychoanal Dyn Psychiatr 2010; 38(4):675–83.
50. Rubin J. Be careful what you wish for: going beyond compliance. J Am Acad Psychoanal 2007;35:203–10.
51. Erikson E. Identity, youth and crisis. New York City, NY: W. W. Norton; 1968.
52. Tolpin M. On the beginnings of a cohesive self. Psychoanal Study Child 1971;26: 316–54.
53. Wolf E, Terman D. On the adolescent process as a transformation of the self. J Youth Adolesc 1972;1:257–72.
54. Floresch J, Townsend L. Adolescent experience of psychotropic treatment. Transcult Psychiatr 2009;44(1):157–79.
55. Floresch J. The subjective experience of youth psychotropic treatment. Soc Work Ment Health 2003;1(4):1–32.
56. Oldani M. Deadly embrace: psychiatric medication, psychiatry and the pharmaceutical industry. In: Singer M, Baer H, editors. Killer commodities: public health and the corporate production of harm. Plymouth, UK: Alyamira Press; 2009. p. (10) 283–311.
57. Harmon A. Talking about sexual side-effects: countering don't ask, don't tell. Adolesc Psychiatry 2007;12:147–59.

Index

Note: Page numbers of article titles are in **boldface** type.

A

Adolescence
  brain structure reorganization in, 303–304
  emerging BPD in, 304–307
    features of, 303–304
Adolescent(s)
  mentalizing-based treatment with, **295–330**. *See also* Mentalizing; Mentalizing-based
    treatment, with adolescents and families
  mentalizing cycle among caregivers and, 307
Aggression
  psychotropic medications for children and adolescents and, 361
Anxiety
  psychotropic medications for children and adolescents and, 361
Arousal
  mentalizing effects of, 298
Attachment disorganization
  emerging BPD in adolescence and, 305–306
Attachment system
  mentalizing and, 299–300
Attachment theory
  in historical foundations of dyadic psychotherapy with infants and young children,
    218–219

B

Board games
  in psychodynamic psychotherapy, **283–293**
    choice of play, 287
    countertransferences in, 291–292
    developmental context of, 284–285
    not following rules, 286–287
    ordinary games, 285–286
    style of play, 287–289
    therapeutic games, 285
    therapist's techniques, 289–291
    treatment progress with, 291
Borderline personality disorder (BPD)
  emerging
    in adolescence, 304–307
      attachment disorganization and, 305–306
      dissociation and, 306–307

Child Adolesc Psychiatric Clin N Am 22 (2013) 367–374
http://dx.doi.org/10.1016/S1056-4993(13)00012-6
1056-4993/13/$ – see front matter © 2013 Elsevier Inc. All rights reserved.

Borderline (*continued*)
       familial/heritable, 305
       features of, 303–304
BPD. *See* Borderline personality disorder (BPD)

   C

Caregiver(s)
   mentalizing cycle among adolescents and, 307
Caregiving-related disturbances
   dyadic psychotherapy with infants and young children for, 224–225
Child and adolescent psychiatry
   recent trends in, 351–352
Child-guidance model, 356
Child-parent psychotherapy
   dyadic
      with infants and young children, 226–234. *See also* Dyadic psychotherapy, with infants and young children, evidence-based interventions
Compliance
   with psychotropic medications for children and adolescents, 363
Confidentiality
   in family therapy, 256
Constitutional challenges
   dyadic psychotherapy with infants and young children for, 223
Control
   psychotropic medications for children and adolescents effects on, 362
Countertransference(s)
   board games in psychodynamic psychotherapy and, 291–292
   in play technique in psychodynamic psychotherapy, 270–272

   D

Developmental psychodynamic therapy
   family therapy as, **241–260**. *See also* Family therapy
Dissociation
   emerging BPD in adolescence and, 306–307
Dyadic psychotherapy
   with infants and young children, **215–239**
      empirical foundations of, 219–221
      evidence-based interventions, 226–234
         child-parent psychotherapy, 226–234
            addressing traumatic reminders, 230–231
            efficacy of, 227
            insight-oriented interpretation, 231–233
            interventions, 228–233
            modeling appropriate protective behavior, 230
            offering crisis intervention, case management, and concrete assistance, 231
            offering unstructured reflective developmental guidance, 229–230
            ports of entry, 233–234
            in practice, 227–228
            promoting developmental progress, 229
            providing emotional support, 230

features of, 221–226
    unique aspects, 225–226
historical foundations of, 215–221
    attachment theory, 218–219
    attention to very young child and caregiver, 216–217
    birth of parent-infant psychotherapy, 219
    psychoanalytic stirrings, 217–218
indications for, 221–225
    caregiving-related disturbances, 224–225
    constitutional challenges in child, 223
    traumatic stress, 223

E

EBPs. *See* Evidence-based psychotherapies (EBPs)
Ethical issues
    family therapy–related, 256
Evidence-based psychotherapies (EBPs)
    for children and adolescents
        state of evidence base for, 149–152
    in psychodynamic psychotherapy for children and adolescents
        state of evidence base for, **149–214**. *See also* Psychodynamic psychotherapy, for
        children and adolescents, state of evidence base for

F

Family(ies)
    mentalizing-based treatment with, **295–330**. *See also* Mentalizing; Mentalizing-based
    treatment, with adolescents and families
Family therapy
    addressing immediate needs in, 251–252
    antecedent history of, 242–243
    conceptual issues related to, 243–246
    confidentiality in, 256
    defined, 241
    as developmental psychodynamic therapy, **241–260**
    ethical issues related to, 256
    indications for, 248–251
    individual intervention in, 253
    intervention in family process in, 252
    managing process in, 256
    marital/couple interventions in, 253
    overview of, 241–242
    parent management training in, 252
    preparing for, 246–248
    process of, 251–256
    research related to, 256–257
    sibling-related interventions in, 253
    in special situations, 257
    stabilizing crisis in, 251–252

G

Game(s)
  in psychodynamic psychotherapy, **283–293**. *See also* Board games, in psychodynamic
    psychotherapy

I

Infant(s)
  dyadic psychotherapy with, **215–239**. *See also* Dyadic psychotherapy, with infants and
    young children
Intrusion
  psychotropic medications for children and adolescents and, 361–362

L

Listening
  to play
    in psychodynamic psychotherapy, 264–266

M

Maturation
  natural
    psychotropic medications for children and adolescents effects on, 362
MBT-A. *See* Mentalizing-based treatment of adolescent breakdown and emerging BPD
  (MBT-A)
Medical issues
  psychotropic medications for children and adolescents and, 362
Mentalizing
  among adolescents and caregivers
    cycle of, 307
  arousal effects on, 298
  attachment system and, 299–300
  automatic/implicit–controlled/explicit, 297
  cognitive–affective, 298
  described, 296–299
  developmental antecedents of, 299–302
  disruptions in, 303
  emerging BPD and
    in adolescence, 304–307. *See also* Borderline personality disorder (BPD), emerging,
      in adolescence
  internally focused–externally focused, 297
  neural systems related to, 298
  neurodevelopmental changes and, 303–304
  patient's ability for, 298–299
  psychic equivalence and, 300–302
  self-oriented–other-oriented, 297
  stress effects on, 298
  types of, 296–299
Mentalizing-based treatment. *See also* Mentalizing

with adolescents and families, **295–330**
    introduction to, 296
    described, 296–299
Mentalizing-based treatment of adolescent breakdown and emerging BPD (MBT-A),
    307–310
    features of, 316–323
        mentalizing loop, 319–320
        spectrum of interventions, 320–323
        therapist's stance, 316–319
    mentalizing assessment in organization of, 311–316

N

Neural systems
    mentalizing and, 298
Neurodevelopmental changes
    mentalizing and, 303–304

P

Parent(s)
    attitudes about medications for children and adolescents, 359–360
    of child and adolescent psychotherapy patients
        concurrent psychodynamic work with
            new model of techniques for, **331–349**. See also Psychodynamic psychotherapy,
                for parents of child and adolescent psychotherapy patients, new model of
                techniques for
        reasons for working with, 331–332
    talking with
        about play, 276–278
Parent-infant psychotherapy
    birth of
        in historical foundations of dyadic psychotherapy with infants and young children,
            219
Parent management training
    in family therapy, 252
Personality
    psychotropic medications for children and adolescents effects on, 362
Play
    children who cannot
        therapist's interventions with, 272–273
    described, 261–262
    helping children to, 275–276
    listening to
        in psychodynamic psychotherapy, 264 266
    in psychodynamic psychotherapy, **261–282**
        choice of, 287
        disruptions in, 273–275
        enactments during, 275
        equipping playroom, 276
        games, **283–293**. See also Board games, in psychodynamic psychotherapy
        how child plays, 273–275

Play (*continued*)
    introduction to, 261–262
    reasons for, 262–264
    style of, 287–289
    as therapeutic action, 278–279
    therapist's interventions in, 264–273
        children who cannot play, 272–273
        countertransference, 270–272
        helping children to play, 275–276
        how to talk to parents about, 276–278
        listening to play, 264–266
        transference, 270–272
        turning passive into active, 268–270
        working within play displacement, 266–268
    talking to parents about, 276–278
    therapeutic action of, 278–279
Play disruptions, 273–275
Play enactments, 275
Playroom
    equipping, 276
Psychic equivalence
    mentalizing and, 300–302
Psychodynamic psychopharmacotherapy, 357–360
    child and adolescent, 358
    parental attitudes about medications, 359–360
    symptom relief by, 358–359
    therapeutic alliance in prescribing, 358
Psychodynamic psychotherapy
    for children and adolescents
        state of evidence base for, **149–214**
            EBPs in, 149–152
            limitations of, 174–175
            observational studies, 170–174
                case series studies, 172–174
                clinic-based studies, 170–172
            RCTs in, 149–152
            review of outcome studies, 153–174
                data extraction in, 155
                methods used, 153–155
                quality rating in, 155
                quasi-experimental and comparison group studies, 166–170
                RCTs, 158–166
            studies related to, 176–207
    developmental
        family therapy as, **241–260**. *See also* Family therapy
    for parents of child and adolescent psychotherapy patients
        new model of techniques for, **331–349**
            components of, 337–338
            development approach, 332
            establishing therapeutic alliance, 337
            parent-child relationship in, 332–333

parents and child as unit of assessment and treatment, 335
psychoanalytic thinking leads to multimodal technique, 335
seeing parents and child as whole people, 335
self-regulation in, 333–334
therapeutic alliance as organizer of techniques, 339–347
therapeutic alliance in determining outcome, 334
therapist's conviction, 336
reasons for working with parents, 331–332
success related to, 332
play in
games, **283–293**. See also Board games, in psychodynamic psychotherapy
play technique in, **261–282**. See also Play, in psychodynamic psychotherapy
Psychopharmacologist
pediatric
described, 352
Psychopharmacotherapy
psychodynamic, 357–360. See also Psychodynamic psychopharmacotherapy
Psychotherapy
evidence-based. See Evidence-based psychotherapies (EBPs)
parent-infant
birth of
in historical foundations of dyadic psychotherapy with infants and young children, 219
psychodynamic. See Psychodynamic psychotherapy
Psychotropic medications
for children and adolescents
compliance with, 363
intrusion related to, 361–362
loss of control related to, 362
loss of personality related to, 362
meanings of, 361–362
medical issues related to, 362
natural maturation effects of, 362
psychodynamic perspectives on, **351–366**
child-guidance model, 356
developmental models, 353–355
dynamic common goals, 356–357
family therapy models, 355
methodological issues in research and practice related to, 353
psychodynamic psychopharmacotherapy, 357–360
realities of, 355–357
recent trends in, 351–352
split-treatment models, 355
meaning of medication to therapist and psychiatrist in, 357
sex and aggression anxieties related to, 361
social stigma related to, 362
symbolic value of, 363

R

Randomized controlled trial(s) (RCTs)
in psychodynamic psychotherapy for children and adolescents

Randomized (*continued*)
    state of evidence base for, 158–166. *See also* Psychodynamic psychotherapy, for
        children and adolescents, state of evidence base for
        active treatment comparisons, 160–163
        comparison with TAU, 158–160
        integrative applications, 163–166
Randomized Controlled Trial Psychodynamic Quality Rating Scale (RCT-PQRS), 153,
    156–157
RCT-PQRS. *See* Randomized Controlled Trial Psychodynamic Quality Rating Scale
    (RCT-PQRS)
RCTs. *See* Randomized controlled trial(s) (RCTs)

    S

Self-regulation
    in psychodynamic psychotherapy for parents of child and adolescent psychotherapy
        patients, 333–334
Sexual anxiety
    psychotropic medications for children and adolescents and, 361
Social stigma
    psychotropic medications for children and adolescents and, 362
Split-treatment models, 355
    meaning of medication to therapist and psychiatrist in, 357
Stress
    mentalizing effects of, 298
    traumatic
        dyadic psychotherapy with infants and young children due to, 223

    T

Therapeutic alliance
    in prescribing psychodynamic psychopharmacotherapy, 358
Transference
    in play technique in psychodynamic psychotherapy, 270–272
Traumatic stress
    dyadic psychotherapy with infants and young children due to, 223

    Y

Young children
    dyadic psychotherapy with, **215–239**. *See also* Dyadic psychotherapy, with infants and
        young children

Moving?

Make sure your subscription moves with you!

To notify us of your new address, find your **Clinics Account Number** (located on your mailing label above your name), and contact customer service at:

Email: journalscustomerservice-usa@elsevier.com

800-654-2452 (subscribers in the U.S. & Canada)
314-447-8871 (subscribers outside of the U.S. & Canada)

Fax number: 314-447-8029

Elsevier Health Sciences Division
Subscription Customer Service
3251 Riverport Lane
Maryland Heights, MO 63043

Printed and bound by CPI Group (UK) Ltd, Croydon, CR0 4YY

03/10/2024

01040436-0001